Calling an Ambulan

■ **Dial 119** (Fire Department) 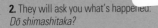 *ichi*)

1. Distinguish between a fire and an emergency: vell-

Kyūkyū desu (This is an emergenc
Kaji desu (Fire! Fire!)   *xaku
desu.*

2. They will ask you what's happened:
Dō shimashitaka?

5. They will ask your name:
O-namae wa?

bleeding *shukketsu*
broken bone *kossetsu*
burn *hidoi yakedo*
chest pains *mune ga taihen kurushii*
convulsions *keiren*
difficulty breathing *kokyū konnan*
high fever *kō netsu*
injury *kega*
poison *dokubutsu*
sick *byōki*
unconscious *ishiki fumei*

6. They will ask your telephone number:
O-denwa bangō wa?

Do not hang up until the control center confirms your address and telephone number. You will be taken to the nearest hospital that is able to treat you. If you wish to be taken to a specific hospital, contact that hospital for permission to go there (you'll need the doctor's name). If you receive permission, write down the name and address for the ambulance crew.

3. They will ask your address:
Nani-ku, nani-machi, nan-ban desu ka?
Give your address in Japanese order:
e.g., Bunkyo-ku, Otowa 1-17-14 (*ichi-no-jū-*

See page 45 for more details on handling an emergency.

In the tension of an emergency you may forget even the most familiar numbers and information. Make a copy of these endpapers to keep near your phone.

Address:	
Phone:	
Family Doctor:	
Emergency Clinic:	

Japan Health Handbook

Japan

Health

Handbook

REVISED EDITION

Meredith Enman Maruyama
Louise Picon Shimizu
Nancy Smith Tsurumaki

Kodansha International
Tokyo · New York · London

Distributed in the United States by Kodansha America Inc., 114 Fifth Avenue, New York, N.Y. 10011, and in the United Kingdom and continental Europe by Kodansha Europe Ltd., 95 Aldwych, London WC2B 4JF. Published by Kodansha International Ltd., 17-14 Otowa 1-chome, Bunkyo-ku, Tokyo 112-8652, and Kodansha America Inc.

98 99 00 01 02 10 9 8 7 6 5 4 3 2 1

ISBN 4-7700-2356-1

Foreword *6*
Introduction *7*
Acknowledgments *8*
How to Use This Book *9*

Contents

At the end of 1993, the Ministry of Justice announced that over 1.32 million foreigners were registered residents in Japan. An additional 300,000 foreigners were estimated to be living here illegally. These numbers came as no surprise to the staff of the AMDA International Medical Information Center, a group offering free consultations of a medical nature over the telephone. Since it was set up by the Association of Medical Doctors for Asia (a nongovernmental organization) in 1991, the group has received over six thousand calls. The callers came from a variety of different countries and backgrounds, but the one thing they had in common was problems caused by lack of information about the Japanese medical system. As health care is very complex in Japan and very different from the medical systems in Europe and the United States, I soon saw the need for a guidebook explaining how to use the Japanese health system.

About a year ago I was delighted to hear that some members of the Foreign Nurses Association in Japan were proposing just such a guidebook. These three American health care professionals are the perfect authors for a guidebook of this type, not only because of their professional background and participation in voluntary activities in the medical field, but also because they have lived a long time in Japan and fully understand Japanese beliefs and customs. I have long believed that health systems and medical practices are heavily influenced by cultural and religious beliefs, and the authors' wide experience makes them the ideal guides to the Japanese system.

In my experiences at the AMDA center I have for a long time been painfully aware that health problems can be doubly distressing to foreigners surrounded by a foreign culture and a seemingly incomprehensible medical system. With wide-ranging information, handy tips, and extensive listings of facilities and resources, *The Japan Health Handbook* finally makes it possible for non-Japanese to utilize this country's medical system with comfort and ease.

I am deeply convinced that the *Japan Health Handbook* will become the health bible for the foreign community. In addition, I hope that this indispensable book will make a real contribution not only to the foreign community, but also to the internationalization of Japan itself.

Note to the second edition: Bravo! Having now experienced the usefulness of this book, I can only say that it has certainly met my expectations. I congratulate the authors on a truly marvelous book and a remarkable contribution not only to the foreign community in Japan but to Japanese caregivers as well.

Yoneyuki Kobayashi, M.D.
President of Kobayashi International Clinic
Director of AMDA International Medical Information Center, Tokyo

We are all members of the Foreign Nurses Association in Japan (FNAJ) and also long-term residents of Japan. With our Japanese husbands, we have raised and are still raising our children here using the Japanese health care system. Nancy Tsurumaki and Meredith Maruyama are nurses and Louise Shimizu is a childbirth educator.

The inspiration for the *Japan Health Handbook* came from the valuable work carried out by the members of the FNAJ in helping non-Japanese make the best use of the extensive health care and health facilities available in Tokyo. We believe that this book extends that perspective to cover the health care system throughout Japan. Although this book cannot begin to give all the answers to all medical and health-related questions, it does include a description of Japanese health care, a wide variety of possible problems and solutions, and handy tips on how best to make use of the system.

We offer choices whenever possible. We try to be non-biased, while at the same time giving as realistic a picture as possible. This book is aimed not only at those who would like to, or who must, use the system as it is, but also at those who use the more international clinics and hospitals. We are not doctors, and cannot prescribe medications or recommend medical treatments, nor do we endorse any of the medical facilities or resources listed in this book. Health care is a very personal issue—care that one person considers to be excellent may not suit another. Likewise, treatments in Japan may sometimes be different than what you expect, but they are not necessarily wrong. We hope that the information in this book will enable you to make informed choices and to use the Japanese system with increasing confidence. There will be other resources in your area that are not included in this book, and we encourage you to research them now. Don't wait until you get sick.

We are especially indebted to Nancy DeVries for writing sections of the chapter on mental health, to Dr. Alice Cary for sharing her knowledge of nonprescription drugs, and to Ritsuko Toda for researching the information on traditional childbirth.

Note to the second edition: In response to the many encouraging comments and helpful suggestions from our readers, this revised edition contains numerous changes, including a greatly enlarged glossary and more detailed index. In particular, we have expanded the sections on choosing a caregiver, health insurance, children's health, managing specific conditions, and mental health. We now have chapters on health checkups, sexual and reproductive health, and the disabled and the elderly, as well as a new section of regional resources (with many local contact numbers). Again, all efforts were made to ensure that the information in the *Japan Health Handbook* is correct. We hope that our readers will continue to find this book a valuable guide to the health care system in Japan.

Meredith Enman Maruyama
Louise Picon Shimizu
Nancy Smith Tsurumaki

The first edition of *Japan Health Handbook* could not have been completed without the enthusiastic help of the following:

Association of Foreign Wives of Japanese members; Ruth Beebe, psychologist; Dr. Alice Cary, formerly of Japan Baptist Hospital, Kyoto; Christian Academy in Japan families; Elena de Karplus, CCE, Tokyo Childbirth Education Association; Nancy DeVries, clinical specialist in Psychiatric-Mental Health Nursing and former president of the Foreign Nurses Association in Japan; Kayoko Fuketa, chief pharmacist, Bosei Tsukiji Pharmacy; Prof. Yasuko Iida, Tokyo Metropolitan College of Allied Medical Sciences; Prof. Yutaka Inaba, Department of Epidemiology and Environmental Health, Juntendo University School of Medicine; Sakae Kikuchi, maternity coordinator; Prof. Rihito Kimura, professor of Bioethics and Law, Kennedy Institute of Ethics, Georgetown University and Waseda University; Kirsten Kjellberg, RN, director of Program Committee, FNAJ; Dr. Yoneyuki Kobayashi, director of AMDA International Information Center; Rita Kubiak, founder of Metamedical Forum, Kyoto; Library Staff, Tokyo Metropolitan College of Allied Medical Sciences; Paula Madsen, principal, Tokyo International Learning Community; Dr. Mariko Makino, psychiatrist, Toho University Hospital; Dr. Hisami Matsumine, obstetrician/ gynecologist, Toho Women's Clinic; Michitaro Morita, director of International Training Services, Kobe; Elizabeth (Ebb) Morris, RN, director of Membership Committee, FNAJ; Rev. Dr. Shuhei Nakajima, chairman of Newhope Hospice Study Society Int'l.; Mio Nemoto, Japanese health care consumer; Dr. Hiroshi Nishida, neonatologist and professor, Tokyo Women's Medical College; Virginia Pieters, nurse practitioner, Walk-In Clinic Department, St. Luke's International Hospital; Dr. Jeanne Scott, family practitioner; Sandra Shigeno, RN, Japan Helpline volunteer; Dr. Michiko Suwa, pediatrician, Suwa Pediatric Clinic; Ritsuko Toda, childbirth educator; Women's Conference participants; Prof. Kaoru Yamaguchi, Research Institute for the Education of Exceptional Children at Tokyo Gakugei University; Yumiko Yamaguchi, Japanese health care consumer, telephoner extraordinaire; and Peter Yates, oriental medical therapist.

For help with the second edition we express our sincere gratitude to: The Art of Light; Janine Beichman, long-time consumer of Japanese health care; Jean Tiffany Cox, R.D. licensed nutritionist; Naoko Hattori, R.N., Medical Coordinator, JICA Office, Asunción, Paraguay; Kelly Lemmon-Kishi, MSW CTS, Resolutions Counseling Service, president of International Mental Health Providers; Joan Matthews, aromatherapist; Dr. Jim McRae, clinical psychologist; Dr. Masafumi Nakakuki, Tokyo Psychotherapy Center; Dr. Yasushi Odawara, Odawara Women's Clinic; Dr. Morio Tonoki, Tokyo Shika Daigaku Ichikawa Sogo Byoin; and most especially, Elizabeth Ogata, our very talented, enthusiastic and conscientious editor, as well as Executive Editor Michael Brase, and the staff at Kodansha.

We also truly thank our parents, our children and our devoted husbands, Tad, Masaharu, and Hogaku, for all their support and patience during the long haul through both editions.

Welcome to *Japan Health Handbook*! To help you get the most out of this book, we'd like to point out a few of its many useful features.

Besides a wealth of descriptive information on health care in Japan, specific resources are plentiful throughout the book. They are primarily organized according to topic, and are located in their appropriate chapters or sections. Resources referred to frequently in various sections of the book are gathered together in the endpapers inside the back cover. Emergency resources are listed on the front endpapers.

Please note that although we cannot provide a resource on every topic for every area of Japan, a telephone call to a resource outside your area can often result in obtaining a contact nearer home for the same or a similar service or product.

To help you find resources in your area, this edition also contains a whole chapter on regional resources (pages 339–52). This chapter organizes the eight general regions of Japan—Hokkaido, Tohoku, Kanto, Chubu, Kinki, Chugoku, Shikoku, and Kyushu—from north to south. Each region's resources are divided into four sections: Section A contains foreigner information services (almost all of which have English speakers on staff), which will lead to more specific local health care information; Section B has regionally-published pamphlets and booklets about local health care, as well as other local information; Section C gives telephone numbers and web sites for finding doctors and hospitals that treat patients at night or on weekends or holidays; and Section D provides a few examples of large hospitals that offer many specialties. Remember, the information services listed in section A and the printed guides in section B will also yield information on many other hospitals and clinics in your area.

Hospitals and clinics are also listed in several other places in our book, but there they are mainly limited to the Kansai and Kanto regions. Clinics with more than one specialty may be found in the list of clinics and small hospitals on pages 33–34. Clinics and hospitals which we introduce for just one specialty are found in the related chapter—for instance, dentists and dental hospitals are in the chapter on "Caring for Your Teeth."

The bilingual Glossary contains many terms useful for discussing health matters, obtaining services, or locating products. However, for greater ease of use, the terms related to childbirth (pages 146–48), the types and forms of medications (pages 252–53), and laboratory test names (pages 90–91) have been placed within the chapters on these topics. You'll also find many other useful words and phrases in English and Japanese within each chapter.

When you are far from home and need more information in your own language, the Internet can be an invaluable reference. Whenever possible, we have given web sites for resources introduced in this book. A word of caution is in order, though—some medical information on the Internet is misleading, untested, incomplete, or outdated. Take note of the date, author, source of information, sponsor, and domain. (The names of the various domains are com (commercial), org (organizational), edu (academic), and gov (governmental); in Japan these are co.jp, or.jp, ac.jp, and go.jp respectively). Check with a doctor before acting on any medical advice you find online.

We encourage you to scan the entire book at least once before carefully reading and tagging the sections that are most helpful to you. You'll want to pay special attention to the first four chapters detailing the system and its use. Be sure to look through the Health Insurance and Public Health chapters even if you do not expect to use these programs yourself. Since they form the cornerstone of the Japanese health care system, understanding them will help clarify any of your encounters with it.

We have tried to use abbreviations sparingly, but you will notice the following throughout the book:

Insurance

Pub. Ins.:   Japanese public health insurance
             (whether national or employees')

Languages

J.	Japanese	*Kor.*	Korean
Eng.	English	*Rus.*	Russian
Camb.	Cambodian	*Sp.*	Spanish
Ch.	Chinese	*Swe.*	Swedish
Fr.	French	*Tag.*	Tagalog
Gr.	German	*Thai*	Thai
Indo.	Indonesian	*Viet.*	Vietnamese

The Health Care System

"I'd been living in Osaka for five years before I finally began to figure out how the health care system worked. At first I thought that the doctor wasn't interested in seeing me, but I gradually discovered that the three-minute visit was determined by the insurance system and not the doctor. When I got an infection, I was mystified as to why I was given a prescription for just three days. When I went back for more medicine, the doctor explained that the reason that he wanted to see me frequently was to check that the medicine was effective and to make sure that I was fully recovered.

"In the end, once I'd got used to the system, my frustration decreased and my family has been able to find good medical care."

A System in Transition

The fundamental philosophy of the Japanese health care system is equal access to health care for all. Every citizen is enrolled in a public health insurance plan, jointly financed by the national and local governments, employers, and individuals. Public welfare covers anyone financially or physically unable to contribute to the system.

The Japanese medical system has been successful in achieving universal health care coverage at an apparent low cost while enjoying some of the best statistics in the world, including the lowest infant mortality rate. However, two other factors should also be taken into account. One is that this success is possible largely because Japanese society is relatively wealthy, well-educated, and homogeneous. The other is that although health care is universally available, it often lacks quality and comfort. Long waits in hospital waiting rooms, overcrowded wards, three-minute consultations—the list goes on.

Presently, the system is in a state of transition. Appointment systems are more common, informed consent is more widely practiced, and private extra insurance plans provide for better care and amenities. The insurance system, which is responsible for many of the negative aspects of Japanese health care, has been partially revised and is still under review.

However, the increasing number of non-Japanese residents with cultural and physical differences, including the uninsured, and the rapidly increasing population of elderly Japanese in particular are putting added strain on the system. It is estimated that by the year 2025 more than one-quarter of the Japanese population will be aged sixty-five or over. Already health care expenditures have jumped from 6.7 percent of the gross national product in 1990 to 12.7 percent in 1996. It will be interesting to see how Japan meets these challenges.

Types of Facilities Available

To know what kind of hospital to visit, you first need a general understanding of the different types of medical facilities that are available.

Clinics *i'in* 医院, *kurinikku* クリニック, *shinryō-jo* 診療所

A clinic is a medical facility with less than twenty beds, where a patient may be hospitalized for up to forty-eight hours. It may not advertise itself as a hospital. Any qualified registered doctor may notify the prefectural or city health department and then set up a clinic. The requirements for staffing (for example, the ratio of professional nurses per number of patients) and equipment are lower than for hospitals. Because of this, and because of a trend toward restructuring unprofitable hospitals into clinics, the number of clinics has increased greatly in recent years.

Your neighborhood clinic, which may be staffed by just one doctor or several, is probably just the place to frequent for treatment for everyday illnesses such as simple colds or intestinal problems. The advantages of these facilities are the comparatively short waiting times, longer outpatient hours, and the proximity to home. Note, however, that most do not offer after-hours care, and should you need hospitalization in a larger hospital, your doctor will not be able to follow you. If your symptoms have not improved within a reasonable amount of time, it is worth finding a larger facility with a specialist on staff who can care for your problem.

Midwifery clinics (*josan'in* 助産院), supervised by a midwife, may have up to nine beds. These clinics have gradually been decreasing in number as young midwives have chosen to work in maternity hospitals or other facilities. Most recently this decline has been offset by younger midwives setting up independent or group practices.

Hospitals *byōin* 病院

A facility with twenty or more beds where physicians or dentists treat patients is designated as a hospital. It must meet the standards established by the Ministry of Health and Welfare regarding facilities, equipment, and staffing ratios. One way to distinguish among hospitals is by ownership—national, public, or private. A survey in 1994 reported 392 national hospitals, 1,375 public hospitals, and 7,108 private hospitals. Any individual or body can establish a private hospital after receiving permission from the prefectural government, but the hospital director must have medical qualifications. Most hospitals are small and privately owned.

The latest figures from the Ministry of Health and Welfare show that Kochi Prefecture, with 2,038 beds, has the largest number of hospital beds per 100,000 people; Hokkaido has 1,519 beds, and Tokushima Prefecture 1,474. In contrast, the figures for Saitama Prefecture show only 693 beds, Chiba Prefecture 702, and Kanagawa Prefecture 737, accentuating the problem of crowding in the suburbs of Tokyo.

Small Hospitals

With between twenty and ninety-nine beds, small hospitals offer various specialties such as internal medicine, surgical medicine, and pediatrics. They are usually equipped with X-ray facilities and surgical wards, and will also have an outpatient clinic. For ordinary family health needs, small hospitals are often ideal, as they are conveniently located, have the specialties commonly used, and, once you learn the weekly or daily flow, can provide a comparatively speedy route to a doctor as an outpatient.

On the other hand, small hospitals may not have the most modern equipment. You may find that the specialty you need is not offered or that a particular specialist is not on duty every day. Doctors at some small hospitals, in order to increase the hospital's income, may be slow to admit that you need to be referred to another hospital for further treatment, may prescribe too many medications, or may even order superfluous tests.

General Hospitals *sōgō byōin* 総合病院

This type of hospital has more than a hundred beds and must provide a minimum number of specialties, including internal medicine, general surgery, obstetrics and gynecology, ENT, ophthalmology, and laboratory and pathology facilities. These hospitals may be national, public, or private. The majority of your health care needs can be taken care of at this type of hospital and all your records will be in one facility, although it will still be your responsibility to report your health history to every doctor you see.

The disadvantages of visiting a general hospital include longer waits, less chance of seeing the same doctor each time you go for the same illness, more confusion, and more walking from window to window. Although many specialties are offered, it can be difficult to develop a personal relationship with your doctor.

Generally, *sōgō byōin* are staffed by full-time medical personnel. If you have to be hospitalized, your private practitioner may visit but not treat you in the hospital—a staff member of that hospital will become your attending physician. Interestingly, the Japan Medical Association has been encouraging local medical associations to establish community hospitals in which local physicians can admit and treat patients with the aim of providing good community health coverage. Unfortunately, this type of community hospital is still rare.

University Hospitals   *daigaku byōin*   大学病院
University hospitals are affiliated with medical or dental universities or colleges and come under the jurisdiction of the Ministry of Education. Their aims are threefold: undergraduate and graduate medical and dental education, research, and patient care. Patients at these facilities must expect to become part of the education process.

University hospitals are generally large, with modern and sophisticated equipment for diagnosis and treatment, and those affiliated with prestigious medical schools have a particularly good reputation. Because of the focus on education at these hospitals, the doctors keep up-to-date in their medical knowledge, and the size of the staff means there is a good chance of finding someone who speaks English or other foreign languages. Even if the university hospital does not have a twenty-four–hour emergency room, regular patients will be seen after-hours if they phone in advance.

On the other hand, with all the technology come all the inconveniences of large hospitals: long waits in the outpatient department and less chance of seeing the same doctor each time. You may be seen by a professor on your first visit and thereafter by new doctors, some of whom may still be learning basic medical techniques. Without a personal connection, there may be long waits for planned surgery.

Patients at university dental hospitals must expect that treatment will be performed by new dentists and that although it will be well done, it will take longer than usual.

National Hospitals   *kokuritsu byōin*   国立病院
Under the general banner of national hospitals come national university teaching hospitals, national hospitals, and national specialist centers focusing on research and

treatment of a particular disease or group of diseases, such as tuberculosis, Hansen's disease, communicable diseases, psychiatric diseases, heart disease, or cancer. You may be referred to these hospitals by your own doctor, or you can call the hospital directly and inquire (in Japanese) about the specialties offered, whether a referral is required, and/or if an appointment is necessary.

Company Hospitals *kaisharitsu byōin* 会社立病院
Some companies provide hospitals for the health care of their employees and their families; the general public may also use these facilities. Employees and their dependents sometimes receive care at a slight discount. Examples are the Japan Rail Central Hospital in Tokyo and the Kansai Power Plant Hospital in Osaka.

Geriatric Hospitals *rōjin byōin* 老人病院
Japan has various health facilities to care for the elderly. See "Help for the Disabled and the Elderly" for a description of different types.

Specialized Function Hospitals *tokutei kinō byōin* 特定機能病院
This is a special designation given to hospitals (usually university hospitals and national cancer centers) which develop new treatments and diagnoses and train doctors in advanced techniques and treatments in at least one designated field of medicine. Unfortunately, other fields at that same hospital may not be as advanced. The best way to use these hospitals is to have a letter of introduction from another medical practitioner to a specific doctor at the center. The practitioner will probably charge a fee for this letter, but you'll be charged an extra ¥1,500 or so on your first visit if you go without a referral. Some very famous doctors absolutely require a letter of introduction. Note that advanced experimental treatment—for example, an artificial ear implant—is not covered by Japanese insurance since by definition it hasn't yet been approved by the Ministry of Health and Welfare. However, whereas at other facilities patients must bear the total financial burden for such care if available, at these centers you'll be charged the full cost only of the treatment itself, while all other fees (hospitalization, etc.) are covered as usual by insurance. Japanese hospital guidebooks (see page 353) usually contain a list of the advanced procedures *kōdo senshin iryō* 高度先進医療 and the designated hospital departments.

Regional Support Hospitals *chiiki shien byōin* 地域支援病院
General hospitals with 200 beds or more may elect to become regional support hospitals. These hospitals are intended for patients with conditions or diseases which cannot be treated adequately at neighborhood clinics. Patients are expected to come with a letter of introduction from a physician at another medical facility and (hopefully) with a record of treatment and tests done to date. Sometimes the hospital has an appointment system.

This is a relatively recent addition to the Japanese medical system. Patients who come without a letter of introduction cannot be turned away, but can be charged an extra initial fee.

Public Health Centers *hoken-jo* 保健所
Public health centers are located in nearly every city or locality in Japan and are the cornerstone of the Japanese medical system. The functions of these centers are explained in "The Public Health System."

Hospices (see page 329)
Home Care (see pages 217, 225, and 330)

Health Care Professionals in Japan
Just like back home, you will find health care personnel in Japan who pride themselves on keeping up-to-date in their fields in order to give the best care possible, as well as those who do as little as possible and yet still manage to keep their jobs. The following will give you an idea about the types of health care personnel you may encounter during your stay in Japan.

Physicians, Doctors *ishi* 医師
At the end of the Second World War, the national health system was reorganized, and a single standard established for medical education. To practice medicine, a physician must complete six years of science and medical coursework at one of the country's eighty medical schools, and must pass the national medical examination administered by the Ministry of Health and Welfare.

It is recommended that newly licensed physicians continue with at least two years of graduate training in a hospital affiliated with a medical school or in a designated teaching hospital. Most new physicians do choose this graduate training; depending on the medical school, a few choose a general program (combining internal medicine, surgery, pediatrics, and emergency medicine), but most opt for more specialty-oriented programs. As in most other countries, reexamination of physicians is not required, so that once a medical school graduate has passed the national medical examination, he or she is a physician for life. (Physicians very rarely have their medical licenses revoked for unprofessional behavior.) The Japan Medical Society actively encourages individual physicians to stay abreast of new developments in their field.

Further graduate programs for physicians include a four- or five-year course leading to a doctorate in medical science (*igaku hakase*). Without this degree it would be difficult to become a teacher in a medical school or president of a large hospital. These physicians' nametags read *hakase* 博士 rather than the usual *ishi* 医師. Although most medical specialties (for instance, internal medicine) have their own academic societies which promote their own programs of specialty training, including examinations, the results of these examinations are not made public. The individual physician undertakes further study to become a better doctor and gain recognition from other doctors. However, the only way a patient will ever know about any such training is to ask the physician directly. In fact, it is illegal for a physician to advertise either the name of the medical school attended or any graduate studies completed.

Physicians educated abroad must have completed at least five years of medical education and passed the Japanese national medical examination in order to practice here. Foreign doctors must also have permanent residency in Japan and pass the top-level *ikkyū* 一級 Japanese Language Proficiency Exam. However, some foreign physicians are allowed to practice in designated clinics catering to the foreign community without having to pass the Japanese medical exam. These physicians are restricted to these specified facilities and are not able to practice in other hospitals to which their patients may be transferred. In such cases the patient would be placed under the care of a physician working at the hospital.

Registered Nurses *sei-kangofu* 正看護婦

Registered nurses are educated in a variety of two-, three-, and four-year programs in nursing schools and colleges following graduation from high school. Upon passing a national exam administered by the Ministry of Health and Welfare, they are qualified to work under doctors in hospitals, clinics, public health centers, industry, schools, visiting nurse stations, etc. Less than three percent are male.

Public Health Nurses *hoken-fu* 保健婦

Public health nurses are educated in one-year public health nursing courses for professional nurses or in a specialized four-year college program. After passing the national examination, they are qualified to work in public health centers, schools, hospitals, clinics, visiting nurse stations, etc.

Midwives *josanpu* 助産婦

Midwives are educated in a one-year midwifery course for professional nurses or in specialized four-year college programs. After passing the national examination they are qualified to work in midwifery clinics, maternity hospitals, obstetric units of general hospitals, public health centers, etc.

Assistant Nurses *jun-kangofu* 准看護婦

Assistant nurses are educated in a variety of programs following junior high school. After passing a prefectural examination they are qualified to work under the direction of a doctor, dentist, or professional nurse. In the hospital there is often no difference in the uniforms of the professional and assistant nurses; likewise, their responsibilities may be virtually indistinguishable.

Pharmacists *yakuzai-shi* 薬剤師

Pharmacists must complete a four-year university pharmaceutical program with a major in pharmacology. After passing the national examination administered by the Ministry of Health and Welfare they are qualified to work in hospital pharmacies, outside dispensing pharmacies (see page 254), and neighborhood drugstores. Every two years they must re-register with the Ministry of Health and Welfare.

Clinical Psychologists *rinshō-shinrigaku-sha* 臨床心理学者

After four years of university, psychologists in Japan study theory and train in a psychology graduate program. They offer various types of counseling and mental health treatments. They cannot prescribe medications but should be working in coordination with a psychiatrist *seishinka-i* 精神科医, a medical doctor who can. The number of students of this specialty has increased dramatically in recent years, reflecting a possible change in attitude toward the value of mental health care. There is no licensing system for psychologists in Japan, but there is Board certification for clinical psychologists.

Speech Therapists *gengo-ryōhō-shi* 言語療法士

Speech therapists work in large general or university hospitals that have rehabilitation units, rehabilitation centers, children's hospitals, etc. Since 1991, a professional support association has given certificates of proficiency to speech therapists who fulfill its education requirements and pass its qualifying examination. The Ministry of Health and Welfare will administer the first national examination for licensure in December, 1998.

Physical Therapists *rigaku-ryōhō-shi* 理学療法士

Physical therapists must complete a three- to four-year degree program and pass a national examination in order to be recognized by the Ministry of Health and Welfare. They are then qualified to work in general and university hospitals, rehabilitation centers, geriatric hospitals, homes for the elderly, etc., under the guidance of a doctor.

Occupational Therapists *sagyō-ryōhō-shi* 作業療法士

Occupational therapists must complete a three- to four-year degree program and pass a national exam in order to be recognized by the Ministry of Health and Welfare. They are then qualified to work under a doctor in facilities that provide rehabilitation services.

Vision Therapists *shinō kunren-shi* 視能訓練士

Vision therapists must complete three or four years of specialized training after high school or complete one year or more of specialized education after college or nursing school. After passing a national examination, they then work with an ophthalmologist, doing vision testing and teaching eye-strengthening exercises, especially to children.

Optometrists *kengan-sha* 検眼士

There are no educational requirements or examinations for optometrists. They are free to prescribe correctional lenses and to sell them to customers in eyeglass stores. Optometrists may also fill prescriptions for corrective lenses written by ophthalmologists.

Podiatrists (foot specialists)

There is no podiatry specialty in Japan. See page 193 for foot care and foreign podiatrists.

Dentists and Dental Hygienists (see pages 265–67)
Alternative Medicine Practitioners (see pages 275–90)

Areas of Medical Specialty

The following are just some of the specialties that you may see posted outside clinics or hospitals. Legally, a physician can list on the signboard any specialty that he or she feels comfortable treating. The sign may or may not mean that the physician has done lengthy postgraduate study in that specialty. When one doctor lists several specialties, the first one or two are likely to be his or her real specialties. In a university hospital, on the other hand, the specialty listed will be the one in which the doctor has done or is doing extra study.

Cardiovascular (Circulatory) Medicine
junkanki-ka 循環器科
Heart disease and circulatory problems.

Dermatology *hifu-ka* 皮膚科
Skin diseases, including male genital rashes.

Otolaryngology (ENT [ear, nose, and throat])
jibi-inkō-ka 耳鼻咽喉科 (*jibi-ka* 耳鼻科)
Privacy is often nonexistent in the ENT office. Allergies such as hay fever are also treated here.

Gastroenterology *shōkaki-ka* 消化器科 or
ichōka 胃腸科
For diseases of the stomach, intestines, and related structures like the esophagus, liver, etc.

Internal Medicine *naika* 内科
For diseases not usually treated surgically, including AIDS. The internist is often used as a family physician or a G.P. If you cannot pinpoint your problem, or if you want a referral, start by seeing an internist.

Neurology *shinkei-naika* 神経内科
For diseases of the nervous system like Parkinson's disease or multiple sclerosis. Might be a subdivision of the Internal Medicine Department.

Ob/Gyn *sanfujin-ka* 産婦人科
Concerned with women's health in general, including childbirth and menopause, and with diseases of the genital, urinary, and rectal organs, including sexually transmitted diseases. In Japan, women go to a surgeon for breast problems.

Ophthalmology *ganka* 眼科
For eye problems, including vision testing.

Orthopedics *seikei geka* 整形外科
For correction of disorders of bones, joints, and muscles. Most sports doctors are orthopedic specialists.

Plastic Surgery *keisei geka* 形成外科
For the restoration and repair of external physical defects (caused by serious burns, accidents, birthmarks, large moles, etc.) including bone and tissue grafts. This surgery is covered by public insurance, but purely cosmetic surgery is not.

Pediatrics *shōni-ka* 小児科
For children up to 15–17 years of age. In Japan, a pediatrician may often work as a G.P., seeing all members of the family. Check when preven-

tive pediatric care is offered. You may be referred to an ENT for children's ear, nose, or throat problems. See a surgeon for cuts, etc.

Psychiatry *seishin-ka* 精神科
Diagnosis and treatment of mental illnesses.

Respiratory Medicine *kokyūki-ka* 呼吸器科
For problems of the lungs and the larger respiratory system, including asthma.

Surgery *geka* 外科
Operative procedures for correction of deformities and repair of injuries. You would go to a surgeon to have a child's cut stitched up, or if you found a lump in your breast.

Urology *hinyōki-ka* 泌尿器科
Concerned with the urinary tract in both sexes

and the genital tract in the male. Also treats male venereal diseases and impotency.

Venereal Disease (V.D.) Medicine *seibyō-ka* 性病科
Counseling and treatment of sexually transmitted diseases. HIV/AIDS patients are cared for by internists or infectious disease *densen-byō* 伝染病 specialists.

Other specialties may include:
Pain clinics *pein kurinikku* ペインクリニック
Allergies *arerugī* アレルギー
Diabetes *tōnyō-byō* 糖尿病, etc.
Check in advance to see if a facility can treat your problem.

Patient Rights and Informed Consent

"I dropped my husband off at our city hospital for a gallbladder test, but the surgeon insisted that I return for a family/doctor conference before the test began. My husband had already been admitted to the hospital, had been started on an intravenous drip, and was scheduled to have the test in 45 minutes. At the conference, the surgeon drew a picture of the gallbladder and explained the testing procedure in detail, telling us about possible complications and how any complications would be handled. He gave us the risk percentages worldwide and his own personal success rate—100 percent in over 500 procedures. He answered all our questions. Then we were asked to sign an informed consent form stating that we had received and understood all the information. Thirty minutes later my husband underwent an uneventful test. I call it 'informed consent in the nick of time.'"

The concepts of patient rights and informed consent are not mandated by law in Japan. Traditionally, Japanese patients have been content to leave most decisionmaking to the doctor and have not asked for a thorough explanation of the diagnosis or treatment.

Back in 1994, the Japan Hospital Association instructed member hospitals on guidelines for obtaining informed consent from their patients. A 1997 survey by the Federation of Health Insurance Societies revealed that seventy percent of inpatients and fifty-two percent of outpatients said their doctors gave them relatively detailed explanations of their conditions in order to get their informed consent. That still leaves many patients who do not receive an adequate explanation of their treatment.

Japanese doctors have traditionally been hesitant to give the bad news about a terminal illness, such as cancer, directly to the patient. Very often a family member (usually a brother or husband and/or sometimes the wife) will be told, and asked to make decisions about treatment and about whether to inform the patient. The word cancer, or *gan* がん, has a very heavy emotional connotation of impending death, and many Japanese say that they would prefer not to know their diagnosis. However, hiding the truth makes it very difficult for patient, caregivers, and family members to build up a trusting relationship, since everyone involved must be constantly evasive, and the patient gets very little chance to talk about his feelings.

On your first visit, try asking some questions and note how the doctor responds. Particularly if you need long-term therapy, it's important to feel comfortable with your doctor. Japanese doctors are aware that foreigners expect to be told their diagnosis, and they may be more willing to speak frankly. Try to understand that doctors are not used to talking about death or terminal illness in their own language, let alone in English, and so may tell you in a manner that seems blunt or unfeeling.

Malpractice

Relatively few Japanese complain about their medical care or go to the trouble of filing a suit, even if they feel mistreated. However, not all cases of malpractice are ignored. The Sanitation Department (*eisei-kyoku* 衛生局 or *eisei-bu* 衛生部) of every prefecture has a section (in Tokyo, it is called the Medical Affairs Section *imu shidō-ka* 医務指導課) which handles complaints about facilities. If you find a facility dangerously dirty, understaffed, poorly equipped, etc., you can report it to this department of the prefectural office where the hospital is located. If your complaint appears valid, a formal investigation will be made. If the facility is found at fault, a warning will be given, with follow-up monitoring. If you're having trouble contacting the appropriate office, the AMDA Centers (see the endpapers) can help you.

If the problem is inappropriate medical treatment rather than hospital management, you'll need to confirm first with a medical lawyer that the care was indeed malpractice, and then file a suit. For more information, consult the organization below.

Consumer Organization for Medicine and Law (COML)
Iryo Jinken Senta
医療人権センター
06-314-1652 (J. only)

2

Choosing a Caregiver and Using the System

"When my husband is ill, he's either seen by a nurse in his company or he goes to a large general hospital near his office. The one time he needed surgery, the problem was identified at his annual physical, and the doctor in charge recommended a hospital and arranged for his admission.

"When I have a cold I go to a neighborhood clinic which I discovered after talking to neighbors. The doctor's English is not fluent but he's patient in listening to my concerns. For health testing I go to the public health center and a clinic downtown that's geared toward working people —it accepts insurance and uses an appointment system. The children go to the neighborhood doctor for simple problems and to the ENT clinic nearby for ear infections; checkups and vaccinations they get at the public health center. However, for specialty checks like developmental evaluations, I take them to a university hospital outpatient clinic. The one time my son needed a doctor late at night, we called ahead to that university hospital's emergency room and got permission to be seen there."

Choosing a Caregiver

Where to Start

The Japanese tend to choose their caregivers on the basis of a facility's reputation, or through introductions to specific professionals by friends, relatives, or a family doctor. Public health centers may also provide information on facilities treating specific conditions. Once the selection is made, the Japanese patient usually feels secure and rarely questions the choice further. Japanese doctors—especially those working in hospitals—don't usually display licenses or diplomas, and Japan has no official statement of patient rights. Like so many other parts of Japanese society, the system has worked on this kind of trust. Only very recently has the media begun to give Japanese patients more details on the care offered at different facilities, so that people can make informed choices.

As a foreign resident, especially if you are a newcomer, you are most likely limited in your access to this kind of information or such introductions. It also may be harder for you to rely on this kind of trust. We suggest that you get names from several different sources. Read the sections on different healthcare facilities and personnel in the previous chapter, to familiarize yourself with the options provided by the system here. Note that although there are a few foreign GPs practicing in Japan, there is no general practitioner system in which a family doctor treats all basic conditions and then refers you to a specialist when necessary. In the Japanese system, you go directly to the specialist yourself (check the list on page 20). Some conditions may be treated by different specialists than would be the case in your own country. Note also the difference between the care at clinics and that at the different types of hospitals.

Keep in mind, too, that certain fields that require licensing or certification in your own country may not in Japan. For example, Japan has no official qualifying exam or surveillance system for chiropractors, homeopaths, podiatrists, or aromatherapists. In the field of mental health, only psychiatrists need to be licensed. Especially if the caregiver is working in a field which is not licensed in Japan and is working independently, don't hesitate to ask about background, experience, and approach. If the referring source does not have this information, you can sometimes make these inquiries in a pre-visit phone call, particularly if the caregiver is a non-Japanese. Once care begins, keep evaluating its appropriateness and effectiveness. If the treatment you are receiving does not seem to be meeting your needs, reevaluate your goals with your caregiver or seek help elsewhere.

One other factor that might influence your choice is that Japanese medicine has not traditionally maintained strict confidentiality about services and records. The very layout of most examining rooms makes privacy of this sort almost impossible. Most people learn to live with this, but if you are concerned about confidentiality, you might seek treatment in an area where you are not known. In addition, you should also refrain from using your Japanese employees' insurance if you don't want your employer to learn that you have been seeing a doctor.

With all this in mind, identify the basic needs of you and your family. For simple illnesses, such as a cold, try and find a user-friendly clinic in your neighborhood. However, remember that at most clinics, physicians are not available after hours. For minor surgery and diagnostic tests, try a larger general hospital which is likely to have a full range of specialties and English-speaking doctors. For complicated procedures, such as heart surgery, the English ability of the doctors may not be so important—you'll want the best available.

Some clinics are especially geared to serving the foreign community. They are staffed by foreign caregivers or Japanese able to speak foreign languages and familiar with the medical customs of foreign countries. Even their receptionist will speak English. They provide a welcome oasis to those who can't speak Japanese or who long for familiar medical practices or a familiar bedside manner. If you have foreign insurance, you'll also find these clinics convenient, since they easily provide itemized receipts in English. Note, that most don't accept Japanese public health insurance and are thus not limited to the restrictions set by the Japanese government—the doctor can spend more time with you and provide medications or treatments not yet approved by the Ministry of Health and Welfare. This also means, however, that the facility can charge any fee it thinks reasonable, and because the fee must cover longer consultations, comfortable sur-roundings, stricter appointment systems, etc., it can sometimes be three or more times that set by the government.

Checking into Appointments and Costs

If the facility does not have an appointment system (and most don't), be sure to ask the days and hours of the physician you want to consult, since he may not be there every day. You can then simply go during those hours and, though you may need to wait an hour or two, you will be able to see that doctor. If you don't know a specific doctor but need someone who speaks English, you can call ahead (in Japanese) to see if there is an English-speaking doctor who can treat your ailment.

Considering cost, you'll want to read the appropriate sections in our health insurance chapter. With Japanese insurance, the initial visit to a doctor at a clinic is presently set at approximately ¥2,800 (¥2,500 at a hospital) of which you pay only 20 to 30 percent. Subsequent visits are approximately ¥740. Tests and treatments are additional. If you have foreign insurance, fees may be different. Be sure to read about the point system on page 80. Note that not only specialized function hospitals (see page 16) but any hospital with over 200 beds may charge an extra initial fee (usually ¥1,000–¥3,000) if you visit without a referral from another medical facility. Some very famous doctors absolutely require a letter of introduction, for which you may be charged.

If you have foreign insurance and need an itemized receipt in English, check ahead of time whether the staff can provide one. If you don't have insurance, see our section on Strategies for the Uninsured, page 84.

Resources for Finding a Caregiver

■ Ask friends, coworkers, and acquaintances.

■ Many local government offices have a list of foreigner-friendly clinics and hospitals. See "Regional Resources."

■ Many information services (see the endpapers) and support groups have lists of doctors.

■ Check listings in English-language phone books and magazines. Although they will almost certainly speak some English and be used to dealing with foreigners, not all accept public insurance. Check before you go.

■ **AMDA International Medical Information Centers**
These centers have extensive lists of doctors nationwide (see the endpapers).

■ Check the sections in this book on your specific problem and the lists of clinics (pages 33–34) and hospitals (see "Regional Resources").

■ **International Association for Medical Assistance to World Travellers** (IAMAT)
417 Center Street, Lewiston NY 14092 U.S.
1-716-754-4883

Organization of medical doctors who have agreed to care for travelers to their countries for a set fee. For a donation, the association will send a booklet listing physicians in 500 cities.

■ **American Express Card and Gold Mastercard Information Service, U.S.**
1-202-554-2639 (Amex)
1-303-271-2421 (Mastercard)
Cardholders can call, collect, a 24-hour phone service in the U.S. that gives information on doctors, hospitals, local interpreters, etc.

■ **Medical Access: A Foreigner's Guide to Health Care in Kobe**
Order from Community House and Information Center (CHIC) in Kobe
078-857-6540, fax 078-857-6541
An excellent guide to health care in the Kobe area.

■ At your local bookstore you will find several books in Japanese introducing hospitals and specialists. See "References and Further Reading."

Making the Most of Your Time with the Doctor

The Japanese health care system is a patriarchal system in which the doctor is believed to be the expert, and his advice is almost unquestioningly accepted by the patient.

Doctors who work under the public health system are on a strict time schedule, with just a few minutes allotted to each patient, so there's not a lot of time to discuss symptoms and possible treatment. Try to research your problems as completely as possible so that you can ask intelligent, specific questions. Ask, "Should I eat any special foods?" or "What is my cholesterol level this week?" Note that some large hospitals keep their patient charts filed according to specialty, which means that the dermatologist you visit may not see your chart from the surgical specialist. It is your responsibility to tell your doctor if you are being treated for another condition, or have another condition which may affect your present problem. *It's of vital importance that you tell your doctor about any other medications that you are taking now or that you sometimes take.* If the doctor listens and responds to your concerns, you've crossed the first hurdle and are well on the way to building a trusting relationship. In a good relationship you should be able to discuss your current diagnosis, proposed treatment, and options.

If you are hospitalized, wait to ask your questions until the doctor is doing his rounds and you have his complete attention—don't run up to him in the hall or send messages through the nurses. Sometimes it helps to appoint one member of the family to communicate with him if there are many concerns or complications, as doctors get tired of explaining the same thing over and over again as each family member visits. For a discussion of Patient Rights and Informed Consent, see page 21.

Getting a Second Opinion

"My son had ear infections that seemed to affect his hearing. He was too young to be tested accurately with the regular hearing test, so I asked his doctor at a university hospital to refer him to another university hospital where I knew they had testing equipment for young children. The doctor wrote out his medical history (for a fee) but wouldn't say that it was a referral to the other hospital, and didn't seem to think it was necessary to go there. I've since learned that doctors are very loyal to doctors from their own medical school and rarely make a referral to a doctor from a different school."

"During my recent illness I was first hospitalized at a large medical center. After tests, my doctor told my wife that I only had another two or three months to live. She immediately asked a friend for advice and he recommended a university hospital. It was very lucky that I moved there, as I subsequently found out that my real condition, while rare, was easily cured by an operation. Getting a second opinion saved my life."

The practice of getting a second opinion is not established here. However, if you are not getting well and/or your doctor will not discuss alternatives, you probably need to get a second opinion. Some contact a physician in their own country for another view or confirmation. You may elect not to tell your first doctor (even if the second diagnosis agreed with the first), since this may make the doctor feel that he has failed to inspire confidence. In order not to alienate the first doctor, Japanese patients often simply go to another hospital, repeat the same tests, and compare the diagnoses. Although this system is a waste of time and money, it seems there is no alternative.

If you are hospitalized and really need a second opinion, not only will a spouse or friend have to do the research, but it may be harder to find another doctor willing to see you. This may also entail discharging yourself from the hospital without the original doctor's permission. But despite the hassles, it's often worth looking until you are satisfied.

Outpatient Care

When you go for an outpatient visit, there will be a lot of other people there too. The high number of outpatient visits made by the Japanese can be ascribed to the low cost of health care under public insurance plans and the prescribing of medications for only two or three days, requiring repeated return visits for more medications.

Preparing for an Outpatient Visit

■ Telephone the facility to find out whether your problem can be treated, and whether an appointment is necessary.

■ Find out the outpatient hours. First-time patients are often seen only in the morning, for instance, from 9:00 to 11:00. If you arrive after that time you will not be seen. Not all specialists are on duty every day, so check if you can be seen that day for your problem.

■ Get your identification cards ready. If it is your first visit, you'll need to fill out a registration form in Japanese. If this presents problems, bring something with your name and address written on it in Japanese (your insurance certificate or a business card) or ask a Japanese friend to help with interpreting. If you are enrolled in a public health insurance plan (see pages 68–78), you must bring your insurance card on the first visit and on the first visit of every month thereafter. If you are going to a different specialty in that outpatient department, you'll need to show your insurance certificate again.

■ Cash is essential. Credit cards are not accepted, nor are personal checks, except at some of the clinics catering to foreigners. Even under public insurance plans, there is still a fee, although it's usually modest. ¥10,000 should more than suffice. If you're not insured under Japanese public insurance, you will be charged the full fee. If you are privately insured, it is your responsibility to get reimbursed; take at least ¥30,000.

■ Before you leave the house, take your temperature.

■ Women should wear a very full skirt if they plan to have a gynecological examination. Gowns and/or drapes are not always provided and the skirt can be used to provide some privacy.

■ Prepare a written description of your illness or problem. Make a list of the questions you wish to ask. Although some Japanese doctors do speak and understand spoken English, written English is often a good way to communicate.

Information for the Doctor

■ Name, age, address.
■ History of present illness.
■ Use the correct medical term wherever possible. A non-native English speaker is much more likely to know the word "vomit" than "throw up."
■ Past medical history.

■ Any medications you are currently taking.
■ Allergies.
■ Family history: Note only things that you've been advised may be hereditary—for example, not "My mother died of old age" but "My father died at forty-two of a heart attack."

Questions for the Doctor

■ What is my diagnosis?
■ What should I do at home if … happens?
■ What medications are you giving me?
■ When should I take them?

■ What are the expected results?
■ Are there any side effects?
■ When should I stop taking them?
■ Do I have to come back?

See "References and Further Reading" for books that give terms and phrases that you'll need to
speak to a caregiver in Japanese.

At the Outpatient Facility

The procedure for an outpatient visit at a doctor's office, clinic, or hospital varies according to facility—at smaller clinics one desk may handle all the various stages, while hospitals may use computers to cut down on paperwork and walking. In any case, the closer you arrive to the starting hour, the shorter will be your wait to see the doctor.

If you are still unsure whether your condition merits an outpatient visit, go! If your condition worsens during the night or over the weekend, it will be much more difficult to find appropriate medical care.

The First Visit

■ Fill out a registration form (*shinsatsu mōshikomisho* 診察申込書) and present it with your public insurance certificate (if you have one) at the reception desk (*shoshin uketsuke* 初診受付). Ask at the registration desk if you need help filling it out. Some facilities have forms translated into English. If you have a letter of introduction, present it at this time.

■ Usually you will be asked to sit down and wait for your patient identification card (*shinsatsuken* 診察券) and your medical chart (*karute* カルテ) to be prepared.

■ When your name is called, go to the relevant department and hand in the chart at the reception desk there. You may be issued a number to indicate your turn for consultation, or your chart may have been sent by computer.

■ Sit down in the nearby waiting area until your name is called. A nurse may come over to ask you why you want to see the doctor. You may also be asked to take your temperature while you wait (place the thermometer under your arm, not in the mouth) or you may be asked to provide a urine sample.

■ In very large hospitals you may be asked to move along to several different waiting areas before you actually see the doctor. This can be very frustrating because with each move you expect to meet the doctor, and instead find that you are just seeing a different part of the outpatient area.

■ Eventually your name will be called when it is your turn to see the doctor. Listen carefully, since the pronunciation of foreign names by non-English speakers may be quite different, and you may be called by your first name with *-san* attached.

■ If laboratory tests or X-rays are needed, you will be directed to the relevant department, and even given a map if it is a large hospital. At each department, hand the test request to the nurse or secretary on duty and wait for your name to be called. Outpatient clinic staff are usually cheerful about directing you (or even taking you in person) to the next department or desk.

■ When your tests have been completed, return to the original clinic, announce your presence to the nurse or secretary again, and wait to be called in to see the doctor. Ask or show your prepared questions, and write down the answers. You should ask the doctor at this time for any necessary copies of lab tests, etc. A fee will be charged for this service. If you need to take time off from work to recover, ask the doctor for a medical certificate (*shindansho* 診断書). Also ask the doctor for a business card (*meishi* 名刺) so that the next time you go for an outpatient visit you can check ahead of time if he or she will be on duty.

■ After seeing the doctor, go back to the reception area of the hospital. If you're carrying your chart, place it in the appropriate container (sometimes a large box) near the accounting department's window. Sit down and wait.

■ When your name is called, settle your account at the payment window (*kaikei* 会計). Your insurance certificate and patient ID card may be returned to you at this time. Private insurance forms are usually completed here. Expect another wait, and possibly a charge for this service.

■ If your doctor has written a prescription for you, sit down near the pharmacy window (*yaku zaibu* 薬剤部) and pick up your medications when your name is called. Check that the pharmacist has noted the name and dosage of each medication on each envelope. See pages 254–57 for further information about obtaining medications.

■ Make sure that you have your patient identification card and insurance certificate before you leave.

■ Go home, have a well-deserved rest, and congratulate yourself on having survived an outpatient visit in Japan!

The Examination Room

"I chose a private physician for general care for our family. She didn't speak much English, but always had several medical dictionaries handy for when we got stuck. Her manner was competent, and her care excellent. The only thing that surprised me was that there was inevitably another patient in her office when she examined me or my children. One time it was a child receiving an intravenous drip, and another time it was a child with a communicable disease."

The examination room may be cluttered with books, assorted equipment, and furniture. This is normal. However, if the equipment is dirty and the doctor doesn't seem to be concerned about cleanliness, it may be time to look for another hospital. Be warned that there may be another patient in sight or at least within earshot. Japanese people seem to be adept at curtaining off space mentally to ensure their own privacy—the best solution is to try to "do as the Japanese do" and learn to screen out distractions.

During a gynecological exam, a woman may be surprised to find a short curtain in place to hide the doctor from her view. This is evidently to protect Japanese women from the embarrassment of looking directly at a doctor when in this uncomfortable position. However, Japanese doctors seem to take it in their stride if a foreign woman whips the curtain aside to talk to the doctor face-to-face while the procedure is in progress.

Follow-up Visits

■ Expect to make return visits—often every three days or so—until the doctor states that you are completely recovered.
■ With the exception of international clinics, very few facilities have a real appointment system. Some facilities use block appointment systems, whereby a certain number of patients are given appointments for a single time-slot. A wait is still involved, but it's usually shorter than the first-come, first-served system. Your next appointment is made at the end of each visit, or when you call ahead to the outpatient department.
■ Present your patient identification cards at the reception desk and follow the outpatient

procedure. If it is your first visit of the month, you will also need your health insurance certificate, if you have one.

■ In large hospitals, it is sometimes difficult to see the same doctor each time you visit. Try to arrange your visit to coincide with the doctor's time on duty by consulting his schedule, which is usually displayed in that outpatient department. At the next visit, tell the nurse which doctor you want to see when you reach the specialty area. In smaller clinics, the chances of seeing the same doctor are of course much greater.

Record Keeping

"When I moved and had to see a new doctor for cancer treatment follow-up, she really scared me when she gave me the frightening news that my blood levels were high and the cancer might have returned. When I called my previous doctor, I found that this level was normal for me. My new doctor had not seen my old records. I hadn't known that it was my responsibility to actually bring a copy of my medical history to my new doctor."

"My son had a CT scan and an EEG at the age of eighteen months. When we went back for a checkup when he was four, the hospital had already destroyed all his old records. There was no way to compare his progress. I should have asked for a written report of the test results to keep myself."

Medical records belong to the clinic or hospital, and you are usually not allowed to read them. However, it is up to you to keep track of the information in those records.

■ Ask your doctor for a written summary of your condition, treatment, and test results to date if you are moving, want to see another doctor, or if you have a condition requiring only occasional checkups, yearly or bi-yearly, for example. Hospitals destroy records periodically, because of the lack of storage space—or so we are told.

■ Doctors see only records from their own specialty area. You must be sure to tell every doctor that treats you if you are receiving treatment or medications for a different condition.

■ Make it a practice to keep your own health and medical history notebook, making entries for each disease and outpatient visit for each member of the family.

Tips for Better Time Management

■ Get sick on slow days. Never take a child to a pediatrician on Monday morning!

■ You may be able to place your patient ID card in the appropriate box before the hospital opens for business and then be one of the first to be called when the facility opens.

■ Be prepared to spend at least half a day on an outpatient visit. Bring books and games for you and the kids. Getting angry and upset merely raises your blood pressure—remember that the Japanese don't like the long wait either.

■ Get to know the flow pattern of your outpatient facility, and plan accordingly.

Clinics and Small Hospitals

These facilities are general practice or multi-department facilities specifically suggested to us as "foreigner-friendly" by non-Japanese who have used them. Other specialty "foreigner-friendly" clinics are scattered throughout the book under the specific specialty. Call in advance, since appointments may be needed. Not all provide care after-hours, even in emergencies. Even if the doctor speaks English, the office receptionist and nurses may not.

✻ Specially serving the English-speaking foreign community.

C: Cardiovascular (Circulatory) diseases; *Ca:* Cardiology; *Cos:* Cosmetic surgery; *D:* Dermatology; *Di:* Diabetes; *E:* Endocrinology; *ENT:* Ear Nose Throat; *G:* Gastroenterology; *GP:* General Practitioner; *H:* Holistic Health; *I:* Internal medicine; *N:* Neurology; *Ns:* Neurosurgery; *O/G:* Ob/Gyn; *Op:* Ophthalmology; *Opto:* Optometry; *Or:* Orthopedics; *P:* Pediatrics; *Pod:* Podiatry; *PS:* Plastic Surgery; *Psy:* Psychiatry; *PT:* Physiotherapy; *R:* Rehabilitation; *Rad:* Radiology; *Res:* Respiratory diseases; *S:* Surgery; *U:* Urology; *V:* Venereal Disease.

Takagi Skin Clinic [Cos, D]
Takagi Kurinikku Shibuya
高木クリニック渋谷
Kuken Bldg. 3 Fl., 36-1 Udagawa-cho
Shibuya-ku, Tokyo
03-3462-2807/03-3461-8178 (Eng.)
(Dr. Chieko McKinstrey)

✻The King Clinic [GP]
ザ キングクリニック
Olympia Annex 4 Fl., 6-31-21 Jingumae
Shibuya-ku, Tokyo
http://member.nifty.ne.jp/the-king-clinic
03-3409-0764 (Pub. Ins., Eng., Gr., Ch., Rus.)
(Dr. Theodor King)

✻Tokyo Medical and Surgical Clinic
[Ca, D, ENT, I, N, O/G, Op, Opt, Or, PT, PS, Pod, Psy, Rad, U]
32 Mori Bldg. 2 Fl., 3-4-30 Shiba-Koen
Minato-ku, Tokyo
03-3436-3028 (Eng.)

✻Tokyo British Clinic [GP]
東京ブリティッシュクリニック
Daikanyama Y Bldg. 2 Fl., 2-13-7 Ebisu-Nishi
Shibuya-ku, Tokyo
03-5458-6099 (Eng.)
(Dr. Gabriel Symonds)
(Dr. Evelyn Lewis)
Includes pediatric care. 24-hour availability.

✻National Medical Clinic [P, I, ENT, D, Breast Exams]
ナショナル メディカル クリニック
#202 5-16-11 Minami-Azabu, Minato-ku, Tokyo
03-3473-2057 (Eng.)
Family medicine.

✻International Clinic
1-5-9 Azabudai, Minato-ku, Tokyo
03-3583-7831 (Pub. Ins., Eng., Rus., Fr., Swe.)
Long-time, family practice with all foreign doctors.

Hibiya Byoin [I, S, Or, PS, U, D]
日比谷病院
1-3-2 Uchisaiwaicho, Chiyoda-ku, Tokyo
03-3502-7231 (Pub. Ins., Eng.)

Kaijo Clinic [I, Or, O/G, Op, ENT, D, C, E]
Kaijo Biru Shinryo-jo
海上ビル診療所
Shinkan 3 Fl.,1-2-1 Marunouchi
Chiyoda-ku, Tokyo
03-3212-7690 (Pub. Ins., Eng.)

✻Dr. Claudine Bliah
Seino Clinic
Minato-ku, Tokyo
03-3400-9942 (direct to Dr. Bliah; Eng., Fr.)
General practice.

Kobayashi International Clinic
(Dr. Yoneyuki Kobayashi: S, G
 Dr. Shiei Kobayashi: P)
小林インターナショナル クリニック
3-5-6-110 Nishi-Tsuruma, Yamato-shi
Kanagawa-ken
0462-63-1380 (Pub. Ins., Eng., Ch., Kor., Viet., Camb.)
Dr. Y. Kobayashi is director of AMDA International Medical Information Center, Tokyo (see the end-papers).

Isanuma ENT Clinic
Isanuma Kurinikku Jibi Inko-ka Shinryo-jo
いさぬま クリニック耳鼻咽喉科診療所
27-1 Furuya-Kami, Kawagoe-shi, Saitama-ken
0492-35-0100 (Pub. Ins., Eng.)
(Dr. Nobuhiro Tokita)

Shinjuku Mitsui Bldg. Clinic [G, Di, C]
新宿三井ビルクリニック
2-1 Nishi-Shinjuku, Shinjuku-ku, Tokyo
03-3344-3311 (Pub. Ins., Eng.)

Sakakibara Kinen Clinic [I, P, Ca, D, C]
榊原記念クリニック
NS Bldg. 4 Fl., Nishi-Shinjuku, Shinjuku-ku, Tokyo
03-3344-3313 (Pub. Ins., Eng.)

Ikoma Clinic 生馬医院 [I]
Ikoma Byoin
Silk Center 1 Fl., 1 Yamashita-cho, Naka-ku
Yokohama-shi
045-231-5921 (Pub. Ins., Eng.)

✳**Bluff Clinic** [I, P, PT, Ob/Gyn]
82 Yamate-cho, Naka-ku, Yokohama-shi
045-641-6961 (Pub. Ins., Eng.)

✳**Dr. Geoffrey Barraclough** [GP]
Kobe Int'l. Hospital & Medical Services
Association
Ninomiya Pearl Mansion 4 Fl.
4-23-11 Ninomiya-cho, Chuo-ku, Kobe
078-241-2896 (Eng., J., Fr., Gr.)
Long-time Kobe resident, British general
practitioner; makes house calls in emergencies.
Will also make referrals.

Gracia Byoin [I, S, Or, Op, R]
ガラシア病院
6-14-1 Aomadani-Nishi, Minoo-shi, Osaka-fu
0727-29-2345 (Pub. Ins., Eng.)

Otani Clinic [I, P]
大谷クリニック
1-9-9 Kyomachibori, Nishi-ku, Osaka-shi

06-441-1980 (Pub. Ins., Eng.)
(Dr. Noboru Otani)

Oba Byoin [I, C, Res, G, D, P]
大場病院
1-1-9 Shikanjima, Konohana-ku, Osaka-shi
06-463-1022 (Pub. Ins., Eng.)
(Dr. Kisaburo Oba)

Sakabe International Clinic [I, S, N, G]
さかべインターナショナルクリニック
435 Yamamoto-cho, Nijo-Sagaru, Gokomachi-dori
Nakagyo-ku, Kyoto-shi
075-231-1624 (Pub. Ins., Eng., Ch.)
(Dr. Yoshio Sakabe)

Hatano Clinic [I]
Hatano Naika
波多野内科
Sakae Dai-ichi Seimei Bldg. 3 Fl., 2-13
Shinsakae-machi, Naka-ku, Nagoya-shi
052-951-1432 (Pub. Ins., Eng. [no Eng. on Thurs.])

Ichinose Byoin [G, S, N]
一ノ瀬病院
1-5-11 Kokutaijimachi, Naka-ku, Hiroshima-shi
082-243-6223 (Pub. Ins., Eng.)

Kotoni Naika Icho-ka Clinic [I, G]
ことに内科・胃腸科クリニック
Hokko Bldg. 2 Fl., Kotoni 2-jo 5-1-3
Nishi-ku, Sapporo-shi
011-643-5311 (Pub. Ins., Eng.)
(Dr. Minoru Yoshida)

Kita-Kanto Cardiovascular Hospital
[C, H, I, *ningen dokku*]
Kita-Kanto Junkanki Byoin
北関東循環器病院
740 Shimohakoda, Hokkitsu-Mura
Seta-gun, Gunma-ken
0272-32-7111 (Pub. Ins., Eng.)
(Dr. Shuichi Ichikawa)
ichikawa@mail.wind.co.jp

Planned Hospitalization

Admission may be necessary for a variety of reasons—to take a series of diagnostic tests, to undergo surgery or medical treatment such as chemotherapy, or even to help stabilize a chronic medical condition such as diabetes mellitus. Most hospitalizations are arranged through outpatient departments.

If you know you're going to need hospitalization, start investigating your condition in the outpatient or affiliated clinic of a hospital where you would like to be hospitalized. This way, if any diagnostic tests or treatment are started, all your records will be in one place.

Choosing a Hospital

In selecting a hospital the basic consideration is medical, such as specialities offered, the range of diagnostic equipment available, and the attending physicians who practice there. However, in Japan, other important considerations should be taken into account, such as the amount of nursing care provided, dietary services, languages understood (especially by the doctors), distance from home, cost of care, and hospital policies.

Does It Look Clean?

The word "hospital" denotes a wide variety of institutions, not all of which may meet your expectations of a high-tech, sterile environment. In Japan, the outer appearance of a medical facility is not necessarily an indication of the care you receive—some of the most prestigious hospitals have rundown-looking buildings and shabby furniture. Many institutions don't seem to have money left over from their limited funds to give their facilities a facelift. Inside, too, Japan's crowded living and working conditions are reflected in the equipment and supplies stored in hallways and large communal wards. Don't confuse clutter with uncleanliness. But if you see dirty instruments, dust under examining tables, and personnel in stained uniforms and with poor personal hygiene, you may want to consider another hospital.

How Are the Medical Services?

Choosing a hospital with experienced doctors is an obvious priority, but some Japanese, perhaps with the recession in mind, recommend a few discreet questions to confirm that the institution is well established—that is, financially stable. Prospective patients are also advised to check that doctors make regular daily rounds, as some doctors often work at several other clinics and may only be available for consultation once or twice a week, which could affect treatment.

On the other hand, in a university hospital or other teaching institution, doctors usually make their rounds with a team of residents, interns, and students. You may find people other than your own doctor asking questions and examining you. Try to think of it in a positive sense, with your illness being used as a teaching tool to train younger doctors. However, if you don't relish the thought of being repeatedly poked and probed, then maybe a teaching hospital is not the best choice for you.

Check the services your hospital offers. Is there an intensive care unit? Are there doctors specializing in your disease? Is support care available? Be sure to check that a full range of equipment—both diagnostic and for treatment—is available. A large percentage of hospitals have CT scans, ultra-sound equipment, and fiberscopes for examining stomach and lungs, but only a small percentage have magnetic resonance imaging (MRI) or mammography equipment.

Is the Nursing Staff Adequate?

According to the Japanese, polite, cheerful nurses and office staff who "move about in an energetic manner" are a sure sign of a good hospital.

For a long time the traditional system of hospital nursing care involved the family's staying in the hospital with the patient to provide physical care, and the nurse acting mainly as a reference person. As a patient, you might have considered this an attractive arrangement since you would have been able to avoid the stress of being separate from family, dependent on strangers for your daily needs. However, for long hospitalizations or serious illness, it could have been an exhausting experience for your family, especially if they had to provide unfamiliar care or treatments normally expected of a nurse in a Western country.

An alternative was to hire a "sitter" *tsukisoi* 付き添い on a private basis to take the place of a family member. However, nursing and Health and Welfare Ministry leaders long considered this practice an added financial burden to the patient and the system, and the practice was officially abolished in 1997. The present official policy is that the number of nurses should be adequate to provide round-the-clock hospital nursing services without depending on family assistance.

The total number of hospital nurses is indeed rising every year. In general, university hospitals, large private hospitals, national hospitals, and city hospitals provide complete nursing care. But since this law has so recently gone into effect, it would not be surprising to find smaller hospitals in which the family might be strongly encouraged to remain for hours at a time at the bedside when the hospital is understaffed (for instance, during the night).

Social customs are also not so quickly changed, as the following story relates.

"I stayed overnight in my nearby city hospital to have some diagnostic tests performed. I couldn't sleep well and was up early, wandering up and down the hallway. Much to my surprise, through the open doorways, I could see feet sticking out from under the curtains in several rooms. It turns out they belonged to family members who had slept on pallets on the floor next to their hospitalized relatives, even though this city hospital provided full nursing services!"

If you are in a position to choose your hospital, and don't have family or friends to care for you, be sure to choose one offering full nursing care.

Getting an Introduction shōkai 紹介

One way of expediting your admission to a large hospital and being sure you get to see the appropriate doctor is through an introduction. In Japan, a common way of finding a hospital is through private or business contacts:

"My six-year-old daughter had become self-conscious about a mole on her nose, so we began to search for the best place to have it removed. By chance, the doctor associated with my husband's company was a graduate of a university hospital famous for its dermatology department. A letter of introduction from the company doctor, although not strictly necessary, seemed to expedite the screening process—on our first visit, the doctors gave us a surgery date within six weeks and performed all the pre-admission tests. However, the hospital was a two-hour train ride from home, so the commute was tiring. Complete nursing care was offered, but as we wanted to stay with her for the first three days after the operation, we had to reserve a private room, at ¥30,000 per day. Although I felt that the treatment was actually excessive for this minor operation, the doctors did an excellent job, her nose healed beautifully, and we were thankful for the introduction."

An introduction may be the best way for you to find good care, but be aware that once you ask for it you are fairly committed. If a doctor goes to the trouble of making an introduction, backing out afterwards will cause embarrassment to both doctors involved. Try to be as thorough as possible in explaining your needs and expectations to the doctor from whom you are requesting the introduction.

Hospital Policies
Hospital stays in Japan tend to be comparatively long—up to three or four times those in many Western countries—and hospitalization is often recommended for conditions which are often treated at home or on an outpatient basis in Western countries. The length of stay seems to be determined by several factors including Japanese housing conditions, relatively low hospitalization costs, and limited visiting nurse/home health care systems. Another major reason is the worry that an empty bed will not be available if a patient is discharged too soon and needs an emergency readmission.

Since the length of stay is determined by hospital policy, it may be impossible to negotiate for a shortened hospital stay before admission. However, if you recover quickly, you may be able to arrange for early discharge.

Many hospitals have set policies regarding visiting hours, particularly at night. One drawback of the complete nursing care system is seen in pediatrics, where parents may stay with their child only during visiting hours and not at night. Since language may be a problem, parents may feel hesitant about leaving a child alone. If you are given permission to remain with your child at night, you may be requested to complete a form explaining your reasons for wanting to stay, such as "to help with communication and cultural differences." Neonatal Intensive Care Units (NICU) are very strict about visiting and about touching the newborn, because of the danger of infection. If you have a child in a NICU, you can try negotiating to lengthen your visiting time, but it may be difficult.

Some hospitals issue a daytime pass *gaishutsu kyokasho* 外出許可書, giving written permission from the doctor to be away from the hospital. An overnight pass *gaihaku kyokasho* 外泊許可書 is sometimes available for long-term patients. If you need a pass or are recovering quickly and need to be discharged earlier than previously planned, try to discuss it with your doctor in advance, as arrangements can take time.

Finally, be ready to compromise. Organize your priorities amd remember that you are in a foreign country and that things are bound to be different. Remember too that even among people from the same country, not everyone has the same priorities.

Preparing for Hospitalization

A two- or three-month waiting time for non-emergency surgery (tonsillectomy, etc.) is not uncommon. You will usually be notified by telephone about two weeks to a month in advance of your admission date. You may be asked to come to the outpatient department for pre-admission examinations (blood tests, electrocardiogram, chest X-ray, etc.), or these tests may be performed after you've been admitted.

Most hospitals have a detailed booklet explaining hospital policies and the supplies that the patient should bring. Typically included are:

pajamas	tea/coffee cup	tissues	slippers
robe	glass	washbowl	chopsticks
towels	cutlery	toiletries	
patient ID	personal seal		

If you don't have a personal seal, your signature will usually be accepted. Sheets are usually provided, but you may prefer to bring your own soft pillow. We also suggest that you bring along:

dictionary	small change	laundry bag	socks
calendar	novel	small clock/watch	clothespins
hangers	washcloth	note pad/pencil	telephone card
address book	this book	coins	

The coins are for vending and washing machines.

If you are having chest or abdominal surgery you may be asked to make and bring a couple of binders made of cotton sheeting, known as *sarashi*, which are used for holding a dressing in place.

If your spoken English is not understood and your Japanese communication is strained, remember that written English is often easier for Japanese to understand. Remember that if you misunderstand and the proper preparations are not carried out, tests may have to be rescheduled, resulting in a loss of time and money. Don't be shy about asking for further explanations or clarifications. If you have forgotten something from home, personal items are generally available at the hospital store.

Admission to the Hospital

For admission to a hospital, take note of the following:

■ You'll need your patient ID card, health insurance certificate, personal seal (if you have one), a deposit and, depending on the hospital, the name, address, telephone number, and personal seal of a guarantor who will guarantee your payment. This person could be a relative, your employer, or a financially independent friend. If your hospital stay will be long (more than a month), periodic payments may be required. After you've paid your final bill, the deposit will be refunded.

■ If you're to undergo surgery, you must sign a surgical permission form (*shujutsu shōdakusho* 手術承諾書) giving the hospital legal permission to perform the surgery. This is not usually a detailed "informed consent" that outlines possible complications, but just a standard, printed form with space for the type of surgery and your signature. If you have any questions or concerns about the procedure, speak to your doctor before you sign.

■ In spite of all the nametags and name cards used in Japan, except for the obstetric floor, hospitalized patients are rarely given identity bracelets, possibly because a family member has traditionally always been present to speak for the patient. Foreigners are usually conspicuous enough not to need a bracelet. For children it's easy to make a small badge showing name and bed number, which can then be pinned to the child's sleeve or back.

In the Hospital

Most hospital rooms have three or more beds separated by curtains. General hospital beds are typically classified into three categories: private rooms; semi-private rooms with two to six beds; and wards with more than six beds.

The curtains are closed at night and left open during the day to give everyone access to sunlight. Usually a bedside table and over-the-bed table are allocated to each patient. Some rooms have a wardrobe or locker for clothes. A small cot, designed to fit under the patient's bed when not in use, is generally available for family members on request. A chair or small stool for visitors may be provided, depending on the space—in general, patients are encouraged to meet with visitors in the patients' lounge.

Many hospitals have at least a few private and semi-private rooms, sometimes with private baths. The cost of these rooms, however, is not covered by public insurance, and at a rate of about ¥10,000 to ¥30,000 per day, can raise a hospital bill considerably, unless you have private insurance. These rooms are available on a first-come, first-served basis, so there may not be one free when you are admitted. If you are requesting one, you will be transferred as soon as a private room becomes available.

Bathing Facilities

Private baths may be available, but most hospitals have Japanese-style tubs. A bath time—not usually daily—may be assigned each patient. As with Japanese baths elsewhere, you're expected to soap and rinse outside, before relaxing in the tub. Remember not to pull the plug when you are done. Access may also be limited by medical necessity, and also by tradition:

"After having a cesarean, I was looking forward to taking a shower. When my dressing was removed on the sixth day, I was informed that cesarean section patients have to wait until the day before discharge (the thirteenth day) before being allowed a bath. I assured the nurse that I would take full responsibility if I got sick or caught a cold, and after negotiating with the head nurse, I was finally allowed to take a shower."

If you don't care to get into the bath with other patients, there are usually hand-held showers around the tub area where you can wash. If you're unable to take a bath for some reason, the nurses will probably bring you warm water for a bed bath. Hot water is often not available from all faucets, so you may need to ask where to find it.

Typical Daily Schedule

The day usually begins at six o'clock with a wake-up chime or announcement. Nurses begin then to take underarm temperature, pulse, respirations, and blood pressure (and, when necessary, to do blood tests), and to ask the following questions:

- How many times did you urinate yesterday?
  Kinō o-shosui wa nankai desu ka?
- How many bowel movements yesterday?
  Kinō o-tsuji wa nankai desu ka?

- Did you sleep well?
  Yoku nemurimashita ka?
- Are there any changes in your condition?
  O-kawari nai desu ka?

The rest of the day will probably be something like this:

7:00– 8:00	Breakfast	11:30	Lunch
8:30	Distribution of medications	1:00	Visiting hours begin
9:00–11:00	Doctor's rounds	3:00	Teatime
	Diagnostic tests	5:00	Supper
	Bed baths	8:00	Visiting hours end
		9:00	Overhead lights off

Questioning the Treatment

"We had been in Japan less than a year when my ten-year-old son fell and broke his leg. He was in a lot of pain when we arrived in the emergency room of a large university hospital. A Japanese orthopedic surgeon said that he would put the leg in traction for a few days until the swelling had gone down and the leg muscles relaxed. This way, the bones would realign well and his leg could then be easily put in a cast. My husband and I had never heard of such treatment. When my cousin had broken his leg a few years

before, his doctor had put a cast on immediately and it healed well. Even though the doctor tried to explain that it would be difficult to get the bone aligned correctly, we didn't feel we could take the risk of treatment we had never heard of, and we insisted the surgeon put on a cast immediately. With some difficulty, our son's leg was put in a cast. That night we were dismayed and very embarrassed to learn from a call to our family doctor back home that the treatment the Japanese surgeon had recommended was correct."

If you consult a physician in your home country and he convinces you of a different diagnosis or treatment, you have the choice of presenting his argument to your Japanese doctor for his reaction or looking for care elsewhere. Changing hospitals once you have been admitted, though, is not always easy. It can mean repeating certain diagnostic tests and added expenses. Remember that just because something is "different," it's not always "wrong." There may be a very good reason why it's different. Make sure that a change is really worthwhile. If you decide that it is, read the section on Transferring to Another Hospital, page 45.

Medications

Adult patients may be handed the whole day's medications in the morning and then be expected to take the prescribed dosage at designated times—so don't forget to take a watch.

If you are having side effects from medications, or you have any questions about dosage or planned duration of the treatment, make sure to clarify this information with your doctor during his daily visits.

Also talk to your doctor before surgery about his plans for pain relief, including your cultural or individual inclinations, to make sure he has something on order, especially for nights. Depending on your height, build, and stress level, the amount of medication prescribed may not be effective. Let your doctor know if you are feeling discomfort. He may be able to increase the dosage.

Meals

Generally, only Japanese food will be available. Japanese are accustomed to eating foods cold or at room temperature, so don't be surprised to receive lukewarm meals. Microwave ovens, refrigerators, freezers, and hot water are sometimes available for use. Unless you are on a restricted diet, family and friends are free to bring food to you, except in pediatrics, where it may not be allowed. If Western food is available, there may be an extra charge. This probably means no raw fish, raw eggs, fermented beans, etc., and bread instead of rice, but otherwise the meal may be very similar to the regular menu.

Don't forget to tell the nursing staff if you are vegetarian or if you have any food allergies or religious taboos. The hospital nutritionist may be able to adjust your menu or at least understand why you don't finish your meals. A Cambodian who refused to eat the bland diet he was prescribed was hospitalized for longer than expected because his leftovers were taken as a sign of a poor appetite. In fact the real reason was his preference for spicy foods, which in Cambodia are considered healing.

Rice gruel (o-kayu) is usually served to patients on a soft diet. The amount of rice added to the water is gradually increased as the patient's condition improves.

Your meal tray may not be brought to your bed. You may be expected to take your tray from a cart at meal times and put it back on the cart when you're through. Since each tray is identified by name, you'll need to be able to read your name in *katakana*.

Drinks are not usually served with the meal. The nurses may distribute tea, but will not provide ice water before each meal. You may be expected to boil your own water if you want a hot drink. Many patients bring a thermos from home. Juice vending machines are commonly available throughout the hospital.

Housekeeping

At most hospitals, simple dusting is done daily. You'll probably be asked to separate your garbage into burnable and non-burnable items.

Bedding is usually changed only once a week, unless it is really soiled. Your family can probably bring extra bedding and linen if you want, but make sure it is marked with your name. You'll also need someone to do your laundry, as you'll be using your own pajamas, and towels, etc. Coin-operated washing machines may be available in the hospital or neighborhood, often near the public bath. The roof of the hospital is usually available for hanging up wet wash; clotheslines are usually provided, but you'll need clothespins or a hanging rack.

Special Hospital Services

Physical therapy is generally available, but occupational therapy, social services, dietary counseling, and religious counseling are not very common. Some hospitals have interpreters for some languages. One hospital in the Tokyo area which has a group of foreign volunteers who visit its foreign patients is Seibo Hospital. Other hospitals which have been mentioned for particularly extensive inpatient services are St. Luke's in Tokyo (page 344), Kameda General Hospital in Chiba (page 343), and Kobe Kaisei Hospital (page 348).

Getting Along with the Nurses

Typical Japanese hospital guides shed light on the atmosphere of Japanese hospitals, with their lists of the types of patients that nurses hate to nurse:

Unpopular patients are those who:

■ pester nurses with questions.
■ ask and talk about the same topic over and over.
■ don't listen.
■ don't talk about things directly.
■ are egotistical and self-centered.
■ don't obey hospital rules.
■ favor only certain nurses.

- demand results immediately.
- treat the nurses like maids.
- don't believe what the nurses tell them.

- take out personal frustrations on other patients or nurses.
- take liberties or are overly familiar.

Tips for Getting Along with the Nurses

- Don't overuse your call bell.
- Try to learn nurses' names—write them down in your notebook for quick reference.
- Be patient when communicating—speak slowly or write down questions and requests.

- Don't use the nurse as a go-between with your doctor, asking her for test results, etc.

Suggestions for Being a Good Roommate

In many Japanese hospitals, communal wards make it necessary to live in close contact with a group of strangers. Remember that everyone is in the same situation, and try and get along. As you can see from the following list, it's sometimes a fine line between being labeled friendly or nosey, and reserved or withdrawn. You don't have to be overly friendly, but try to greet everyone in the morning, and be polite.

Don't:

- feel you must answer personal questions.
- refuse to converse with others.
- set the TV too loud.
- be pessimistic or gloomy.

- talk nonstop about your own illness.
- expect exceptions to be made for you. Regulations concerning visitors, noise, bedtime, etc. are made for the comfort of all.

Leaving the Hospital *tai-in* 退院

Your doctor will probably tell you your discharge date a few days ahead of time so that you can make plans for payment and transportation. Note that some hospitals have regulations about the number of patients that can be discharged on one day, which could mean that your preferred date will not be open.

Payment *kaikei* 会計

Your hospital bill must be paid in cash before you leave. If your initial deposit exceeds your final bill, the excess amount will be refunded. Plan ahead if your discharge date falls on a day when banking facilities and the hospital office are closed. After paying in full, you must provide any necessary insurance forms and be prepared to wait for the return of the completed forms. There is often a fee for preparation of English-language forms and letters. The discharge slip is then brought back to the charge nurse on your floor, indicating that you've paid your bill. Your insurance card and patient identification card will be returned to you at this time.

Gifts for the Staff *sharei* 謝礼

At the time of discharge, especially in smaller hospitals, Japanese often give a gift to the nurses and attending doctor to thank them personally for the care received. As a foreigner, you may be excused if you choose not to follow this custom. However, if you have been referred to the hospital and doctor by a Japanese friend, correctly following the local customs will reflect well not only on you but also on your friend—which is an important consideration in Japan. Ask a roommate or nurse about how the custom is followed in your particular hospital. Unless notices are posted stating that no gifts can be accepted, after initial hesitation your gift will be graciously received. Some Japanese go so far as to disregard these notices, ascertain the doctor's home address through physician acquaintances, and send gifts directly there to make sure that their sense of gratitude is clear.

When the Japanese give gifts, a set of cakes or jellies is usually considered appropriate for the nurses, and whiskey or gift coupons for the doctor. It is not uncommon for Japanese to give ¥100,000 in thanks for an operation requiring a two-week stay. There are stories of patients giving up to ¥500,000 or more after a life-saving procedure. For the Japanese, this is considered a form of "insurance" in case the doctor's skill (and goodwill) should be needed in future. We repeat that this probably won't be expected of non-Japanese. Though monetary gifts will be welcomed, a nice letter and a special homemade item or a gift from your country may be equally, or in some cases even more, appreciated.

Visiting a Patient in the Hospital   *o-mimai* お見舞い

When you visit a Japanese friend or acquaintance, it is customary to bring a small gift *o-mimaihin* お見舞い品 or an envelope of money *o-mimaikin* お見舞い金 to show you wish the person a speedy recovery. The patient will make a note of your gift, and upon discharge, either send or bring you a return gift worth approximately half the price. This is called *kaiki iwai* 快気祝い. This is not always done or expected these days, since it places a burden on the newly discharged patient.

Keeping this custom in mind, some inexpensive ideas for gifts are books and magazines, food items like canned fruit which can be eaten later or small cakes which can be shared with roommates, cut flowers, or a telephone card. Inappropriate for Japanese patients are potted plants, which are considered bad luck since the roots are viewed superstitiously as suggesting that patients will become "rooted" to the hospital in a similar way and have their discharge postponed. Other taboos are flowers with a strong perfume, chrysanthemums (associated with death since they are usually placed as offerings on Buddhist altars), and white flowers (also associated with death). Avoid flowers or any gifts in sets of four or nine, as the Japanese terms for these numbers are homonyms for the words meaning death and pain.

Follow-up Care

You will probably be given follow-up care in the outpatient department of the hospital. Depending on your diagnosis and condition, the doctor may want to follow your progress carefully. Once your condition has stabilized, the doctor may suggest that you continue treatment at a smaller clinic with a location and hours more convenient to you. Home visit systems are not yet well developed in Japan, although some hospitals do have nurses who make periodic home visits to help with the treatment of bedridden patients.

Transferring to Another Hospital

If you are very unhappy with the care you are receiving, or are in a hospital far from home, you may want to transfer to another hospital. You will need your attending doctor's permission and the hospital to which you'd like to be transferred must also be willing to admit you. In addition, you (or a friend or family member) must make all the arrangements. Reasons easily accepted and which would facilitate a smooth transfer would be a desire to be nearer home or for ease of communication with staff in your own language. Smoothing things over in this way will ensure that your old and new doctors discuss your treatment, and will make the transfer easier all around. To change hospitals, you will need to hire a private ambulance or get a friend to drive you, since the fire department ambulance service is not available for this type of transfer.

Private Ambulance Services

Ask your hospital for a referral. Expect no English. These ambulances are not allowed to use sirens or ignore traffic rules. They may not provide medical staff or equipment.

Japan Emergency Service
Nihon Kyukyu Sabisu
Setagaya-ku, Tokyo
03-3700-6088

Zen Nikkyu Patient Transport
Chiyoda-ku, Tokyo
0120-34-0560

Tokyo Kyukyu Toranomon Transportation Center
Minato-ku, Tokyo
03-3434-0609

Tokyo Private Emergency Service
Tachikawa-shi, Tokyo
0425-35-1199

Tama Emergency Transportation
Higashi-Murayama-shi, Tokyo
0423-97-3123

Kobe Nada Transport
078-452-5121

Sapporo Private Ambulance Kyukyu Kanri Center
011-864-1199

Emergency Medical Care

Medical emergencies can be frightening when you are in a foreign country—regardless of the seriousness of the injury or illness, matters are often taken completely out of your hands by strangers, whose skills you can only hope are adequate to the task.

Even if you do arrive at your favorite health care facility, a familiar doctor will probably not be available, and the unfamiliar emergency care system may leave you feeling baffled, angry, and powerless. Being unfamiliar with the language and customs will only compound the frustrations.

However, preparing in advance for possible emergencies can make all the difference.

"Within days of our move to Tokyo, our five-year-old son dropped a sharp rock and severed the end of his finger. It happened at suppertime, just after the local clinic had closed. I had no idea where to go. Our Japanese neighbors came running to help: we jumped into the car and careened through rush-hour traffic to the nearest hospital—but it had no emergency facilities. We were directed to a small, dingy emergency room about five minutes away, which was staffed with one doctor and a nurse. The doctor examined my son's finger and snipped off the dangling fingertip. When I sputtered something about reattachment surgery, the doctor laughed and said I would have to go to a much larger facility for that kind of treatment. He said that if we kept the wound clean it would heal naturally. Of course, I didn't believe him.

"When we arrived home, another neighbor came running up waving a magazine. In it was an article which said that in small children, severed fingertips tend to grow back if the wound is kept clean. I immediately believed the author of the article, because he was an American doctor writing in English. I felt guilty about making such a fuss with the Japanese doctor who had been right. And yes, the fingertip did grow back!"

The Japanese Emergency Medical System

The nationwide availability of good twenty-four–hour emergency medical care has long been a goal of government and health care planners. Since the 1970s, efforts have been made to improve the system of emergency care all over Japan. The resulting three-tiered system of emergency medical care is an attempt to steer patients to one of three levels of care (primary, secondary, or tertiary) according to the seriousness of the illness or injury. The control of emergencies arriving at each of the three different types of facilities has been a boon to medical personnel, as it allows for efficient purchasing of equipment and supplies and assignment of medical and nursing personnel. In addition, patients, especially those who are severely injured or sick, can be seen more quickly by the appropriate medical staff. However, determining and finding the proper emergency care facility can be a challenge, even for the Japanese themselves.

Primary Emergency Care *shoki kyūkyū iryō* 初期救急医療

"My Japanese husband had to make three phone calls before he found our local primary emergency care facility one Saturday afternoon. First he talked to a physician in a twenty-four–hour secondary emergency care facility, who decided our son was not ill enough to go there. We were referred to two local doctors whose turn it was to see patients on Saturday (as part of the primary emergency care system). The second doctor we tried was able to see our son."

Primary care clinics offer after-hours treatment of non-urgent medical problems, such as flu for those who can travel to the clinic on their own or with the help of family.

There are various types of primary care facilities. Night and Holiday Medical Service Centers (*yakan kyūjitsu no shinryō* 夜間休日の診療) are permanent clinics with local doctors taking turns being on call. The hours of these clinics are limited, for example 7:00–11:00 P.M. during the week and 10:00 A.M.–3:00 P.M. and 7:00 P.M.–11:00 P.M. on weekends. There seem to be no consistent standards for these clinics and you'll probably find a wide variety, from minimal to luxurious. Take the time now to locate the one in your area and jot down its operating hours.

Depending on the area, primary emergency care may also be provided at a regular doctor's office, designated an After-Hours Clinic in Rotation (*kyūkyū tōban-sei* 救急当番制). The local doctors take turns being on call. The schedule of these clinics is usually printed in the local paper or health news bulletin. You can also call your local fire department's telephone number (not 119) in Japanese. Also see the emergency information telephone numbers on the front endpapers and in "Regional Resources."

Primary emergency care is also available in some registered emergency hospitals. In all these facilities, the doctor on duty or on call will act as a general practitioner, although in his normal practice he will specialize in some area. The selection of medications available may be limited (to pain medication, for example) and you may be asked to return (or go to your usual doctor) the next day for tests and further treatment. Always call ahead to let the facility know you are coming. Immediate referral to a facility with a specialist on duty (for instance, to a different hospital with an orthopedic surgeon on duty to look at a dislocated finger) is rare. Instead you will be asked to return the next morning during regular outpatient hours when a specialist in that area will be at the hospital. In all the above situations, you may be asked to leave your insurance certificate or money as a deposit, and be asked to settle the bill during regular hours.

Although it is not part of the regular system, another way to obtain primary emergency medical care is at the large general hospital where you or a family member have already been seen in the outpatient department. Even though the hospital may not be on "emergency duty," doctors will usually see their own patients. As always, call ahead first.

Secondary Emergency Care *dainiji kyūkyū iryō* 第二次救急医療

"When my husband fell through a window early one Saturday morning and cut his arm badly, I immediately telephoned our local community hospital, which is a registered emergency hospital, to check if there was a surgeon on duty. When we arrived by car about ten minutes later, the surgeon examined the arm and stitched up the cuts. Healing was normal and follow-up care was conscientious."

Secondary emergency care is for those who are more seriously sick or injured and need more intensive care. This care is given in the emergency rooms *kyūkyū gairai* 救急外来 of both public and private hospitals which have been designated by the government as registered emergency hospitals *kyūkyū shitei byōin* 救急指定病院. These hospitals have facilities for caring for more seriously injured or ill patients offering a variety of specialties and inpatient care. However, as with primary emergency care clinics, facilities vary widely. Some may be twenty-four–hour permanent registered emergency hospitals, while others accept patients on a rotating basis as scheduled by the fire department. Some may be prepared to treat most injuries and illnesses, while others accept only one type of patient, for instance, orthopedic or geriatric. These facilities, too, may offer only palliative care, and may ask you to come back at regular outpatient times. In fact, if you arrive, as an emergency, during outpatient clinic hours, you may be shuttled through the clinic if your injury or illness is not life-threatening. One foreign patient remarked,"You get treated more quickly if you haven't washed off the blood!"

Usually patients are brought to the registered emergency hospital by fire department ambulance. Call 119, and the fire department will send an ambulance to take you to the nearest registered emergency hospital which is equipped to treat your condition. The ambulance service is free of charge, and is usually the fastest way to get to the appropriate hospital.

Tertiary Emergency Care   *daisanji kyūkyū iryō*   第三次救急医療

Tertiary emergency care is for patients with life-threatening illnesses or injuries, not the casual walk-in patient, and is available at life-saving emergency centers *kyūmei kyūkyū sentā* 救命救急センター, or trauma centers. There are 115 of these centers in Japan, at least one in each prefecture. Specialists in traumatology and acute-care medicine are on duty twenty-four hours a day, and facilities are equipped with high-tech life-saving devices. These are permanent facilities and may be located in either public or private hospitals. In principal, patients are taken to trauma centers by ambulance referred through the fire department ambulance service. The trauma team will have been alerted to the imminent arrival of the patient and will be standing by, ready to give emergency care.

Ambulance Service   *kyūkyūsha*   救急車

"I had been in Japan for about one year and couldn't speak much Japanese when my brother came to visit us. One night he had an epileptic seizure and fell unconscious. I called for an ambulance. I couldn't understand the operator, but said my name, address, and phone number and then just kept repeating 'keiren, keiren' (convulsions, convulsions). It worked fine and my brother was taken to a hospital where some staff spoke English. I've since heard the saying, 'If you can order a pizza in Japanese, you can certainly call for an ambulance!' and I believe it."

"Our thirteen-year-old son was attacked by a dog and suffered many deep cuts and tears on his face and arm. Someone called 119. He was given immediate first aid by the ambulance crew and then taken to a large hospital only after the ambulance crew leader made sure that a plastic surgeon would be standing by. He had three hours of surgery. His follow-up care took place over a weekend and a holiday, and even then a doctor was always available. His cuts are healing well. The ambulance service worked beautifully for him."

A recent survey revealed that nearly four out of five foreigners living in Tokyo did not know the emergency number for fire and ambulance. The number is 119.

119, 119, we'll all be fine with 119

After practicing this ditty a few times, even children should be able to make that important telephone call. See the front endpapers for phrases to use when calling an ambulance.

Calling for an Ambulance

Even if you are alone and cannot speak, call 119 and leave the phone off the hook (if possible, tap the receiver twice), and your call will be traced. If you're away from home, call from a green or purple phone by pressing the red emergency button and dialling 119. No coin or card is required. For pink and red phones, drop in ¥10 and dial 119. Pink telephones also have a special key to unlock the phone so that calls can be made for free—tell the shop attendant that you wish to call an ambulance (*kyūkyūsha ga yobitai*).

■ If there is a hospital you wish to be taken to, call that doctor and get permission. Do this before you call an ambulance because once you call 119, your phone line may be locked open until the ambulance arrives.
■ Call 119 and speak to the controller.
■ Send someone outside to look for the ambulance crew.
■ Start CPR or first aid if necessary.

■ Collect doctors' names and phone numbers.
■ Gather together insurance certificate, patient ID card, and medical history.
■ Take at least ¥30,000.
■ Take the name of a guarantor in case you have to be hospitalized (see Admission to the Hospital, page 39).
■ If you receive permission to go to a certain hospital, show the ambulancemen your patient ID.

Secondary and tertiary emergency care facilities are served by ambulances supplied and organized by the fire department. A call to the nationwide emergency number 119 will bring either a fire engine or ambulance or both to your home. Be sure to ask for an ambulance (the word *kyūkyū* will do) if you don't want a fire engine to arrive at your door. A three-member ambulance crew will arrive at your home within minutes (six minutes is the national average). The specially trained crew will assess the patient's condition and report their findings to the 119 control center, who will then decide which hospital can give appropriate care and will also make sure that emergency care staff and a bed are available. Japanese know it is usually the quickest way to get medical care, although there is no guarantee that it will be at the hospital of your choice. Meanwhile, the ambulance crew may give first aid. By law they are *not* paramedics and cannot start intensive medical treatment. However, all fire department ambulance crews in Tokyo now include an emergency medical technician (EMT), and this service is gradually being extended nationwide. Under the guidance of a doctor (by direct telephone communication), the emergency medical technician can insert more sophisticated airways, start an intravenous drip, electronically monitor the heart, attach and run a semiautomatic defibrillator, use an automatic cardiac massage machine, and apply shock pants.

The ambulance can be used for:
■ Accident victims (traffic, fires, typhoons)
■ Home emergency victims when there is no other means to transport the patient to medical facilities
■ Those suffering from acute illnesses (not psychiatric)
■ Pregnant women in abnormal labor

The ambulance cannot be used for:
■ Acute psychiatric illnesses (call police, 110)
■ Pregnant women in normal labor
■ Drunk people who can't get home by themselves (this becomes a police matter)
■ Elderly or handicapped people who simply need transportation
■ Hospital-to-hospital transfer patients (non-emergency)
■ Hospital-to-home transfer patients.
■ Hospital-to-airport transfer patients.
■ Obviously dead bodies

Troubleshooting

You may find you have to wait a long time before the ambulance arrives, or that the ambulance is slow to leave the house once it does arrive, or that you are taken to a hospital other than the one you had in mind. There may be several reasons for this other than traffic conditions.

■ All nearby ambulances are in use and more distant units have to be called.
■ More serious cases will be picked up first.
■ Rural or remote areas have fewer ambulances and longer distances to travel.
■ The hospital you wish to go to is not prepared to treat your condition.
■ The 119 control may have to contact several hospitals before locating one that can treat your condition. (The ambulance will not move until it has the name of a registered emergency hospital prepared to accept you.)
■ The staff of the hospital you wish to go to may be busy with another emergency, or there may be no bed available.
■ Your condition may be too serious for a long drive.

Tips for Handling an Emergency Smoothly

"My college-aged son went snowboarding over Christmas vacation, on a mountain several hours away from our home. On the first ride down the hill he fell and broke his collarbone. Fortunately we had a fax machine, and when he called to tell us the news, I was able to fax our family health

insurance card directly to the hospital. Next time, I'll make sure he carries a copy with him."

"Mrs. S. took her children to a friend's birthday party. In the space of two hours both children had cut themselves badly enough to need stitches. Without the insurance card, the bill came to over ¥30,000, which she had to borrow from her friend. Mrs. S. later sent the insurance card to the friend, who returned to the hospital and was reimbursed for 70 percent of the bill, a nuisance which could have been avoided by better planning."

■ Place health insurance certificates and patient IDs, in a spot that your family knows about.
■ Place phone numbers of emergency hospitals and clinics by the phone.
■ Prepare a first-aid kit (below; also see the nonprescription drug list on pages 257–61).
■ Have all members of your family practice the dialogue for calling an ambulance.
■ If you're single, tell a friend where your health records are kept.
■ Whenever you go out, even for a short trip, take your health insurance card (or a copy of it) with you. Have every member of the family keep a copy of your health insurance card in their wallets. (With a copy, some facilities may still require you to pay the bill in full and then be reimbursed, but the likelihood of being turned away will be less.)

Children's Emergencies (see page 164)
Elderly Emergencies (see page 227)

First-Aid Kit

See also the nonprescription drug list for the names of specific products that you may need to complete your kit.

Gauze *gāze* ガーゼ
Sterile gauze pads *genkin gāze* 滅菌ガーゼ
Band-Aid *bando eido* バンドエイド
Tape *kami tēpu* 紙テープ
Long rolled bandage *hōtai* 包帯
Bandage clips *hōtai dome* 包帯止め
Scissors *hasami* ハサミ
Tweezers *pinsetto* ピンセット

Thermometer *taionkei* 体温計
Hot water bottle *yutanpo* 湯たんぽ
Chemical hot packs *onshippu* 温しっぷ
Chemical cold packs *shippuyaku* しっぷ薬
Cotton buds *membō* 綿棒
Large all-purpose triangular bandage
  sankakukin 三角巾
Packets of ready-to-mix isotonic sports drinks

Nonprescription Medications

Pain and fever reliever of your choice
Antihistamine tablets for allergic reactions
Antiseptic lotion for cleaning minor cuts
  and scrapes

Antibiotic ointment for minor cuts and scrapes
Insect sting/bite reliever medication
Burn ointment

Classes in Cardiopulmonary Resuscitation (CPR) *shinpai sosei* 心肺蘇生

Knowing how to do CPR might save the life of someone you love or a stranger who needs your help. Fire departments around Japan have started offering CPR classes. Language may not be such a big barrier as you practice the demonstrated techniques, but you'll probably want to read an English text as well. CPR instruction books published by the American Red Cross can be ordered from English-language bookstores. For class information, call your local fire department in Japanese.

Canadian Academy, Kobe
078-857-0100
CPR and first-aid courses. Call for schedule.

Foreign Nurses Association in Japan (FNAJ)
CPR and first-aid courses. Call TELL for the telephone number of the current FNAJ president. Can also write or email FNAJ (see endpapers).

3

"A neighbor started finding a strange type of insect in her apartment. She captured one and took it to her local public health center. A specialist there not only identified it for her but told her which kind of insecticide she needed. He also suggested she try to coordinate everyone in her apartment building to use a fog-type insecticide on the same day so the insects would have no escape and be eliminated."

"A very noisy alleycat had begun to frequent my veranda. At first I ignored it, but each day it became increasingly bothersome, and it was obviously suffering from some kind of disease. Finally it had weakened to the extent that I could coax it into a box. A neighbor told me to take it to the local public health center, which I did."

The Public Health System

With the possible exception of the imperial family and perhaps a few extremely wealthy individuals, all Japanese use the public health services. To begin with, every citizen is obliged to enroll in one of the public health insurance plans, all of which are administered under the umbrella of the public health system. The public health system also directs Japan's preventive health resources, making available free or low-cost health checks and childhood immunizations. Other major functions are administrating public assistance to those who suffer from disabling conditions and providing a noncommercial source of information on all kinds of health-related matters.

In Japan, the public health care system is administered by the Ministry of Health and Welfare, the prefectural governments, and the local city or ward governments. Each works in cooperation with affiliated institutions and other governmental agencies.

Local Government Health Departments

Local government systems vary, but generally public health programs are administered by welfare divisions, public health divisions, and public health centers. Until very recently, the ministry and the prefectural governments controlled many of Japan's public health programs. The trend now is toward decentralization, to allow local governments to provide services geared to the needs of their own communities. This means that services provided in one locality increasingly may differ from those even in neighboring areas, with the systems in larger cities offering more services than are available in other areas. The booklet which you receive from your government office when you first apply for alien registration (titled something like *A Survival Guide to Living in* ....) usually explains the system and general services in your area.

Foreign residents are most likely to encounter the public health system at this local level. Those enrolled in a National Health Insurance plan (see pages 74–77) will find that it is administered by local government offices, although supervision comes from the ministry. Those taking care of a disabled or elderly family member may use some of the various programs run by local governments (see "Help for the Elderly and the Disabled"). Of particular interest, though, are the public health centers, which provide numerous services for the surrounding community, some of which may be used regularly by foreign residents.

Public Health Centers hoken-jo 保健所

Staffed by government officials, public health nurses, and various other specialists, public health centers are located in every city or ward. They are the cornerstone of the Japanese medical system, the main vehicles of preventive health care. Perhaps because they provide numerous free or low-cost preventive services, Japanese public health insurance has excluded coverage of preventive health care. In some countries, those who cannot afford to go to a private physician make use of public health centers, but in Japan these centers are used by nearly everyone in some way. Their services start from before birth and continue throughout one's life.

"My child received all his vaccinations through the public health system. It was a bit time-consuming, but at least I made friends with the other mothers while I waited in line."

Each city or ward sets its own schedule of services and publicizes it in the local health bulletin distributed either to all households or to all households who subscribe to a Japanese newspaper. If you aren't receiving one, a call in Japanese to the local center will put you on the mailing list. The schedule is also available at the city or ward office or at the public health center. Some cities print the schedule in English; resident foreigners—and those with young families in particular—would be advised to occasionally check up on what's going on at the health center. You'll probably find the staff friendly and eager to assist you.

The following, based on wards in Tokyo, will give you an idea of what to look for at your public health center. Don't forget: services vary greatly, with systems in large cities tending to be more extensive. But even in large cities, you'll probably need to speak Japanese or bring someone who does. Some local governments have registered volunteer interpreters (usually housewives who have lived abroad) and can arrange for one to be there if you call ahead. If the public health center doesn't know about volunteers, try the office where you registered as a resident.

"From the time my daughter was eighteen months until she was three years old, she had quarterly dental check-ups at the public health center. The dental hygienist applied fluoride (it only cost four hundred yen a visit) and showed us proper brushing techniques."

Personal Health and Welfare Services

- General health examinations (see pages 87–88) and counseling
- Health check-ups and counseling for pregnant mothers and for infants (see pages 118, 120, and 144)
- Health check-ups and dental examinations for children (see page 158)
- Coordination of childhood immunizations (see page 159)
- Consultation on public financial assistance and/or medical care for:

  those with mental or physical disabilities (see page 214)

  those with designated contagious or incurable diseases (see page 62)

  pregnant women and new mothers with certain circumstances/conditions (see pages 61–62)

  mothers of premature babies (see page 140)

  those with emotional problems

  alcoholics and their families

  those taking care of senile family members

- Testing for STDs (see pages 110–112)
- Anonymous testing for and counseling for HIV/AIDS (see page 206)

- Consultation on all kinds of health matters, including health maintenance for the elderly
- Birth control consultation
- Lectures and classes in Japanese on, for instance, cooking for health, diabetes control, living with asthma, prevention of adult diseases, tips on care of the elderly
- Group therapy for those recovering from mental health problems
- Home visits for those who are bedridden or confined
- Free use of center equipment (e.g., blood-pressure machines)
- Introduction to area medical facilities

"I take advantage of the free cancer checks held every year through the public health department. One year, when it was discovered that I had blood in my stools, the public health department referred me to a large hospital where further testing was done almost free of charge, because I had been referred by the center."

Household and Environmental Sanitation Services

- Pet dog registration and rabies vaccination
- Water testing
- Consultation on household pest control
- Assistance with stray animals
- Disposal of dangerous materials, e.g., mercury from a broken thermometer

"A stray dog started hanging around the neighborhood park. As time went by, he became increasingly thinner, and a bit sick-looking. A lot of mothers were worried about letting their small children play there while the dog was around. Finally, someone called the public health department and a truck came to pick him up."

The public health center also conducts demographic surveys and collect statistics on all kinds of health- and sanitation-related matters. This makes it an appropriate place to inquire about the prevalence of pests, a particular disease, or a source of pollution in your area.

Prefectural Government /Departments of Public Health

"My son's speech was delayed, so I consulted with the public health nurses. They asked me if he'd had a complete hearing test yet. When I said that he hadn't, they telephoned and arranged for an appointment at a prefectural hospital noted for its treatment of children with hearing problems. Although the hospital was nearby, I hadn't known that this was one of its specialty areas. My son was able to get a complete checkup."

Prefectural governments focus on the health and welfare needs in their area and administer prefectural health institutions, many of which specialize in specific fields of medicine. These institutions train health personnel, inspect businesses, and monitor health-related aspects of the environment in their area.

"When sixty students from my daughter's kindergarten got food poisoning from egg salad sandwiches while on a school excursion, the public health department quickly arranged for medical care and hospitalization of the children who needed it. They also checked the food-processing plant that had provided the sandwiches, while the kindergarten teachers went around visiting each sick child and apologizing to the parents."

Prefectural governments run a variety of health centers. For example, the Tokyo-to Kenko Plaza (Hygeia) in Shinjuku-ku, Tokyo (03-5285-8015) is a health maintenance center with fitness centers, machines for measuring blood-pressure, health literature and videos, and computer terminals for locating health facilities in Tokyo. The Maternal and Child (Boshi Hoken) Health Services Center at Tokyo Metropolitan Otsuka Hospital provides an information hotline (03-3941-8818 Mon.–Fri. 5:00–9:00 P.M., in Japanese only), as well as counseling and computerized information on allergies and child development. Other prefectural centers are introduced throughout this book. The Tokyo government publishes a Japanese-English bilingual guide to the functions of the Tokyo Bureau of Public Health (03-5320-4347), *Health Care for Tokyo Residents* (*Tokyo no Hoken Iryō* 東京の保健医療). Other prefectures may have similar publications.

Ministry of Health and Welfare

This ministry (*kōsei-shō* 厚生省) is naturally at the top of the hierarchy. It designs laws on, for instance, standards for health professionals, control of communicable diseases, and bioethics. The ministry also accredits medical facilities and personnel and sets national health standards on medical equipment, food businesses, the nation's blood supply, pharmaceuticals, and the control of poisonous substances. In addition, it administers various nationwide programs, including those for the elderly and the disabled.

The ministry also oversees national medical institutes and facilities for research and development. Some of these R&D centers are the National Cancer Center, the International Medical Center, the National Rehabilitation Center for the Disabled, and the National Institutes of Health, all of which have home pages in English linked to the ministry web site given below.

Internal ministry bureaus coordinate the insurance and pension systems. The affiliated Social Insurance Agency (*shakai hoken-chō* 社会保険庁) is in charge of the government-managed insurance programs (*seifu kanshō kenkō hoken* 政府管掌健康保険), seamen's insurance (*sen'in hoken* 船員保険), and the employees' and national pension systems (*kōsei nenkin* 厚生年金 and *kokumin nenkin* 国民年金 respectively).

Individuals rarely have direct dealings with the ministry. However, for example, foreign health professionals might contact the Examining Board (*shiken menkyo-shitsu* 試験免許室) for information on the licensing or authorization of health care professionals in Japan. Foreign companies might contact the Pharmaceutical and Medical Safety Bureau (*igaku anzen-kyoku* 医学安全局) for information on government approval of drugs or medical equipment. Inquiries on approval of foods and other products related to health would go to the Environmental Health Bureau (*seikatsu eisei-kyoku* 生活衛生局).

"As an Iranian doctor temporarily doing research here, I thought I could use my spare time to care for my countrymen who have had difficulty using the Japanese medical system. I called the ministry to see if I could take the exam for licensing in Japan, but was politely told that I would not only have to pass the highest level of the Japanese-language proficiency exam, but also be a permanent resident, before I could sit for the board exam."

Ministry of Health and Welfare
1-2-2 Kasumigaseki, Chiyoda-ku, Tokyo
03-3503-1711
http://www.mhw.go.jp/english/index/html

Government Publications Service Center
Seifu Kanko-butsu Sabisu Senta
政府刊行物サービスセンター
(located in the Ministry of Agriculture, Forestry, and Fisheries/*norin suisan-sho*)

1-2-1 Kasumigaseki, Tokyo
03-3504-3885, fax 03-3504-3889

(and Otemachi Branch, next to the Immigration Office)
Otemachi Godo Chosha Office Building No. 2
1-3-1 Otemachi, Chiyoda-ku, Tokyo
Ask for their *List of Publications*, a quick reference containing English titles of English and Japanese-language publications.

Health Care–Related Laws and Public Assistance

Many of the Japanese health-related laws and assistance systems for those in special situations are administered under the public health system, and most are also applicable to foreign residents.

For details of special assistance for the elderly or the disabled, see pages 214–15, 220.

Workmen's Compensation Insurance rōsai hoken 労災保険

Under the Workmen's Accident Compensation Insurance Law, all employers in Japan (except national and local governments which have separate systems) are required to register and pay periodic contributions to provide compensation in the event that employees should be injured while working or commuting to work, or that they should develop a work-related illness. One-man businesses without any employees, and businesses employing only family members are not eligible. Regardless of whether the company actually contributes, however, all employees in Japan, including foreign workers, full-time or part-time, are eligible for the benefits provided by this law. Note that foreign trainees in Japan on trainee visas are not covered by this law since they are considered "trainees" rather than "employees."

Hospitals included in the insurance plan will bill the insurer directly. If you use other hospitals, you'll have to pay first and then be reimbursed. Workmen's compensation insurance includes the following benefits (a doctor's certificate is required):

■ Compensation for medical expenses for job-related injury or illness, provided that the government recognizes the treatment as necessary.

■ Long-term financial support even after you return to your own country (a physician must certify that you are handicapped) for aftereffects of a work-related disease or injury.

■ Salary compensation for the period in which you are unable to work because of medical treatment for a work-related injury or illness, if that period is a cumulative sum of at least four days. You will receive 80 percent of your average daily income per day starting from day four.

■ Pension (instead of salary compensation) for a serious work-related injury or illness, when the period of medical treatment exceeds a year and a half.

■ Pension or temporary subsidy to be paid to your dependents if you should die of a work-related illness or injury. A funeral subsidy will also be paid.

Procedures for receiving these benefits after returning to your own country are difficult but possible. Benefits can also be received after retiring, but in some cases for only two to five years. Details of this law are complicated—contact a lawyer or the following:

Resource

Kalabaw no Kai
Sanwa Bussan Bldg. Rm 701
3-11-2 Matsukage-cho, Naka-ku, Yokohama-shi
045-662-5699

Assists foreign migrant workers with labor problems. Also serves as a resource center for information on other groups in Japan.

Assistance for Contagious Diseases

Tuberculosis Prevention Law *kekkaku yobō-hō* 結核予防法
Under this law, the government will cover the complete expense of hospitalization and half the expense of outpatient care for treatment of tuberculosis. This applies to anyone with TB in Japan, regardless of nationality or visa status. If the patient's income exceeds a certain amount, however, the cost of hospitalization may not be fully subsidized. If the patient is under 18, school supplies and daily necessities are also provided.

Prevention and Treatment of AIDS
AIDS testing is available at most public health centers free of charge (see page 206). AIDS patients may qualify for disability benefits, depending on the progress of the disease. Consult with your doctor and your local public health center.

Other Contagious Diseases
Laws also exist to prevent the spread of other contagious diseases such as cholera, diphtheria, dysentery, epidemic meningitis, Japanese encephalitis, Lassa fever, paratyphoid, plague, polio, scarlet fever, smallpox, typhoid fever, and typhus. If you have any of these diseases you may be isolated in a hospital, and your home sterilized, all at government

expense. Free testing for cholera, dysentery, paratyphoid, typhoid, and syphilis is available at public health centers. Testing for the other diseases must be done at a medical facility.

Assistance for Childbirth

Besides the lump-sum "gift" to those with Japanese public insurance, assistance such as free or inexpensive hospitalization and delivery at a designated maternity clinic or obstetric hospital is available to those with an extremely low income. Ask for details at your local welfare office.

Benefits for the Working Mother

The employment equal opportunity law *danjo koyō kikai kintō-hō* 男女雇用機会均等法 states that every pregnant woman must be given time off to attend prenatal visits, once every 4 weeks in the first 7 months, once every 2 weeks during the 8th and 9th month, and once a week after that until the birth. She should also be allowed flex-time commuting schedules and be given appropriate working hours and conditions, allowing for periodic rests during working hours as needed.

The labor standards law *rōdō kijun-hō* 労働基準法 states that any pregnant woman with a job which involves poisonous substances or which otherwise puts her or her fetus at risk, should be moved to more appropriate work during the period of her pregnancy. A pregnant woman also cannot be forced to work overtime against her will. Regarding maternity leave, the law requires that pregnant women be given a 6-week leave (10 weeks for those carrying more than one fetus) prior to her expected date of delivery, at her request. This leave is extended if the baby is late. After the birth, she must take a compulsory 6-week leave of absence and can take 8 weeks if she desires. The woman and her employer are free to extend these times under mutual agreement. The employer cannot discharge the woman during prenatal or postnatal leave, nor for 30 days after, unless the business cannot continue otherwise. If for some reason the woman's condition does not permit her to return after the agreed-upon time, additional leave will be treated as regular company or contractual sick leave. This law applies to any pregnancy which has progressed 12 weeks or longer, meaning that it is also applicable to miscarriage, premature birth, stillbirth, and artificially induced abortion. The law does not state whether any of this leave should be paid or unpaid. However, women enrolled in Japanese employee's insurance plans can receive a certain percentage of their salaries and other benefits (see pages 72–73). Also under this law, during the first year after the birth, the mother is also entitled to two 30-minute rest periods during the working day to take care of her baby.

The childrearing leave law *ikuji kyūgyō-hō* 育児休業法 states that for one year after the birth either the father or the mother can take a leave of absence from work to care for the baby. Employers must also cooperate with parents requesting a short-term leave or shortened work hours during this period after the birth, although they need only pay wages for the hours actually worked.

Assistance for Infant/Child Medical Treatment

Local governments will pick up the co-payment for medical bills of resident children up to age three (in some areas up to age six, if the family's income is low), including registered foreign children who are enrolled in Japanese public insurance. Some programs are limited to hospitalization, low income, etc. Tokyo has no income limits, but the child cannot be receiving any kind of welfare assistance. This assistance is only for treatment covered by Japanese public insurance.

Present your health insurance certificate (and your child's, if different), your personal seal, and both your alien registration cards to the Child Welfare Section at your municipal office. You'll be issued an Infant Medical Certificate *nyūji iryōsho* 乳児医療書証. Show this along with the insurance certificate to contracted medical facilities, and you will not be charged anything for the care your child receives. If your child is treated at other facilities, you must submit your co-payment directly to the facility and then apply to your local government for reimbursement within six months, showing receipts.

Assistance for Children with Special Conditions

Assistance can pay the difference between actual medical expenses and the amount covered by insurance for children with certain nationally designated chronic diseases or disorders *tokutei shōni mansei shikkan* 特定小児慢性疾患: asthma, cancer, chronic blood or kidney disease, collagen diseases, congenital metabolism, heart or intestinal diseases or disorders, diabetes, endocrine diseases, neuromuscular disorders, and mobility, hearing, balancing mechanisms or speech limitations. Both the child and the guardian must be registered residents and one or more family members must be enrolled in a Japanese public insurance plan. Apply at your local public health center.

Children with long-term mental or physical disabilities can also receive other types of assistance including artificial limbs, wheelchairs, etc. Home help, or accommodation for disabled children, can be requested at welfare centers or other public facilities in cases of emergency or other necessity.

Children of single-parent families *hitori-oya no katei* ひとり親の家庭 can receive free medical care and medications covered under insurance until March 31 of their eighteenth year, if the guardian is covered by public insurance and the family income is below a certain level. Apply at your local government office. You will receive a "Welfare Medical Certificate" *fukushi iryō-shō* 福祉医療証 which must be shown when receiving medical care.

Assistance to Patients with Intractable Diseases/ Disorders *tokutei shikan iryō-hi kōhi futan seido* 特定疾患医療費公費負担制度

There are thirty-nine nationally designated diseases *tokutei shikan* 特定疾患 for which the national government provides financial assistance by paying most of the cost of medical care not covered by insurance. These are generally diseases for which the cause is unknown and for which there is no known cure. (literally, "difficult diseases," *nanbyō*. 難病). Patients with other diseases in this category may also receive similar financial assistance from their local government.

To qualify for this additional assistance, you must be enrolled in a Japanese public insurance system and be a registered resident.

(Source: Health Care for Tokyo Residents 東京の保健医療, edited and published by the Bureau of Public Health of the Tokyo Metropolitan Government, 1996.)

Diseases in bold letters are covered by National Treasury Assistance; others are covered by Tokyo Municipal Government assistance for patients who are residents of Tokyo.

Blood Disorders

■ **aplastic anemia** 再生不良性貧血
■ **congenital coagulation defects** 先天性血液凝固因子欠乏症
■ **idiopathic thrombocytopenic purpura (ITP)** 特発生血小板減少性紫斑病

Brain and Nervous System Disorders

■ **amyotrophic lateral sclerosis** 筋萎縮性側索硬化症
■ Creuzfeldt-Jacob disease クロイツフエルト・ヤコブ病
■ hereditary (essential) neuropathy 遺伝性(本態性)ニューロパチー
■ **Huntington's chorea** ハンチントン舞踏病
■ mitochondrial encephalomyopathies ミトコンドリア脳筋症
■ **multilevel spinal canal stenosis** 広範脊柱管狭窄症
■ **multiple sclerosis (MS)** 多発性硬化症
■ **myasthenia gravis** 重症筋無力症
■ myotonia syndrome ミオトニー症候群
■ progressive supranuclear palsy 進行性核上性麻痺
■ **Parkinson's disease** パーキンソン病
■ phacomatosis 母斑症
■ **spino-cerebellar degeneration** 脊髄小脳変性病

■ **subacute myelo-optico-neuropathy (SMON)** スモン

Cardiovascular Disorders

■ **aortic arch syndrome (Takayasu's arteritis)** 高安病
■ **Buerger's disease** ビュルガー病
■ **idiopathic dilated (congestive) cardiomyopathy** 特発性拡張型心筋症
■ idiopathic portal hypertension 特発性門脈圧亢進症
■ malignant hypertension 悪性高血圧
■ **Shy-Drager syndrome** シャイ・ドレーガー症候群
■ **spontaneous occlusive disease in circle of Willis** ウイリス輪閉塞症

Digestive Disorders

■ cirrhosis of the liver, hepatoma 肝硬変ヘパトーム
■ **Crohn's disease** クローン病
■ chronic hepatitis 慢性肝炎
■ **fulminant hepatitis** 劇症肝炎
■ lipidosis リピドーシス
■ **primary biliary cirrhosis (PBC)** 原発性胆汁性肝硬変
■ **severe acute pancreatitis** 重症急性膵炎
■ **ulcerative colitis** 潰瘍性大腸炎

Genito-urinary Tract Disorders

- dialysis　人工透析を必要とする腎不全
- nephrotic syndrome　ネフローゼ症候群
- polycystic kidney　多発性嚢胞腎

Multisystem and Miscellaneous Disorders

- **Behcet's syndrome**　ベーチェット病
- hypereosinophilic syndrome　好酸球増多症候群
- **primary amyloidosis**　アミロイドーシス
- **primary immunodeficiency syndrome**　原発性免疫不全症疱侯群
- **retinitis pigmentosa**　網膜色素変性症
- **Wegener's granulomatosis (WG)**　ウエゲナー肉芽腫症

Musculoskeletal and Connective Tissue Disorders:

- ankylosing spondylitis　強直性脊椎炎
- **dermatomyositis, polymyositis**　皮膚筋炎・多発生筋炎
- **idiopathic osteonecrosis of the femoral head**　特発性大腿骨頭壊死症
- **malignant rheumatoid arthritis**　悪性関節リウマチ

- **mixed connective tissue disease (MCTD)**　混合性結合組織症
- **ossification of the posterior longitudinal ligament of the spine**　後縦靱帯骨化症
- **periarteritis nodosa (PN)**　結筋性動脈周囲炎
- **progressive systemic sclerosis (PSS)**　汎発性強皮症
- Sjögren's syndrome　シェーグレン症候群
- **systemic lupus erythematosus (SLE)**　全身性エリテマトーデス

Skin Disorders

- **epidermolysis bullosa**　表皮水疱症
- **pemphigus**　天疱瘡
- **pustular psoriasis**　膿疱性乾癬

Respiratory Disorders

- diffuse bronchiolitis　ひまん性汎細気管支炎
- **idiopathic interstitial pneumonia**　特発性間質性肺炎
- **sarcoidosis**　サルコイドーシス

Although you may never need to use the system, it can be reassuring to know that these services, facilities, and assistance programs exist. For whatever health problem or concern you have, you can start at the public health center, and nurses and other staff members there can direct you to the appropriate resources. As we note in other chapters, the actual preventive health services are assembly-line–style and would be hard to utilize unless you speak some Japanese, but they are available, practically free of charge, to all residents.

Health Insurance

"After calling every emergency hospital in Shinjuku-ku, the ambulance squad finally received a positive response from a hospital in neighboring Chiyoda-ku. The foreign worker they were transporting should have been operated on two days earlier after being diagnosed with acute appendicitis at a neighborhood hospital. Instead, he had been turned away when it was discovered he had no health insurance. A Japanese friend took him to the local public health department, where an official called his embassy, only to find his government could take no responsibility. The official called an ambulance as a last resort, but by the time the man arrived at the hospital, his condition had progressed to full-blown peritonitis. Not only had his life been endangered, but the care he now needed would be several times the cost. And who would pay?"

Health Insurance

If you are young and healthy, paying insurance premiums may seem an extra and unnecessary expense. But with the present high cost of medical and dental care, being caught without health insurance could be disastrous.

The Japanese insurance system aims at universal coverage and equal opportunity. The law states that all citizens are obliged to join an insurance program and that those not insured through the workplace must enroll in the public National Health Insurance system. Local governments interpret "insurance through the workplace" as referring to enrollment in the public Japanese Employees' Health Insurance system. Virtually all Japanese are enrolled in one or the other of these public insurance systems, or in a public welfare program. Private Japanese insurance companies offer only supplementary health insurance. Public insurance coverage is relatively generous even of chronic conditions, at least within Japan, and is accepted by the majority of medical and dental facilities throughout the country. Although originally designed for Japanese, this law and insurance have been extended to include the majority of foreign residents as well.

For some foreign residents, admission to the system is a blessing, giving them the same access to medical care as the Japanese. Without health insurance, care in Japan can be extremely costly. This is because the Japanese government sets only the cost of care covered by Japanese public insurance. If you are not covered by a Japanese public insurance plan, or if you receive treatment which is not covered by this insurance, facilities are free to set the fee themselves (see Point System, page 80). Moreover, it may not be just a matter of paying the bills—finding a hospital willing to treat you could also be an arduous task—especially, but not only, in areas away from large cities.

But some foreign residents still have complaints. For example, the salary-based premiums can be relatively high, especially for young, high-income individuals; this may pay off for Japanese when they reach old age and are eligible for highly-subsidized care, but this benefit will not apply to people who are here for only a few years. People who are paying very high premiums in Japan may find they they have no coverage whatsoever during overseas trips home. Moreover, since Japanese insurance only serves residents of Japan, if you develop a chronic condition while in Japan and have not maintained lifetime global insurance, you may have trouble finding an insurer in your next country of residence. This is particularly true if you are self-employed and reside in a country like the U.S., which doesn't have socialized medicine. On top of this, if you have already joined the National Health Insurance, but decide that you want global insurance instead, you'll usually find that your NHI insurer will refuse to terminate your membership, since private insurance is not recognized as a legitimate primary form of insurance. Maintaining both global and Japanese insurance can be quite costly. You should also be aware that NHI insurers are free to charge people who are eligible for, but who fail to join, the NHI, for the equivalent of up to two years of back premiums (see NHI, page 74).

Though we can't advise you on what insurance choice may be best for you, we will try to explain the types of health insurance available in Japan. The majority of foreign residents qualify for and maintain Japanese public health insurance, so most attention is given to this. Others will find coverage under private plans (see pages 80–82).

Note, however, that the insurance situation in Japan is in a state of flux. Watch especially for the possible abandonment of the present government-mandated pricing system for drugs, the expansion of a fixed-sum payment system to cover common chronic diseases, and the creation of a completely separate health insurance system for those over seventy. Already a 1997 law to go into effect in April 2000 requires virtually all residents aged forty or over to join a public nursing care insurance system, in order to support care for the elderly (see pages 78–79).

Public Health Insurance

Japanese public insurance plans can be divided into two main categories.

■ Employees' Health Insurance—for employees and their dependents
■ National Health Insurance—for the self-employed, the retired, and others not covered by Employees' Health Insurance, including most foreign students. Also, the dependents of people in these categories.

Retirees and the elderly are enrolled in one or the other of these plans, but are also eligible for special benefits or subsidies.

Register in one of these plans, and you'll be issued a large, plastic-laminated health insurance certificate (*hoken-shō* 保険証) which you must be ready to show whenever you visit a medical facility. If you don't have this health insurance certificate with you, you may be asked to pay the full fee; you can usually be reimbursed by the facility or the insurer if you present your certificate later.

The system is designed so that wherever you go, if you're covered by Japanese public insurance, you can expect to pay about the same amount for the same care. In practice, you may find that the fees for care are more expensive in large cities because of higher overhead and personnel costs. Note also that you pay more for treatment after hours, on holidays, or if a doctor makes a house call, but even these extra fees are set and regulated by the government and are covered by insurance if the situation was unavoidable or an emergency.

Employees' Health Insurance (EHI) *shakai hoken* 社会保険 (*kenkō hoken* 健康保険)

QUALIFICATION: If you work full-time, or at least more than three-fourths the hours of a full-time worker, for a company or organization which has joined an EHI plan, you are eligible for this type of insurance. However, since membership is usually combined with the company pension system, in practice, some companies and their foreign, relatively short-term employees find it mutually beneficial to exclude foreign employee membership. If you do become a policyholder (*hi-hokensha* 被保険者), your dependents (*hi-fuyōsha* 被扶養者) will also be covered. Those who are "dependent" on you for their livelihood must meet the following qualifications:

■ Dependents eligible for coverage even if they don't live with you: spouse (even in a common-law marriage), children, grandchildren, younger siblings, parents, grandparents, great-grandparents.

■ Dependents who must be living with you to receive coverage: older siblings, aunts, uncles, nephews and nieces (and their spouses), spouses of younger siblings, your spouse's parents (even in a common-law marriage), stepchildren, great-grandchildren, and any other dependents related to you within three generations.

■ If your dependent has an income, it must be less than ¥1,300,000 a year (less than ¥1,800,000 if he or she is disabled or over sixty). If your dependent lives with you, his or her annual income should also be less than half of yours; otherwise, it must be less than the amount of financial support received from you.

ENROLLMENT: Submit the form *hi-fuyōsha todoke* 被扶養者届 to your employer, who will register you and your dependents with your EHI office. Report any change in dependents within five days. If both parents are working, children become the dependents of the parent with the larger salary. Once you are registered, your portion of the premium (*hoken-ryō* 保険料) will usually be deducted automatically from your monthly paycheck.

PREMIUMS: Under EHI plans, the employer and employee generally split the cost of the premium, usually fifty-fifty. The premium is based on the employee's average monthly income, and does not change with the number of dependents or the number of claims you make. The rate varies among different plans, but currently stands at around 8.5 percent of the employee's standard monthly income—with "income" being defined as salary including benefits such as commuting allowance and housing allowance. Biannual bonuses are either not included, or calculated at a lesser rate. A list of standard income categories should be available from your company. Note that with the recent change from 10 percent to 20 percent in the amount which the policyholder must co-pay for outpatient care, some EHI societies have slightly lowered the percent for calculating the premium, in order to lighten the burden on the individual employee.

BENEFITS: Japan has various employees' societies and associations including hundreds of insurance societies for workers in large enterprises; several mutual aid associations such as those for private school teachers, local government employees, and national government employees; and a government-managed health insurance program for workers in small companies of more than five but less than 300 employees. Benefits differ somewhat among different health insurance societies or associations, but are generally as outlined below.

Partial Cost Sharing *ichibu futan* 一部負担

Outpatient Fees: The policyholder pays twenty percent, and the insurer eighty percent. A dependent pays thirty percent, and the insurer seventy percent. Patients pay the co-payment (*jiko futan* 自己負担) to the medical facility at the time of treatment; the facility then bills the insurer for the rest. For outpatient medications, the same percentages apply (to anyone except children under six or to the low-income elderly), but in addition, patients bear an extra portion of the cost, as follows. [Please note that throughout this chapter, "low income" refers to income that is so low that municipal taxes are not required.])

■ Internal medications (*naifuku-yaku* 内服薬)

No extra cost burden for one type of medication; ¥30 per day for 2–3 medications prescribed in the same dosages and on the same schedule, ¥60/day for 4–5 medications, ¥100/day for 6 or more medications.

■ External medications (*gaiyō-yaku* 外用薬)

¥50 extra cost burden per prescription for 1 type of topical medication, ¥100 for 2 medications, ¥150 for 3 or more. Includes compresses, ointments, eye drops, etc.

■ PRN medication (*tonpuku-yaku* 頓服薬)

¥10 extra cost burden per prescription for prescribed medications to be taken only if symptoms arise. This includes medications for nausea, fever, itching, pain, and stomach gas or acidity.

Inpatient Fees: Policyholders and dependents pay twenty percent; the insurer pays the remainder. The patient pays the facility his co-payment before discharge and the facility bills the insurer for the rest. These percentages also apply to inpatient medications; patients bear no extra cost burden. For hospital meals (*nyūin-ji shokuji ryōyō-hi* 入院時食事療養費), patients bear an extra cost of ¥760/day (those with low income can apply for a reduced fee).

Infant/Child Medical Fees: Local governments will pick up the co-payment for medical bills of resident children up to age three (in some areas up to age six, if low income), including registered foreign children, who are enrolled in EHI. See page 62.

Care Not Covered

Fees for Treatment of Injuries Caused by Another: The patient should report to his insurer before settling with the responsible party. Fees for treatment of injuries from traffic or other accidents caused by someone else should be paid by the party responsible for the accident. If the responsible party cannot pay, or if reimbursement takes too long, the insurer will temporarily cover the cost, and claim the amount later from the responsible party.

Fees for Treatment of Work-Related Injuries/Illnesses: These fees are covered under workmen's compensation insurance (see page 59).

Fees for Other Care: Preventive health care (except company approved annual checkups see pages 88–89); immunizations; cosmetic surgery; luxury items such as private hospital rooms; normal pregnancy and birth; orthodontics; simple fatigue; sterilization or abortion performed for economic reasons; self-inflicted injuries or conditions arising as a result of neglect of a doctor's orders; injuries resulting from criminal acts, fighting, or drunkenness; alcoholism or drug addiction treatment; any treatment not approved for coverage by the Ministry of Health and Welfare, including dental work using precious metals or materials not prescribed within standard treatment.

Reimbursements

Medical Bills Paid in Full: If the patient can show that it was not a choice, but a medical emergency, that caused him to seek care at a facility that would not accept his insurance, he can apply for reimbursement. Note that the amount reimbursed may not be based on the amount paid, but on the government-fixed fee for that service. Some insurance societies will cover care received overseas in this way. To apply, submit an itemized receipt to the insurer with the form *ryōyō-hi shikyū shinsei-sho* 療養費支給申請書.

High-cost Medical Fees (*kōgaku ryōyō-hi* 高額療養費): If within one month, a policyholder or dependent's inpatient co-payments to the same medical facility, or outpatient co-payments to the same department of the same medical facility, exceed ¥63,600, the insurer will reimburse the amount paid over this figure. (Inpatient dental treatment and inpatient medical treatment are calculated separately, even if they are received at the same facility.) This is also true if these co-payments exceed ¥30,000 two or more times within a month if the total exceeds ¥63,600, even if the payments were made by separate persons under the policy. For example, if in one month you pay co-payments amounting to ¥34,000 for your son's broken leg and in the same month your wife is hospitalized and you pay a co-payment of ¥50,000 for her care, you can be reimbursed ¥20,400 (¥84,000 − ¥63,600 = ¥20,400). You would not be eligible for this reimbursement if you had paid only ¥29,000 for your son's care, even if you had paid a total of, say, ¥20,000 to another department in the same month. If reimbursement for high-cost treatment is received four or more times within 12 months, from the fourth time on, reimbursement will be for the amount paid over ¥37,200. Extra fees paid for inpatient hospital meals, private or semi-private rooms, etc. cannot be included when calculating these amounts. The amounts can vary among different societies. Amounts are less for those with low income.

Note that maximum monthly co-payments will be no more than ¥10,000 for long-term, high-cost treatment, such as that for diabetes, chronic kidney insufficiency, and other designated chronic conditions.

Interest-free loans for 80–90 percent of the expected reimbursement are available to help until reimbursement comes through (usually about two months later). Apply at the local EHI branch of the Todofuken Shakai Hoken Kumiai 都道府県社会保険組合.

Transportation to Hospital: If a patient is seriously ill or injured and the doctor judges that he must be transported by car, etc. to a hospital, or transferred from one hospital to another, he can be reimbursed for the cost of that transportation (*isōhi* 移送費), although prior permission from the insurer may be required. Reimbursement is based on the most economical and ordinary route and method.

Specified Medical Equipment/Treatment: With prior permission from the insurer, a patient can be reimbursed a fixed amount for plaster casts, corsets, artificial eyes, acupuncture, massage, moxibustion, blood for transfusions, and treatment for bone fractures, etc. by *sekkotsu* therapists (see pages 283–84). Usually, a medical doctor must have ordered the equipment/treatment.

Extra Nursing Care: Since all Japanese hospitals in principle now provide full nursing care, inpatient extra nursing care is no longer considered necessary, and therefore not covered. Home visiting nurse services are covered generally three times a week, but will not be restricted to this if the patient is in the final stages of cancer or certain designated diseases. Home nursing is mainly for patients suffering from dementia or who have been bedridden usually at least six months. There are no age limits. A doctor must have ordered the care and the nurses will follow his instructions. Policyholders must pay twenty percent, dependents thirty percent; the insurer pays the rest. The patient also must pay for supplies (diapers, etc.), housekeeping assistance, and the nurse's transportation.

Allowances

Sickness and Injury Allowance (*shōbyō teate-kin* 傷病手当金): A policyholder who must be absent from work without pay for four or more days due to illness or injury can receive a subsidy equivalent to sixty percent of the standard daily income for his income range for each day absent, starting from the fourth day, for a period of up to eighteen months. If there are no dependents and hospitalization is necessary, the subsidy is only forty percent. Percentages and time periods vary among different health insurance societies and associations.

If a patient receives a reduced income during his recuperation period which amounts to less than the subsidy to which he is entitled as described above, he may receive a subsidy of the difference.

To receive the subsidy, he must submit certification from his employer to his insurer regarding his employment and salary and a written statement of his doctor's recommendations.

Pregnancy and Delivery: "Normal" pregnancy and birth are not covered. If medical interventions such as a cesarean are used, insurance covers the cost of the birth and hospitalization, just as with other medical procedures. Interventions such as an episiotomy, pain-relief medications and sutures may be charged to insurance but usually are not if used simply to facilitate a normal labor and birth. Treatment of complications such as toxemia are covered. The following subsidies are also available. Amounts may vary among different societies or areas, and some societies give supplementary subsidies as well:

■ Lump-sum Maternity Subsidy (*shussan ikuji ichijikin* 出産育児一時金): Following birth, mothers, both policyholders and dependents, can apply to their insurer for a fixed sum, generally of ¥300,000–¥350,000, to help cover childbirth related medical costs. This is paid not only for the birth of healthy, living babies, but also for miscarriages or stillbirths, if the pregnancy lasted eighty-five days or longer. In many cases this can be awarded even if the baby is born outside Japan or if the mother has been a been a policyholder but recently quit working and is no longer enrolled in EHI (it is best to get application forms before leaving the job).

■ Maternity Allowance (*shussan teatekin* 出産手当金): A mother who is a policyholder and is taking a leave of absence without pay from work can apply for an additional allowance through her insurer. This allowance is usually based on 60 percent of the standard daily income for her income range and covers a period of 42 days before her due date (70 days for multiple births) through 56 days after the birth. Percentages vary among different health insurance societies and associations. In some cases you can receive this allowance even if you leave your job (see Leaving Your Job, below).

Funeral Allowance (*maisōryō* 埋葬料): If a policyholder dies, the family can apply for an amount equivalent to his standard monthly income (or ¥100,000, whichever is more) for funeral expenses. Even if no funeral is held and the burial is informal, the family can receive this allowance. If there are no dependents, the person taking care of the arrangements can receive a allowance of up to ¥100,000 to cover expenses. If a dependent dies, the family receives a fixed sum of ¥100,000 for funeral expenses. If the person dies at work, while commuting to work, or from work-related causes, this allowance is not given, since everything will be paid by workmen's compensation insurance (see page 59).

Health Resorts
For health promotion, some insurers will subsidize a stay at specified beach and mountain hot springs or other types of health resorts.

LEAVING YOUR JOB, OR EMPLOYEE RETIREMENT
If you have been an EHI policyholder for at least one year before leaving your job, you and your dependents can still use EHI for continuing treatment of preexisting ailments (*keizoku ryōyō* 継続療養) after you stop working. You will lose this coverage when you reach age seventy (sixty-five if you are bedridden) or five years after the treatment started. Apply for this coverage at your EHI office within ten days of leaving your job. You can also apply for a two-year continuation of EHI coverage (*nin'i keizoku* 任意継続) if you have been a policyholder for more than two months, and if you apply within twenty days of the

termination of your employment. Note, however, that you'll now be responsible for the full premium, although you can deduct it from your taxes (see page 79) at the end of the year. You can extend your coverage beyond the two years, until you reach age sixty (if you retired at age fifty-five or over), or until you join the Retiree Health Care System (see page 77).

In some cases, as when you leave your job while you are still receiving or still eligible for a maternity allowance or illness/injury allowance, or if you give birth within six months of leaving your job, you may still receive the allowances under the same terms as an employee. Cutoff dates vary, so check with your insurer.

Other options for health insurance until you reach age seventy (sixty-five if you're bedridden) and become eligible for the Health Insurance System for the Elderly (see pages 77–78) are to join the NHI system and pay premiums and co-payments, or to become a dependent of a family member and be covered under that person's policy.

National Health Insurance (NHI) kokumin kenkō hoken 国民健康保険

NHI (literally, "Citizen's Health Insurance") is offered by local governments and guilds for residents of Japan who are not covered by other insurance plans. However, since the local governments or individual NHI associations decide the details according to the resources and needs of the population they serve, check the finer details with your local NHI office.

QUALIFICATION: Foreigners qualify for (and are obliged to join) NHI if they are not covered by insurance at their workplace and if they are registered and permitted to remain in Japan one year or more at the time they enter Japan. This includes students and others with visas for less than a year, provided that they can show proof of intention to stay more than one year. Since you will not be able to join NHI until you have determined the place where you will live in Japan and registered with your municipality, it is wise to have travelers' insurance to cover any care you may need until then.

You should also be aware that NHI insurers around Japan have been directed that, as of April 1998, they should charge anyone who is eligible but who has failed to join NHI for the amount equivalent to up to two years of back premiums. Most NHI insurers won't actively seek out non-joiners, but should your case be brought to their attention—for example, if you approach NHI for membership later—you could be charged for these back payments.

All family members who are living in the same house and who are enrolled in NHI will be on one policy. Generally, those living elsewhere cannot be included, with the exception of dependent children away at school.

ENROLLMENT: If you are eligible for NHI, apply within fourteen days of your alien registration at your local government NHI office, which is usually located in the building where you registered as a foreign resident. To enroll or withdraw, you will need your alien registration card, personal seal, and documents such as a housing rental contract, statement of retirement, etc. proving your changed status.

One problem sometimes faced by foreigners is that once a member of the NHI plan, it is impossible to withdraw by choice. As was stated before, Japanese law states that all citizens (this is extended to foreign residents) are obliged to join a health insurance program. NHI offices interpret this as enrollment in NHI, unless one is enrolled in insurance through the workplace (interpreted as EHI) or a welfare program, since Japanese private insurance is only supplementary. Enrollment in foreign insurance has not been a consideration to date, and therefore has not been included as an acceptable substitute for enrollment in NHI or EHI. This makes switching from NHI to foreign insurance difficult if not impossible. If you will be outside of Japan for an extended period and show proof of this to NHI before you leave, some NHI offices will refund your payments when you return. But to withdraw from NHI completely, you'll be asked to prove that you are moving out of the NHI jurisdiction, changing your status to short stay or diplomat, going on welfare, or joining an insurance plan at your place of work.

PREMIUMS: NHI premiums are calculated taking into consideration household income, assets, the number of people covered in one household, and the amount necessary to keep the community's health care functioning. It is not affected by the number of claims you make. Some adjustments are made for households with very high or very low incomes. At present, the highest annual premium which any household in the twenty-three wards of Tokyo may be charged is ¥530,000. The lowest is ¥26,100, the flat rate charged per person. Your premium consists of this basic amount plus the amount equivalent to 187 percent of your last year's municipal taxes. If you did not pay taxes in Japan the previous year, your premiums will be calculated using only the flat rate. Payments are made in installments every four or six months at a bank, post office, or NHI Office. The highest premium, percentages, flat rate, etc., vary in different areas and are subject to change each year. Note that premiums are not necessarily calculated from the date you apply, but from the date on which you became eligible—i.e., moved into the area, registered as a foreign resident, or withdrew from EHI. As was mentioned before, a new national regulation states that if you have been eligible for NHI but did not enroll, you can be charged for up to two years back premiums when you do enroll. In some areas, refusal to pay premiums despite repeated notification can result in seizure of property.

BENEFITS: Householders and dependents are treated equally, with equal benefits. Note that many of the NHI benefits are the same as those of EHI plans (see page 69), and that benefits vary among different areas.

Partial Cost Sharing *ichibu futan* 一部負担
Outpatient Fees: Householders and dependents pay thirty percent; NHI pays seventy percent for care and medications (retirees, see page 77). The person receiving medical care pays the co-payment to the medical facility; the medical facility bills NHI for the rest. Patients bear the same extra cost burden for medications as in EHI plans.

Inpatient Fees: Householders and dependents pay thirty percent; NHI pays the remainder; otherwise, same as in EHI.

Infant/Child Medical Fees: Same as in EHI.

Reduction or Exemption From Co-payment of Medical Fees: If an NHI policyholder is temporarily suffering severe hardship due to disaster, bankruptcy, etc., he may apply to his NHI office for temporary exemption or reduction of hospitalization fees. NHI will examine the application and determine if the need is sufficient. This will not apply to any extra fees such as those for private or semi-private rooms.

Care Not Covered

Fees for Treatment of Injury Caused by Someone Else: Same as in EHI.

Fees for Treatment of Work-related Injury/Illness: Same as in EHI.

Fees for Other Care: Same as in EHI, except that treatment received outside Japan is not covered, unless you are also enrolled in the Health Insurance System for the Elderly.

Reimbursements

Medical Bills Paid in Full: Same as EHI. Within two or three months, NHI will send the insured a card notifying of eligibility for reimbursement. This card should be submitted to your local NHI office, along with itemized receipts, to receive the reimbursement. Interest-free loans are available from NHI for up to ninety percent of the amount to be reimbursed, if necessary.

High-cost Medical Fees: Same as in EHI.

Transportation to Hospital: Same as in EHI.

Specified Medical Equipment/Treatment: Same as in EHI; NHI will reimburse seventy percent.

Extra Nursing Care: Same as in EHI, except that NHI will reimburse seventy percent for both householder and dependents.

Foreign Students can receive an eighty percent reimbursement for the amount paid as co-payment from AIEJ (see page 83).

Allowances

Sickness/Injury: NHI does not provide a Sickness and Injury Allowance.

Pregnancy and Delivery: Same as in EHI, except that the Maternity Allowance for leave from work is not offered. Note also that NHI will not pay the Lump-sum Maternity Subsidy if the mother is still eligible for payments related to the birth from any previously-held insurance. Applications for the subsidy should be submitted to the NHI office.

Funeral Allowance: If an NHI-insured person dies, the person arranging the funeral can receive an allowance of ¥30,000–¥70,000 or more (amount varies with the local NHI plan). Applications are made at the NHI office with the health insurance certificate and personal seal of the deceased, and the bank account number of the person in charge of the funeral.

Health Resorts
Same as in EHI.

RETIREES' HEALTH CARE SYSTEM (RHC) *taishoku-sha iryō seido* 退職者医療制度
The RHC plan is part of the NHI system. You can apply if you are eligible to receive a pension, and have been paying into a *kōsei nenkin* or *kyōsai nenkin* (pension) program for more than 20 years (or after age 40, at least 10 years), and are no longer working but too young for the Health Insurance System for the Elderly (see below). Apply within 14 days of receiving your pension certificate (*nenkin shōsho* 年金証書). Once you have joined, membership continues until you qualify for the Health Insurance System for the Elderly.

The RHC system is generally the same as the NHI system except in a few points. Policyholders and dependents receive a retired person's health insurance certificate (*taishoku-sha [hi] hokensha-shō* 退職者［被］保険者証) instead of the usual certificate. Also, the policyholder pays a co-payment of 20 percent for outpatient and inpatient care. Dependents pay 20 percent for inpatient and 30 percent for outpatient care. Dependents must live in the same household and have an annual income less than half that of the retiree; in addition, the dependent's income must not exceed ¥1,300,000 (¥1,800,000 for dependents who are sixty or over or disabled).

Health Insurance System for the Elderly (HISE) *kōrei-sha no hoken iryō* 高齢者の保険医療
Residents aged seventy or over, or sixty-five or over if bedridden, continue to participate in EHI or the NHI plans as a policyholder or a dependent, paying premiums as required. However, certain additional benefits are also available from HISE.

Those who qualify can receive outpatient care at any one department of any one clinic or hospital for ¥500 per visit, for the first four visits each month. No payment is necessary for the fifth or successive visits to that department during that month. The inpatient co-payment is ¥1,100 per day (less for those who are members of households with low income). This amount is scheduled to rise to ¥1,200 in fiscal 1999. Further increases are likely in future. Inpatient hemophiliacs and those on kidney dialysis are exceptions, and pay no more than ¥10,000 per month. As with EHI and NHI, coverage does not apply to any forms of treatment which are not covered by public insurance.

To receive these benefits, apply for an elderly person's medical care certificate (*rōjin iryō jukyūsha-shō* 老人医療受給者証) at the NHI office or the senior welfare section (*kōreisha fukushi tantōka* 高齢者福祉担当課) of your local government office. You must show this certificate in addition to your NHI or EHI, certificate, when you visit a hospital.

Other assistance is available for low-income or bedridden people in this age group. See "Help for the Disabled and the Elderly."

Note that NHI will reimburse you for treatment received overseas, at a rate based on what insurance would have covered in Japan (unless the overseas fee was lower).

Compulsory Nursing Care Insurance System *kō-teki kaigo hoken seido* 公的介護保険制度

Although details may change before the start of this system in April 2000, the present plan calls for compulsory enrollment and payment of an average of ¥2,500 per month premium (to be raised periodically) by every resident aged 40 or over who is enrolled in Japanese public health insurance, including foreign residents. Excluded will be those who are not enrolled in Japanese public insurance, those who are permanently hospitalized for disabilities, or those who have been specially exempted by the government. The patient's co-payment will be ten percent of the actual cost, and local municipal governments will be the insurers, covering the rest of the cost.

The insured will be divided into two categories. Those 65 and older will be in the primary-level category (*daiichigō hi-hokensha* 第一号被保険者), and those aged 40 through 64 in the secondary-level (*dainigō hi-hokensha* 第二号被保険者). Premiums for primary-level insured persons will be based on income as well as on local government resources. The secondary-level insured will pay premiums combined together with public health insurance payments. Premiums for employees' insurance plans will vary from insurer to insurer, but the employer will pay half of the premium. National Health Insurance premiums will be based on income and community resources.

In return, the primary-level insured (and secondary-level insured with conditions caused by aging) will be entitled to as much as ¥290,000 per month for support/care at home or at Special Nursing Homes for the Elderly, as much as ¥320,000 per month for care/support at Intermediate Care Facilities for the Elderly, and as much as ¥430,000 for care in wards at hospitals that offer skilled nursing long-term care. The insurance will mainly be limited to those who are bedridden or suffer from dementia or those who without support are deemed in danger of becoming bedridden or of suffering dementia.

Home nursing care that will be covered will include home-help services, home bathing assistance, visiting nurses, at-home rehabilitation, meals and baths at day-care centers, rehabilitation at day-care facilities, lending of special equipment, instruction for the family in at-home care, short-term stay at welfare facilities, short-term stay at medical facilities, care at group homes for the senile elderly, and care at designated private nursing homes for the elderly or at moderate-fee assisted living homes (Care Houses) for the elderly. Care will also be covered at Special Nursing Homes for the Elderly, Intermediate Care Facilities for the

Elderly, and wards at hospitals providing long-term skilled nursing care (see pages 224–25).

Applications for this care will be made to the local government office. An examining committee will use a six-level ranking system to assess the need for care, with "level six" being the greatest need, and "level one" the least. The application process is expected to take up to one month, but services may be started before the application is complete, when necessary. Governments will begin accepting applications from October 1999. At the end of the process, the patient will receive an insurance card with the assigned ranking stamped on it.

Next, a care manager (*kea manejā* ケアマネージャー)—probably from a home nursing support center (*zaitaku kaigo shien sentā* 在宅介護支援センター)—will discuss a three- to six-month plan for care (*kea puran* ケアプラン). The plan offers a choice of institutional or home care and public or private services, generally located or operating within the municipality but not limited to it. If the costs of an individual's plan exceed the allotted amount, the individual pays the amount in excess.

Tax Deductions for Medical Expenses

If in one year your household out-of-pocket medical expenses exceed a total of ¥100,000 or five percent of your income (whichever is less), you may deduct the excess amount, up to ¥2,000,000, from your income taxes. If your taxes have been withheld, you will be applying for reimbursement. Out-of-pocket expenses are amounts actually paid minus any reimbursements or assistance (for example, from supplementary insurance). Included are medical fee co-payments for outpatient or inpatient care, medications, prenatal checkups, delivery, transportation to hospital, massage, shiatsu, acupuncture, moxibustion, and *sekkotsu* therapies. These items cannot be claimed, however, if the care was preventive, cosmetic or for the sake of ordinary health maintenance. Note that in order for the fee to be termed "medical," the massage, shiatsu, acupuncture, or *sekkotsu* treatment must have been ordered by a doctor. Fees paid for health checkups may not be included unless the exam diagnosed a condition for which you then sought treatment. If ordered by a doctor, you may also include amounts paid for an at-home blood pressure machine, home-help services if you are confined to bed for an unusually long time after childbirth, and, for the bedridden or senile elderly, home-help services, home nursing, and (if you are bedridden for more than six months) diapers. Also included in this category are amounts paid for exercise therapy or for hot spring therapy prescribed for certain adult disease conditions such as diabetes, high blood pressure, or arthritis. To qualify, you will need a certificate confirming that you have been attending sessions more than once a week for eight weeks at a designated center. Those in a company retiree health insurance program can include the amount paid in monthly premiums by submitting the receipt of payment (*hoken-ryō haraikomi shōmeisho*) 保健料払込証明書 received from the insurer.

To receive the deduction, apply at your local tax office, presenting all receipts and certificates to them, usually when you file your income tax, in February or March.

Government Point System for Medical Fees

The Japanese government uses a point system to set medical fees. All treatments and prescription medications covered under Japanese public insurance have been assigned points representing the relative fee. Medical facilities use these points to calculate the fees they charge. If the care is covered by public insurance (termed *hoken shinryō* 保険診療), the calculation base is always ¥10 per point. This means that the fee for a treatment assigned 100 points will be ¥1,000. Those who have Japanese public insurance will pay the facility administering the treatment a co-payment of ¥200 (20%) or ¥300 (30%) of this amount, and the insurer will pay the rest.

However, if the treatment is not covered by Japanese insurance, either because the patient is not enrolled in Japanese insurance or because the treatment has not been approved by the government for coverage, the patient is considered fully responsible for payment (termed *jihi shinryō* 自費診療), and the facility can set the fee either at this amount (100% of the insurance fee [termed *jū-wari keisan* 十割計算]), or at a multiple of it. When public insurance is not applicable, some hospitals charge 150% of the insurance fee (in this case, ¥1,500 with 1 point = ¥15), 200% (1 point = ¥20; in this case a total of ¥2,000), or even 300% (1 point = ¥30, in this case ¥3,000). All national hospitals (including national university hospitals) provide care at 100% of the insurance fee. Tokyo and Osaka metropolitan hospitals and Chiba prefectural hospitals also use the 100% rate; however, Kobe municipal hospitals and Osaka prefectural hospitals charge 120%, Sapporo 130%, and Chiba municipal hospitals 150%. Matsudo asks for 100% from uninsured residents and 150% from non-residents. Private hospitals and clinics, including Red Cross hospitals, tend to use a higher percentage base (Tokyo Jikei and Nihon University Hospitals charge 200%), but many do not. If cost is a concern, you can check by phone before visiting. To ask for this information in Japanese you might say, *Jihi shinryō ni tsuite kikitai n desu ga, otaku no byōin de wa itten wa jū-en desu ka* (I'd like to ask you about the self-payment rate at your hospital. Is one point ¥10?). The facility will likely say *Hai, sō desu. Jū-en desu* (Yes, it is. It's ¥10.) or give an alternative figure, usually no more than ¥30.

Private Health Insurance

Foreign-based

Foreign-based health insurance is offered in Japan mainly as supplementary insurance to Japanese public insurance. However, some non-Japanese maintain foreign-based travelers' or primary health insurance during their stay in Japan. Most clinics specially serving the English-speaking foreign community do not accept Japanese public insurance. One advantage of a foreign-based plan is the greater affordability of these health facilities, as well as of health care overseas. In choosing a plan, note that some plans do not cover dental or maternity care, or have other limitations. Pay particular attention to deductibles, coverage ceilings, renewability, and whether the plan covers preexisting conditions and outpatient visits. You also may need to check if coverage is adequate in countries which you are likely to visit, and whether it can be transferred to a plan in your home country should you leave Japan.

When using foreign-based health insurance, the patient usually prepays the medical facility the entire fee, then applies to the insurer for a reimbursement. Generally, health facilities will not accept credit card payment or payment directly from foreign insurers. Many foreign-based employers prepay any extremely high medical fees for their employees, to help them out until reimbursement arrives. Nevertheless, some Japanese facilities refuse to treat people who do not have Japanese health insurance. If you have only foreign-based insurance, check which facilities in your area are willing to treat you. You may also want to keep in mind the medical fee point system (explained at left) to help determine affordability.

Foreign-based Health Insurance

IHI danmark Regional Representative Office
Kokaji Bldg. 2 Fl., 3-62-1 Sendagaya
Shibuya-ku, Tokyo
03-3405-0794, fax 03-3405-1294
ihidk@tkb.att.ne.jp
Owned by Denmark's national health insurer, with an 80-year history and an AAA-rating. Lifetime-guaranteed medical and dental policies worldwide which can never be reassessed. Though policyholders have a free choice of treatment and physician, the company keeps updated information on specialists and hospitals around the world, including Japan, from which it can offer suggestions.

AON Risk Services Japan, Ltd.
Mita 43 Mori Bldg. 3-13-16 Mita
Minato-ku, Tokyo
03-5427-2001, fax 03-5427-2052
Insurance consultants with a specialty in health insurance, offering private global policies, both supplementary and primary, including the Medicare International Health Plan. Choose from various types of coverage. Preexisting medical conditions, routine checkups and immunizations are generally not covered.

ALICO Japan (American Life Insurance Company)
International Ikebukuro Office
2-13-2 Ikebukuro, Toshima-ku, Tokyo
03-3590-2331
ALICO has a well-established history in dealing with both Japanese and non-Japanese. Various plans are offered, including insurance to supplement national or private insurance plans in the areas of extra hospitalization, surgery, cancer, hospital discharge, and insurance for disability, death, sickness, and accidents. Contracts written only in Japanese.

Banner Japan, K.K.
Esperanza Ebisu Bldg. 4 Fl., 3-2-19 Ebisu-Minami
Shibuya-ku, Tokyo
03-5724-5100, fax 03-5724-5300
This British-based company offers both supplementary and primary insurance. Choose from various types of coverage from preventive to dental care to overseas accident insurance. However, on-going medical conditions and immunizations are not covered.

All Japan Financial Group
N.V. Koshien, Suite 101, 13-19 Tendocho
Nishinomiya-shi, Hyogo-ken
(toll-free) 0120-634-419, fax 0798-64-3894
British-based company offers both primary and supplementary insurance. Primary plan covers outpatient and hospitalization, emergency dental, travel, and income replacement up to 6 months. Coverage in North America is 90 days per year. Fast claim reimbursement. Preexisting medical conditions, routine health checkups, and immunizations are not covered.

Advanced Insurance
Jeff Tingley CLU, ChFC
3-10-14-202 Tsurumaki, Setagaya-ku, Tokyo
03-3429-2670, fax 03-3434-1171

Blue Cross/Blue Shield of Delaware, IHG and others.

U.S.-chartered life underwriter professional offering catastrophic but comprehensive insurance.

Japan-based

Japan-based private health insurance offers coverage for cancer treatment, extra hospitalization (for instance, a private room), high-tech or advanced treatment, home nursing, and death expenses. It will also cover or prepay a patient's co-payment under public health insurance. Private health insurance is usually offered as an option with the purchase of life insurance, and cannot be purchased separately. Examples of companies offering private health insurance are the Yasuda Fire and Marine Insurance Company, the Nippon Life Insurance Company and Meiji Mutual Life Insurance Company.

Note that the contracts at Japanese private health insurance companies are usually written completely in Japanese, and also that some Japanese companies will sell insurance only to long-term residents.

Accident Insurance

Japanese public health insurance does not cover the treatment of an injury resulting from an accident caused by someone else, since the person responsible is expected to pay. However, if the person is unable to pay for the care you need, or if you cause the accident, then having supplementary accident insurance can help you out. Private accident insurance is available from most insurance companies that sell life insurance. A cheaper option is to join one of the local government-run insurance unions or a union at your place of work.

Schools usually offer parents the option of enrolling their children in school accident insurance. Insurance at international schools may provide worldwide coverage. Note that the school itself is not responsible for accidents occurring at or on the way to school.

Travelers' Insurance

If your company does not provide insurance, and you will be staying in Japan for less than a year, the best form of coverage is usually a global insurance plan (a primary plan covering care around the world), or traveler's accident insurance. Travelers' insurance is only valid in Japan if purchased outside the country. Although these plans generally do not cover ailments preexisting at the time of purchase, they will cover most newly-acquired illnesses or injuries.

For travel insurance for foreign residents of Japan traveling outside Japan, you might try the Yasuda Fire and Marine Insurance Company. It is affiliated with the large U.S. insurance company Blue Cross/Blue Shield and World Access, so you'll find numerous facilities around the world willing to accept its insurance. To be eligible for Japanese travel insurance that offers coverage abroad, you must be a registered resident in Japan. See also the list of companies on page 81.

Special Assistance for Non-Japanese

In the past, uninsured foreigners were granted assistance under the Livelihood Protection Law, but since the revision of this law some years ago an uninsured foreigner must now be a permanent resident, a refugee, or married to a Japanese or to a permanent resident in order to receive this type of welfare. Some local governments (notably those in Tokyo, Gunma-ken, and Kanagawa-ken) have taken temporary measures to assist institutions by appropriating funds to offer medical facilities compensation for unpaid medical bills. However, this is not direct coverage, nor is it consistently available throughout the country. Various private organizations, such as Bright and Minatomachi Mutual Aid, have taken steps to aid foreign workers.

Minatomachi Foreign Migrant Workers' Mutual Aid

045-453-3673

Foreign workers pay a membership fee of ¥2,000 per month and a thirty percent co-payment when they receive medical or dental care at one of the organization's medical centers. Depending on the day, care is available in English, Korean, Tagalog, Persian, French, Spanish, Portuguese, Chinese. Call for an appointment. Japanese public insurance is accepted at all the following:

■ Minatomachi Medical Center
7-6 Kinko-cho, Kanagawa-ku, Yokohama-shi
045-453-3673

■ Yokosuka Chuo Clinic
Suzuman Bldg. 3 Fl., 1-16 Wakamatsu-cho
Yokosuka-shi
0468-23-8691

■ Jujodori Clinic
8-23-8 Minami-Rinkan, Yamato-shi
Kanagawa-ken
0462-74-5884

■ Isezaki Clinic (Ob/Gyn)
K Bldg. Isezaki 2 Fl., 3-107 Isezaki-cho, Naka-ku
Yokohama-shi
045-251-8622

This plan cannot accommodate all medical situations commonly experienced by foreign workers. For example, there is no ophthalmologist available at present. There are also no affiliated hospitals, only clinics. This means that in cases in which patients must be referred to larger hospitals, care will not be covered by insurance.

Bright International Cooperative Society

2-60-2-2FA Higashi-Ikebukuro, Toshima-ku
Tokyo
03-3590-9110
9:00 A.M.–8:00 P.M. daily

To apply for this insurance as a non-Japanese, you'll need two photographs of yourself and two copies of your passport or alien registration card. You will not be asked your address. Any non-Japanese living in Japan who is healthy and does not qualify for Japanese public insurance, regardless of visa status, may apply. Members pay a membership fee of ¥3,000 per month. There is no restriction on the facilities or doctors you may use, but when you receive medical care you must first pay the entire amount, after which 70 percent reimbursement will be paid into your or a friend's bank account. Not all conditions or treatments are covered—for example, chronic conditions, hospitalization, pregnancy, abortions, dental care, and AIDS are not. This organization has branches in Manila and will also help foreigners involved in on-the-job accidents and labor disputes.

Association of International Education Japan (AIEJ)

4-5-29 Komaba, Meguro-ku, Tokyo
03-5454-5213

Those with student visas who intend to be in Japan for one year or more can participate in the NHI system. AIEJ offers foreign students a program which reimburses 80 percent of the student's co-payment. Registration for AIEJ assistance can be made through universities and colleges.

Strategies for the Uninsured

Study the assistance and insurance plans explained in this chapter—you may qualify for one or more of them. If you qualify for NHI and just haven't joined, it is really never too late, though you may be asked to pay back premiums (up to two years) for the time during which you were eligible but didn't join. If you join in the morning, your operation that afternoon will be covered. Just avoid joining on, for instance, the 31st of any month; since you will be charged for the full month in which you join. If you don't qualify and have no insurance, first consider that national hospitals are likely to be less expensive than private hospitals, facilities in small towns less than those in cities, and midwife clinics less expensive than hospitals or obstetric clinics. Call beforehand to check the rates for care which is not covered (see discussion of the point system on page 80). Discuss your situation and the cost of care with your doctor before beginning any treatment. Some doctors are willing to perform a minimum of tests and treatment to help keep costs down. Call one of the helplines in your area, such as AMDA (see the endpapers)—they may be able to direct you to an appropriate facility, or inform you of an insurance or welfare plan which can help.

Keep in mind that under Japanese law, public funds are available to cover the amount not covered by insurance, or the entire amount if necessary, of certain kinds of medical care, regardless of the patient's insurance coverage or visa status. These include provisions under the Tuberculosis Prevention Law, parts of the Child Welfare Act, Assistance for Childbirth and laws relating to certain degrees of mental and physical disabilities (see pages 59–62 for details of these programs). Application procedures are delicate and difficult, so it is best to get the help of a non-governmental organization (NGO) accustomed to the process. The *Manual for Migrants: Information for Living in Japan,* put out by the Catholic Diocese of Yokohama Solidarity Center for Migrants, is an excellent source of information on these programs and on NGOs around Japan. Order this publication from the Center (044-549-7678, fax 044-511-9495), which can also help you find the appropriate NGO.

Health Checkups

"Even though I hate the lack of personal attention, I use the public health facilities for cancer tests and for the health checks available to people over forty."

"Maybe it's because I'm a foreigner, but the staff at the public health center always takes time to make sure I understand the results of any tests that have been done."

"My husband's company insurance plan pays for him to have a thorough annual physical and also for me to have a slightly less thorough one. We take full advantage of the tests, even though I detest the whole atmosphere. I skip the stomach X-rays—at my age and with my racial background they're not worth the risk."

Health Checkups

Preventive health checkups of all sorts are an integral part of the Japanese health care system. Through the public health system these are free or very inexpensive, although they can be quite costly when done on a private basis. Now you may think that the only purpose of a health checkup is to try to detect a disease as soon as possible so that quick treatment will lead to a quick cure. This is only half the story. An even more important objective is to spot where changes in your present life-style (exercise, diet, work, play, etc.) would result in better health now and so prevent future health problems. For example, a rise in blood pressure since the previous year's checkup might signal stress at work, a lack of exercise, or a gain in weight. All of these could be rectified now to prevent dire problems later on (and avoid higher health care costs in the future).

You'll note that Japanese general health checkups include annual stomach X-rays for those over forty, because of the high rate of stomach cancer here (probably resulting from the combined effect of a salty diet, high alcohol intake, and stressful life-style). Pap smears and breast exams for women are not included in the free public health screenings until the age of thirty, when the incidence of these cancers starts to rise.

Yearly General Checkups

Public Health Department Checkups

Taking the recommendations from the Ministry of Health and Welfare into account, every year each city or ward makes up its own schedule of preventive health examinations *yobō kenkō kensa* 予防健康検査 available to residents (whether Japanese citizens or not). The time schedule and optional exams vary according to resources available, but the basic preventive examinations *kihon kenkō kensa* 基本健康検査 are the same. Although the tests are offered through the public health department system, they are not always done at the public health center. The testing schedule is usually published only in Japanese, although a few cities or wards with large foreign populations print the schedule in other languages as well.

Urawa City in Saitama Prefecture, for example, distributes a health calendar in April which lists the preventive tests and exams to be offered during that fiscal year, along with the names of clinics and hospitals where these tests can be performed. In Urawa, these exams are offered at individual clinics and hospitals from August through November. These facilities can be contacted directly, and all tests but stomach X-rays are free. Any resident of Urawa aged forty or over, except the main policyholders of Employees Health Insurance plans (since checkups are available through their insurance), can have the basic preventive checkup. In addition, residents aged between thirty and thirty-nine who are policyholders in a national health insurance plan can have a similar checkup called *kokuho ningen dokku* 国保人間ドック. They must contact their local NHI office to make arrangements.

If a doctor orders further tests after seeing the results of this checkup, the cost of these additional tests will only be between ¥500 and ¥1,000 (at designated facilities). Tests offered in fiscal 1998 include:

■ Brief noting of health history, height and weight, blood pressure measurement, blood tests for liver function, cholesterol, and creatinine, a urinalysis, and lung and heart examination by stethoscope.

Optional tests (undertaken when warranted by the results of the basic tests): blood chemistry, blood sugar, complete blood count, complete urinalysis, fecal blood, electrocardiogram, retinal scan and intraocular pressure test, chest X-ray, stomach X-ray, and manual examination of the vertebrae.

Although the mass screenings may be crowded, and scheduled for inconvenient times, your city or ward may have a similar system to Urawa's, where you can make your own arrangements through individual hospitals and clinics within a set period of time. This kind of exam is unlikely to include much private discussion time with the doctor, a thoroughgoing check of your medical history, or easy communication. But the service is there if you choose to use it, and you can't beat the price!

Workplace Checkups shokuba kenkō shinsa 職場健康診査

These yearly checkups are offered at your place of work. They may be done in the company health room (if there is one), or the company may hire a clinic bus (shinryō basu 診療 バス) to do the checkups in the company parking lot during the working day. For companies with fifty or more employees, the government requires that a minimum of preventive tests and exams, similar to those offered at public health checkups, be offered.

"Human Dry Dock" Ningen Dokku 人間ドック

Another option is a more comprehensive annual physical exam. Ningen dokku (a colorful phrase coined about forty years ago to express the idea of a human [ningen] being pulled into dry dock [dokku] for an annual inspection) has become very popular and a huge business. The ningen dokku is done at selected clinics or hospitals, and expenses are reimbursed under employees' health insurance plans as well as some private health insurance plans.

Exams can be spread over one to seven days. The one-day basic tests are reported in a computerized printout which is reviewed by a physician at the end of the day. Longer versions include more tests (for instance, stress tests or a brain scan) and more time for rest and relaxation away from one's job or normal routine. Of course, the price jumps accordingly for the longer versions. Everything will be done in Japanese, so you may need someone to translate. The general flow of a one-day (actually, three- or four-hour) ningen dokku is something like this:

■ Make an appointment for the exam (expect a one- or two-month wait). Ask whether the clinic can do any extra tests you might want (like a mammogram), as the clinic will not be able to do every possible test.

■ Before your appointment day you will receive a health and medical questionnaire by mail, which you are to complete and bring with you. You will also receive instructions on what to eat (or not to eat) before the exam. It will include foods to avoid for several days before taking your stool sample, as well as a kit for obtaining this specimen. Usually there is to be no eating, drinking, or smoking for eight to twelve hours before the tests.

■ On the day of the exam, present yourself at the hospital or clinic with your completed health questionnaire and your stool specimen. Ask again which tests are to be done. If you want to omit or add any, now is the time to make your wishes known.

■ Once at the hospital or clinic, you will be moved steadily from department to department as different tests are done. Although the facility will be less crowded than a public health center, there is still the feeling of being on an assembly line as, your hospital gown flapping, you wait your turn to have blood drawn or an X-ray taken.

■ When all the tests have been completed, and after a brief waiting period when you may be offered some food, you will receive a copy of the test results, along with any recommendations of further medical tests or changes in life-style. Since you receive a copy of the test results, you can do your own research at home if you have questions that were not answered at the hospital or clinic. Note that the hospital or clinic is not responsible for offering you treatment. If a problem is spotted, it's up to you to go to a specialist, although the clinic or hospital will usually be quite willing to refer you.

■ You will be given a lovely meal or a coupon good for a meal at a nearby restaurant.

■ If the test results were incomplete, within a week you will receive a completed copy of all the test results, with comments from the doctor and suggestions for further tests or life-style changes, if applicable.

If your insurance plan offers a yearly physical for you (and your spouse), use it. If you want to have some of the tests omitted, it's easy to do so. The bill will be sent to your company, or you may be required to pay it yourself and apply for a full or partial reimbursement later. Ask your personnel department or insurance adjuster for details ahead of time.

Tests performed in the *ningen dokku* but not in the public health exams include more detailed blood tests, hearing tests, tests of physical stamina, gynecological exams, and the compiling of a longer health history.

Private Ningen Dokku

A third option is to make an appointment at a clinic or hospital on your own, and pay privately for the same procedures outlined above. The cost of a private *ningen dokku* can range from ¥30,000 to ¥120,000 or more, depending on the number of tests performed and the time spent at the clinic or hospital.

The following is a representative list of tests done during a one-day physical exam at St. Luke's International Hospital in Tokyo (St. Luke's can also give you the test results in English). Each hospital or clinic may vary the type or number of tests.

Tests and Exams Done in the *Ningen Dokku*

General health assesssment

問診 *monshin*, personal history

身体各部 *shintai kakubu*, a complete physical examination by the doctor

心理問診 *shinri monshin*, psychological examination

社会生活 *shakai seikatsu*, life-style questionnaire

家族の状況 *kazoku no jōkyō*, family health history

一般健康状態 *ippan kenkō jōtai*, general health status review

Internist's general physical examination
naika ippan shinsatsu 内科一般診察

General urinalysis *nyō ippan kensa* 尿一般検査

比重 *hijū*, specific gravity

PH (acidity/alkalinity)

蛋白 *tanpaku*, protein

糖 *tō*, sugar

ウロビリノーゲン *urobirinōgen*, urobilinogen

潜血 *senketsu*, occult blood

白血球 *hakkekkyū*, white blood cells

Blood chemistry *ketsueki kagaku kensa* 血液科学検査

尿素窒素 *nyō-sochisso*, urea nitrogen-BUN

クレアチニン *kureachinin*, creatinine

尿酸 *nyōsan*, uric acid

総ビリルビン *sōbirirubin*, total bilirubin

アルカリ P *arukari P*, alkaline P

LDH (lactic acid dehydrogenase)

GOT (glutamic oxaloacetic transaminase)

GPT (glutamic pyruvic transaminase)

r–GTP (r–glutamyl transpeptidase)

総蛋白 *sōtanpaku*, total protein

A/G比 *A/G hi*, albumin/globulin ratio

コレステロール *koresuterōru*, cholesterol

1Pトリグリセライド *toriguriseraido*, triglycerides

Na (sodium); K (potassium); Cl (chloride); Ca (calcium)

HDLコレステロール *HDL koresuteroru*, HDL cholesterol

前立線 *zenritsusen*, PSA (prostatic specific antigen)

空腹時血糖 *kūfukuji kettō*, fasting blood sugar

Complete blood count *ippan ketsueki kensa* 一般血液検査

赤血球数 *sekkekkyū sū*, red blood cell count

ヘモグロビン *hemogurobin*, hemoglobin

ヘマトクリット *hematokuritto*, hematocrit

平均赤血球容積 *heikin sekkekkyū yōseki*, mean corpuscular volume

平均赤血球色素量 *heikin sekkekkyū shikiso-ryō*, MCH mean corpuscular hemoglobin

血小板数 *kesshōban-sū*, platelet count

白血球数 *hakkekkyū-sū*, white blood cell count (WBC)

白血球像 *hakkekkyū-zō*, leukocyte morphology

Blood type *ketsueki-gata* 血液型

ABO式 *ABO-shiki*, ABO factor

RH式 *RH-shiki*, RH factor

Serology *kessei hannō* 血清反応

VDRL venereal disease research laboratory

TPHA treponema pallidum hemagglutination assay

CEA carcinoembryonic antigen

HBS抗原抗体 *HBS kōgen-kōtai*, hepatitis B antigen and antibody

HCV抗体 *HCV kōtai*, hepatitis C virus antibodies

Respiratory system tests *kokyūki-kei kensa* 呼吸器系検査

　肺活量 *haikatsu ryō*, vital lung capacity

　胸部 X 線検査 *kyōbu X-sen kensa*, chest X-ray

Digestive system tests *shōkaki-kei kensa* 消化器系検査

　胃部 X 線検査 *ibu X-sen kensa*, stomach X-ray

　検便（潜血）*kenben (sen ketsu)*, stool test (occult blood)

　腹部超音波検査（肝胆腎）*fukubu-chō-onpa kensa (kan, tan, jin)*, abdominal ultrasound (liver, gall bladder, kidneys)

Circulatory system tests *junkanki-kei kensa* 循環器系検査

　血圧測定 *ketsuatsu sokutei*, blood pressure

　心電図検査 *shinden-zu kensa*, electrocardiogram

Eye tests *ganka kensa* 眼科検査

　視力測定（裸眼 矯正）*shiryoku sokutei (ragan, kyōsei)*, visual acuity (with vision uncorrected, and with vision corrected)

　眼圧測定 *ganatsu sokutei*, intraocular pressure

　眼低写真撮影 *gantei shashin satsuei*, ocular fundus photography

Hearing tests *chōryoku kensa* 聴力検査

　左右の聴力 *sayū no chōryoku*, both ears

Body measurements *shintai teisoku* 身体計測

　身長測定 *shinchō sokutei*, height

　体重測定 *taijū sokutei*, weight

　肥満度測定 *himando sokutei*, body fat measurement

　体脂肪率 *taishibō-ritsu*, percent of body fat

Women's exams *fujin-ka kensa* 婦人科検査

　婦人科診察 *fujin-ka shinsatsu*, internal pelvic exam

　子宮細胞診 *shikyū saibōshin*, Pap smear

　乳房検査 *chibusa kensa*, manual breast exam

Nutritional counseling *eiyō shidō* 栄養指導

General evaluation of test results *sōgō hantei* 総合判定

(Laboratory testing methods are similar to those used in Western countries. Norms for specific tests may vary somewhat from Western norms, but the differences are slight.)

Mobile Checkups for the Bedridden can be arranged through your public health center.

Checkups for Children (see pages 56 and 158)

Cancer Screenings

Cancer screenings are offered during some of the yearly checkups described just above, as well as at other times and places. Of course, if you detect any symptoms of cancer, you should head straight to a physician.

Colon, Stomach, and Lung Cancer Screenings *daichō, i, hai gan kenshin* 大腸, 胃, 肺がん検診

Remember that each city or ward decides how and when it will offer these screenings to its residents. In Urawa, these are offered at the same time and at the same clinics as yearly checkups. There is a charge for stomach and lung X-rays for anyone under seventy. The occult blood test for colon cancer is free. A stomach X-ray is also offered during certain other months of the year to anyone aged thirty-five or over, for ¥500.

In Tokyo's Arakawa-ku, cancer screenings are done for free by the Arakawa-ku Cancer Prevention Center. Postcards are sent to residents in certain age groups to inform them of their eligibility for the tests, and the scheduled dates.

Cervical, Uterine Cancer Screenings   *shikyū (keibu), shikyū taibu gan kenshin* 子宮（頸部）, 子宮体部 がん検診

A yearly gynecological checkup with a private gynecologist is not the custom for a healthy woman in Japan. Women usually go to a gynecologist only when they know that something is wrong. Here, it is interesting to note how women's disease statistics and health practices have influenced Japan's cancer screening programs.

Because the rate of cervical cancer is low in young women, this test is not offered to women through public health screenings until the age of thirty. This contrasts with the U.S., where the rate of cervical cancer in young women is higher, and where the American Cancer Society advises all women who are (or have been) sexually active or have reached the age of eighteen to have an annual pelvic exam and Pap smear. In Japan, Pap smear testing is usually not started until the woman reaches thirty (through public health screenings) or until her first pregnancy. As the main method of birth control is the condom, which requires no doctor's examination, young Japanese women are especially unaccustomed to internal exams.

The Pap smear for cervical cancer (*shikyū saibō-shin* 子宮細胞診 or *sumea tesuto* スメアテスト) is offered free of charge to women aged thirty or over at public health centers, on days announced in the city or ward's health newsletter. Some areas offer the tests free of charge at private clinics during the clinics' regular office hours. Depending on where you live, you may need to get a coupon from the public health center, and present it when you go to a designated clinic for the examination. In other areas, you may only need to tell the doctor's receptionist that you are there for the city or ward's free cervical cancer test. Since regular visits to the gynecologist are not customary here, when you call a health facility to inquire about such exams you should say that you want a Pap smear done (*shikyū saibō-shin o shite moraitai n desu ga*). Note that the phrase "women's health check" (*josei no herusu chekku*) refers to a more general exam that includes no cancer screening (see page 94).

Don't forget to wear a loose skirt, to use as a drape. The examination includes questions by the doctor or health worker, a visual examination of the outer and inner vaginal area, a manual examination of the internal organs, and a cell examination (Pap smear). You may be told that if you are not contacted within about two weeks, this means that the results were normal. If you are contacted and asked to call the clinic or health center back, do it. They will not check back with you. One woman finally remembered three months later to return the telephone call, when it was almost too late. During the annual *ningen dokku* (pages 88–91), women should request this cervical cancer exam. And of course any girl or woman from puberty onward can go to a gynecologist and pay to have this test done. Some private gynecologists who are familiar with Western medical practices will offer a more familiar complete gynecological checkup, including a breast exam. This visit, however, will not be covered by Japanese public health insurance.

If the physician feels there is a need, you will be referred to a hospital for a further uterine cancer screening. In this test, cells are taken from higher up inside the uterus with a long thin tube. It is uncomfortable, but over quickly. You will be asked to make a return visit to discuss the results of this test.

Breast Cancer Screenings nyūgan kenshin 乳がん検診

Japan has a very low rate of breast cancer (about one in fifty) compared with other industrialized countries (one in nine or ten in the United States). However, the rate has been increasing over the last twenty years, possibly due to a change to a diet higher in fat.

Breast problems are usually treated by a surgeon *geka-i* 外科医 and not by a gynecologist, although some gynecologists have recently begun to perform this examination. Should a gynecologist find a breast abnormality, you would be referred to a surgeon.

Public health policy encourages self breast examination, or SBE *jiko kenshin-hō* 自己検診法, by women aged thirty or over as the best and fastest way to notice any sort of change in their own breasts. Examine the breasts every month at the end of the menstrual period or, if you have already passed menopause, every month on an easily remembered day. A diagrammed explanation of the SBE is available from the Akebono Kai (see page 94) and at public health centers. Free manual breast examinations are also scheduled at public health centers when a surgeon will be on hand to visually and manually examine the breasts, or your city may provide the names of gynecologists or surgeons who will do this examination in their offices.

Mammography screening (*manmogurafī* マンモグラフィー) is available for a fee at large hospitals all over Japan, but has not yet been included in the public health centers' free screening tests. If, after the manual exam, the doctor feels that further tests are necessary, you will be referred for a mammogram. If further diagnostic tests are called for, ultrasound imaging (*ekō* エコー) is used in combination with mammography to get accurate images of the breast. CAT (computerized axial tomography; *CT sukan* CTスキャン), thermography (*samogurafī* サモグラフィー), and biopsy are also used in diagnosis.

Since breast cancer rates differ widely, consider your family history, nationality, and ethnic background in deciding how often to be screened. If you find a lump (*shikori* しこり), see a surgeon immediately for further diagnostic examinations.

Akebono Kai
03-3792-1204 (Eng.)
(Contact: Takako Watt)
A network of support groups all over Japan for women who have had mastectomies. Promotes self breast examinations. List (in Japanese) of surgeons and hospitals that do mammograms and support Akebono Kai.

Prostate Cancer Screening   zenritsusen gan kenshin   前立線がん検診

This blood test (PSA) for early discovery of prostate cancer is not provided through any of the public health checkups, probably because of the comparatively low rates of the disease among Japanese men. Make sure that it is on the list of exams done at your yearly *ningen dokku* exam, or see a urologist.

Other Checkups

Women's Health Check   josei no herusu chekku   女性のヘルスチェック

This preventive health check, offered to women aged eighteen through thirty-nine through the public health department, includes blood tests for cholesterol, etc., a urine test, measurement of height and weight, lung and heart auscultation, and counseling on diet, exercise, and life-style. Its purpose is to steer young women toward a lifetime of wise nutritional and life-style choices. It is free, but note that no cancer screenings are offered.

Vision Checkups   ganka kensa   眼科検査

Although vision acuity checks are done during the more thorough *ningen dokku* exams, they are not provided through the public health screenings. And vision testing done at schools ordinarily only checks for distance reading. If you notice that your vision or your child's has changed in any way (even if you have had an eye exam recently), your first visit should be to an ophthalmologist *ganka-i* 眼科医 who will examine your eyes for signs of disease as well as for any changes in vision. If you choose to go to a larger hospital for the exam, you may need to make an appointment. The medical examinations will check for retinal detachment, high blood pressure, diabetes, cataracts, and glaucoma. Drops to dilate the pupils are usually used. Preventive tests are not covered by Japanese public health insurance, but tests done when there is a problem are covered.

The Landort Ring, which looks like a very fat, round C, is often used in vision test charts. Even if you can't read Japanese, you will be able to see this mark and point in the direction of the opening, to indicate whether it's up or down, right or left. If you can see the opening in this 7.5 mm round figure from five meters away in 500 luxes of light, then your sight is said to be 1.0, or normal. If you can only read the top line of the chart, then your vision is 0.1, very nearsighted *kingan* 近眼. Each descending line signifies a 0.1 increase in vision rating until, if you can read the tenth line, your vision is 1.0 or normal. In the annual vision checks at public schools, a result below 1.0 requires further testing to determine the degree of nearsightedness. (Normal vision for children: three years, 0.5 and up; 5 years, 0.7 and up; 6 years, 1.0; over six years, 1.0 and up.)

Many Japanese seem to try to put off for as long as possible the day when they or their child must start wearing glasses. Some feel that poor vision is like a disease that should be kept hidden. Others think that wearing glasses will further weaken the eyes. Fear that their child will be teased for being different is yet another reason given. This cultural bias against glasses is deep enough that at the end of the eye exam, you may find that the doctor asks you, "Have you decided to get glasses?" instead of declaring firmly that you or your child needs glasses.

Vision Measurement Comparison Chart

Japan 5 m.	U. S. 20 ft.	U.K. 6 m.	
0.1 (5/50)	20/200	6/60	
0.2 (5/25)	20/100	6/30	
0.5 (5/10)	20/40	6/12	
1.0 (5/5)	**20/20**	**6/6**	*Normal vision*
2.0 (5/2.5)	20/10	6/3	

If you know your own vision acuity on the 20-foot or 6-meter scale, you can convert it into the approximate Japanese equivalent by changing it to a decimal reading:

20/30 (20 ÷ 30) = 0.66
6/15 (6 ÷ 15) = 0.4

Hospitals Noted for their Ophthalmology Departments

Note that all the following accept Japanese public insurance and have English speakers on staff. See also "Regional Resources" for a list of large hospitals and pages 33–34 for a list of small clinics.

Tokai University Hospital
(Shibuya-ku, Tokyo; see page 344)

Tokyo Dental University Ichikawa General Hospital
(Ichikawa-shi, Chiba-ken; see page 343)

Inoue Eye Hospital
Inoue Ganka Byoin 井上眼科病院
4-3 Kanda-Surugadai, Chiyoda-ku, Tokyo
03-3295-0911

Juntendo University Hospital
(Bunkyo-ku, Tokyo; see page 343)

Tokyo Women's Medical University Hospital, Diabetes (Tonyobyo) Center
(Shinjuku-ku, Tokyo; see page 344)

Kyoto Furitsu Medical University Hospital
(Kyoto-shi; see page 348)

Kyushu University Hospital
(Fukuoka-shi; see page 351)

Buying Glasses or Contact Lenses

After the vision examination, if you need them, an ophthalmologist will write you a prescription for glasses or contact lenses to be filled by an optometrist at an eyeglass store (*megane-ya* 眼鏡屋). An optometrist can also test your eyes with lenses for near- or farsightedness, check if you need reading glasses, and make the glasses for you. He can

Health Checkups

95

also duplicate lenses, even if you don't have the prescription. Glasses are not covered by public insurance plans unless you are severely vision-impaired and have a handbook for the physically disabled *shintai shōgai-sha techō* 身体障害者手帳.

All types of glasses and hard and soft contact lenses are available. Expect to pay about ¥30,000 and up for contact lenses, and about the same for glasses.

Wasin Optical Head Store
6-4-4 Ginza, Chuo-ku, Tokyo
03-3572-3693
English-speaking staff at branches in Ginza and

Shibuya (ask for U.S. optician); other stores in Shinjuku, Ikebukuro, Urawa, Yokosuka (Seiyu Department Store, 2 Fl.), Osaka, etc.

Hearing Testing *chōryoku kensa* 聴力検査

Hearing testing is not done in the public health examinations but it is done during the *ningen dokku* exams and at Japanese public schools and some international schools. If you notice that you or your child is having hearing problems, the first step is to head to an ENT specialist *jibika-i* 耳鼻科医 to be examined and diagnosed. For your hearing test, select a larger hospital, if possible, which will be more likely to have a quiet room. Hearing tests involve donning headphones and being asked to signal as soon as you hear a sound coming from them (the ears are tested one at a time). See pages 164–65 for pediatric specialty hospitals where young children can be tested (with toys that light up, trains that run, etc.).

The problem may just be the buildup of earwax (*mimi aka* 耳垢), which can easily be cleaned out. Or you may find that you need a hearing aid (*hochō-ki* 補聴器). If necessary, the doctor will refer you to a hearing aid shop which can make sure that the appliance you will use fits correctly. Hearing aids are not covered by national or employees' health insurance plans unless you are profoundly deaf and have a handbook for the physically disabled *shintai shōgai-sha techō* 身体障害者手帳.

For Hearing Problems

Azabu Otolaryngology Clinic
Azabu Jibi Inko-ka Kurinikku
Azabu Yano Bldg. 2 Fl., 4-13-5 Minami-Azabu
Minato-ku, Tokyo
03-3448-0248 (Pub. Ins., Eng.)

Osaka Hankyu Dept Store 3 Fl.
8-7 Kakuda-cho, Kita-ku, Osaka-shi
06-361-1381
Hearing-aid room; hearing tests done (no appointment necessary).

Teikyo University Hospital, Tokyo (noted for children's ENT; see page 344)

Tokai University Hospital, Tokyo (see page 344)

Boei Medical University Hospital
(Tokorozawa-shi, Saitama-ken; see page 342)

For a list of large hospitals, see "Regional Resources."

Brain Dry Dock *nō dokku* 脳ドック

Along with cancer and heart disease, cerebral vascular accident (also called CVA, stroke, or cerebral apoplexy) *nō socchū* 脳卒中 is one of the three main causes of death among adult Japanese. In response to these statistics, brain checkups are now offered on a private basis. The purpose is to spot weaknesses or malformations in the brain's blood vessels so that treatment can be started to prevent the CVA. Magnetic Resonance Imaging (MRI) is used to get clear images of all densities of brain tissue without using radiation. Discuss your family health history and health risks with your doctor before deciding that you need this screening.

This screening is safe and painless but can be very expensive—from 30,000–200,000 yen and up—since it is considered a preventive health screening. You can sometimes include this test in your yearly physical exam (*ningen dokku*), if the clinic or hospital has the equipment.

The procedure will take about two hours, including blood tests, health questionnaire, physical exam, and the MRI. An appointment is necessary.

If you are having neurological symptoms such as headaches, dizziness, vision problems, etc. and go to a doctor to try to find out why, the MRI may be done as a diagnostic test; in that case it would be covered under Japanese public health insurance.

Bone Check/Bone Mineral Density Test   *hone dokku* 骨ドック

In response to statistics showing that osteoporosis—a loss of calcium from the bones— is crippling many elderly people (especially women) in Japan, the public health department is now encouraging women aged eighteen and over to have a baseline bone-mineral density test *kotsu soshō-shō kenshin* 骨粗鬆症検診. An image of the bones (in the foot and ankle) is taken by ultrasonography so that the amount of bone calcium can be calculated. On the basis of the test results, you and your doctor can decide if you need to change your present life-style and diet to increase your bone strength.

These inexpensive (¥200 or so) tests are done by public health centers in roving mobile vans or at designated sites for women aged eighteen and over. The schedule for your area will be announced in the city health bulletin. You may need to make a reservation by sending in a return postcard (*ōfuku hagaki*). Two weeks or so after the test is done, another meeting will be scheduled to discuss the results. Similar information can also be acquired through an X-ray of the bones of the back. These procedures are also done at many special menopause clinics *chūkōnen* 中高年 or *kōnenki kurinikku* 更年期クリニック in university and other large hospitals, at your own expense.

Alternatively, you can make an appointment at a private clinic advertising bone tests *hone dokku* 骨ドック or see a gynecologist in a clinic catering to foreigners. See page 194 for osteoporosis.

Health Certificate   *shindan-sho* 診断書

During your stay in Japan, you may well have to present a health certificate for one reason or another. If the company or institution requiring the medical exam does not provide a form, your doctor will fill out an all-purpose one for you. Neither the exam nor the certificate are covered by public health insurance, and completing it in English will cost extra. Japanese schools do not require a health certificate because yearly mini-physical exams are done in the schools. However, one may be needed in certain situations, such as starting at an international school or going to Boy Scout camp, or returning to work from a sick leave or to school after recovering from a communicable disease.

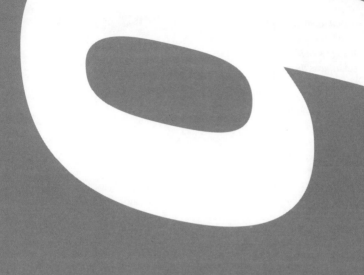

"During my first days in Japan I opened the door to a saleswoman selling some kind of skin cream. Or so I thought, since 'sukin' was the only word I understood from her entire sales pitch. She finally opened her case and proceeded to blow up various condoms, to show me how strong and light her product was. It was only later that I learned that 'sukin' refers to a condom and that it is usually the wife who buys them, hence the daytime door-to-door sales."

Birth Control/Family Planning *kazoku keikaku* 家族計画

According to a 1996 survey by the *Mainichi Shinbun,* up to ninety-six percent of Japanese couples used the condom "at times" as their family planning method. The rhythm method, basal body temperature method, and other similar methods were also used by ten to fifteen percent of respondents, and just a very small percentage used any other means.

Condoms *kondōmu* コンドーム, *sukin* スキン

Japan leads industrialized countries in the use of condoms, which are readily available at drugstores, supermarkets, and automatic vending machines, and from door-to-door sales-women, public health nurses, and family planning clinics. The price may seem expensive (¥1,000–¥3,500 for a pack of twelve), but according to the Japanese Organization for International Cooperation in Family Planning, Japanese condoms are "of good quality and very thin, at .02–.03 mm," resulting in, in the words of one manufacturer, a "super, natural fit." They come in a variety of colors and are lubricated. They are all the same "free" size; for larger sizes (Trojan brand) try the American Pharmacy (see page 255) or the Foreign Buyers' Club (see the endpapers).

Latex condoms say *ratekusu* ラテクス on the package. Water-based lubricants for use with a condom are Ryubu Jelly リューブゼリー or Pearl Lulu パールルル Jelly.

Spermicidal Products

Spermicidal jelly (F.P. Jelly) is only available with a prescription. Mairura マイルーラ, by Taiho Pharmaceuticals, is a thin spermicidal film (like a piece of dissoluble clear wrap) which is placed deeply in the vagina before sexual intercourse and used together with a condom. It is available at your local drugstore.

IUDs (Intrauterine Devices) *hinin ringu* 避妊リング

In 1974, four kinds of IUDs, all inactive types, were approved for distribution in Japan. They are not popular, and only certain gynecologists *fujinka-i* 婦人科医 will insert them. Check by telephone before visiting a doctor.

Diaphragms *pessarī* ペッサリー

Diaphragms can be fitted by some privately practicing midwives *josanpu* 助産婦 who are specially trained in fitting and then teaching the correct way to use a diaphragm. Inquire at your public health center for the names of midwives in your area who fit diaphragms and prescribe contraceptive jelly (this is a prescription product in Japan).

Basal Body Temperature (BBT) Method *kiso taionhō* 基礎体温法

A special thermometer *fujin taionkei* 婦人体温計 for taking daily morning temperatures to determine the time of ovulation and the period of optimal fertility is available in most drugstores.

Ogino (Rhythm) Method   *Ogino shiki*   オギノ式

The Ogino method charts the days of the menstrual cycle to pinpoint fertile days, and is usually used in combination with the BBT method.

Sterilization   *funin shujutsu*   不妊手術

Tubal ligation *rankan kessatsu* 卵管結紮 and vasectomies *paipukatto* パイプカット are not commonly done here, as they are considered drastic forms of birth control. Unless you already have several children or are no longer young, it will be difficult to persuade a surgeon to do these procedures. These forms of surgery are not covered by public insurance plans.

Oral Contraceptives   *piru* ピル, *piru horumon* ピルホルモン

The Pill (which contains a combination of two hormones that work together to suppress ovulation) has not yet been authorized by the Ministry of Health and Welfare for use as a contraceptive, although similar hormones are available for treatment of menstrual irregularity. In spring 1993, the Ministry of Health and Welfare was poised to approve low-dosage contraceptive pills for general use, but scrapped the plan at the last minute, citing fears that use of the Pill would make people stop using condoms and result in increased incidence of AIDS. Women in Japan, who are greatly concerned about possible negative side effects of the Pill, seem to have accepted the decision. Recent news reports have hinted that approval is right around the corner, but as of summer 1998 Japanese women still do not have the option of easily procuring the Pill for use as their birth control method.

Alternatives

The morning-after pill, hormone implants, cervical caps, spermicidal sponges, and female condoms are all unavailable here. Unless you plan to use condoms or one of the natural family planning methods, bring a supply of contraceptives with you from overseas.

Home Pregnancy Tests   *ninshin kensa*   妊娠検査

The directions for all brands of home pregnancy tests state that they can be used from about a week after the missed menstrual period. However, because cycles are not always perfectly regular, a week may not always be long enough. If your test result is negative but you still think that you may be pregnant, repeat the test a week later. Urine from any time of day can be used but the urine first passed after you wake up has the most concentrated hormone levels, and so is the most reliable. Use an early-morning, concentrated urine sample if you test during the first few days following the missed period. Have a watch or a clock with a second hand ready. Open the test pad or stick just before you do the test. Do not expose the urine or tester to heat or direct sunlight.

How to Use Well-Known Japanese Brands

Check One (by Arax)

1. Remove the cap from the tester. 2. Urinate on the entire test pad for *at least* 5 seconds. 3. Cover the tip again, while keeping the tester pointed downward. Then lay the tester down in a horizontal position so that you can see the results (*hantei* 判定) window. The two windows will turn reddish purple as an intermediate stage. 4. Wait three full minutes. A small reddish-purple dot will remain in the completion (*shūryō* 終了) window. If a reddish purple dot also remains in the results window, the test is positive.

Dotest (by Rotto)

1. Remove cap from test stick and urinate on test end for 2 seconds or more. 2.Replace cap and lay test stick on a flat surface. Wait 3 to 5 minutes until the test completion *kensa shūgyō* 検査終了 window turns red. 3. The test result is positive if a reddish line appears in the results (*hantei* 判定) window.

Predictor (by Lion)

1. Remove cap from the tester. 2. Dip tip of tester in cup of urine for at least 5 seconds *or* urinate on tester for 5 seconds or more. 3. Remove from urine, replace cap and wait for 3 minutes. 3. If the test result is positive, a red dot will appear in both windows.

Help With an Unexpected Pregnancy

Resources

TELL (see the endpapers)
Offers crisis counseling.

Ai no Kesshin (Loving Decisions)
愛の決心
1-14-2 Azuma, Narita-shi, Chiba-ken
0476-28-4436
10-15 Hinode-cho, Shizuoka-shi (Shizuoka office)
054-250-0217, fax 054-250-0217
(toll-free help lines) 0120-41-8277 (J. only)
0120-42-8277 (Eng., Tag.)
Private, non-profit Christian organization with English newsletter. Free twenty-four–hour crisis counseling service (with no hassle for women who decide on abortion). Also longer-term counseling, information on adoption processing, birth-mother counseling and follow-up care, foster care for children in need, and placement of babies in Christian homes. However, few babies are available for adoption.

International Social Services
3-6-18-601 Kami-Meguro, Meguro-ku, Tokyo
03-3760-3471, fax 03-3760-3474
Private, licensed organization handling international adoptions. Counseling for birth mothers in Japanese, English, Spanish and Tagalog. Preference is given to adopting couples with at least one partner who is of Asian descent.

Association for Advancement of Family Care
Katei Yogo Sokushin Kyokai
Osaka Shiritsu Shakai Fukushi Senta Rm. 210
12-10 Higashi-Kotsucho, Tennoji-ku, Osaka-shi
06-762-5239 (J. only)
One child introduced each week in *Mainichi Shinbun.* Priority given to couples with at least one partner who is Japanese. Foreign couples planning to reside in Japan long enough to complete all the adoption procedures are also considered (the final adoption decree is usually not given until at least a year after the child is received into the home).

Wa no Kai (Motherly Network)
環の会
4-14-13 Shimo-Ochiai, Shinjuku-ku, Tokyo
03-3951-7270 (24-hour crisis counseling; J. only)
fax 03-3951-9495
Crisis and longer-term counseling on unexpected pregnancy, and infertility, childbirth problems (expenses, etc.). Sometimes has babies available for adoption. Publishes newsletter (in Japanese).

City or Ward Offices
City or ward offices may arrange for adoptions of babies from Japanese orphanages. However, willingness to place children varies from one ward office to another.

Adoption *yōshi* 養子

The most prevalent form of adoption in Japan today is the adoption of a son-in-law by his in-laws. Upon marriage, he takes his wife's surname and becomes the successor to the wife's father as head of the household (and so carries on the family name and often the family business). Men who marry in this way almost always have at least one brother to carry on the name of their own natural parents.

Another type of adoption, which is actually quite uncommon in Japan, is the adoption of a baby or child by someone wishing to become a parent. Even though revision of the adoption law in 1988 now allows adopted children to be treated just like any other children on the family register, the practice is still not widely accepted. The cultural emphasis placed on family blood ties makes it difficult for people to believe that the bond between adoptive parent and child can be as strong as that of a natural parent and child. The wide availability of abortion also keeps the number of unwanted babies low. Children placed in orphanages are rarely put up for adoption.

International adoption by a single adult is rare, but it has been done.

If you are hoping to adopt, or are considering giving up a child for adoption, contact the organizations on this or the previous page.

Becoming a Foster Parent *sato oya* 里親
If you are considering becoming a foster parent, inquire at the child guidance consultation office *jidō sōdan-sho* 児童相談所 at your local city or ward office.

Elective Abortion *jinkō ninshin chūzetsu* 人工妊娠中絶
About 350,000 abortions are performed every year in Japan, which is why this procedure is sometimes referred to as the third most popular method of family planning in the country. Although repeated abortions can damage the lining of the uterus, the surgery itself is safe and accepted. The Eugenic Protection Law, enacted in 1948, aimed at protecting the life and health of mothers and at preventing the birth of children with birth defects. In 1996 this law was amended slightly to remove the eugenics clause. Now known as the Maternal Protection Law; it specifically recognizes concerns about the mother's health or economic situation as legitimate reasons for seeking an abortion. Abortions may be performed up until 21 weeks and 6 days of gestation. Spousal consent

is still required, although a wife can easily put her husband's personal seal on the required document.

For teenagers, the question of parental consent is a concern. Although parental consent is not required by law, large government-supported hospitals tend to require it. Smaller clinics generally do not. So teens are likely to head to the smaller clinics.

Ninety percent of abortions are performed within the first three months. The procedure consists of dilating the cervix and then scraping or suctioning out the uterus. Check that the doctor will be giving you a general anesthesia, as this is not always done. In order to have an abortion, you need to set aside at least two days. On the first day, you will be examined by the gynecologist in order to confirm the pregnancy. Then you will be sent home with instructions to think about your decision. No additional counseling is required or provided. The abortion is performed on the second day. You may be required to stay overnight after the procedure if the pregnancy is your first, or depending on how far along the pregnancy has advanced.

In later abortions, medication that induces contractions of the uterus is given through an intravenous drip. No anesthesia is used, and the procedure requires about a week's hospitalization.

Elective abortions are not covered by public health insurance plans, and costs vary from ¥80,000 to ¥180,000 or more depending on the procedure, the number of days of hospitalization, and the clinic or hospital used. A gynecologist who performs abortions must be a "eugenic protection–designated doctor" *yūsei hogo shitei-i* 優生保護指定医 (this simply means a gynecologist who is permitted by the prefecture to do abortions); this designation will appear on the clinic's signboard.

Miscarriage (see page 138)

Infertility *funin* 不妊

"Even though the doctors there are very good, university hospitals are impersonal and involve long waits. The younger doctors seem to explain more than older ones do. But the hormone treatments seem to be less aggressive than in the West, and there is little psychological support."

"If you can, form your own support group with other women who are undergoing fertility treatments. That's the only way to stay sane!"

Infertility—generally defined as the inability to conceive after two years of unprotected sexual intercourse—is the same heartbreaking problem in Japan as in any other part of the world. In about fifty percent of cases, the cause is unknown, although age is known to contribute. Treatment in Japan involves a combination of the highest modern technology—like that used in other developed countries—with a refreshingly holistic approach. Whether or not the cause is known, treatment can be long and frustrating.

Medical Treatment

Typical fertility treatment involves the following steps. If one step does not result in pregnancy, then you and the doctor come to a decision about proceeding to the next.

■ Physical exam and diagnostic testing of each partner to try to discover the cause
■ Careful monitoring of ovulation and sexual intercourse
■ Medication (hormones) to encourage ovulation
■ *In vitro* fertilization & embryo transfer (IVF & ET) *taigai jusei hai-ishoku* 体外授精胚移植

Other possible treatments include: hormones and vitamins for either partner; corrective surgery for either partner; artificial insemination with the husband's (AIH) *haigūsha kan jinkō jusei* 配偶者間人工授精, which can be done at many clinics (but infertility specialists who can treat sperm beforehand, resulting in a higher success rate, are recommended); artificial insemination by a donor (AID) *hi-haigūsha-kan jinkō jusei* 非配偶者間人工授精 (performed only for married couples, this is said to be done at many university and other large hospitals around the country, but Keio University Hospital (page 343) is the only one which has publicly announced its program); microfertilization *kenbijusei* 顕微授精; freezing of embryos *juseiran no reitō hozon* 受精卵の冷凍保存; gamete intrafallopian transfer (GIFT) *gifuto-hō* ギフト法; or a combination of these techniques.

Surrogate motherhood *dairi haha* 代理母, host motherhood *kari-bara* 借り腹, and the use of donor eggs *tamago no teikyō* 卵の提供 or donor-fertilized eggs *tamago to seishi no teikyō* 卵と精子の提供, are all procedures which have not been accepted by the medical community in Japan. Some couples go to the United States or South Korea for these procedures.

Holistic Approach

Some gynecologists and fertility specialists take a holistic approach to the problem of infertility by combining high-tech treatment with the principles of oriental medicine. Oriental medicine treats the whole body and not just the reproductive organs; this may be of help to couples who have no known structural impediments to conception. For women, the holistic approach starts with an examination of the teeth, diet, and stomach, as it is believed that if the uterus does not receive proper nourishment, it will not be able to function properly. An examination of the whole body follows, after which five or six (of about thirty-five) types of *kanpō* medicine will be prescribed. (Men, too, are prescribed *kanpō* medicines, which are said to be good for increasing sperm production.)

A special diet prepared according to the tenets of oriental medicine is often also prescribed. Black beans, black sesame seeds, and *hijiki* (fine black seaweed) are good, but eggplant and *gobo* (burdock root), which cool the stomach, are not considered good for the uterus. Foods high in water content, such as pineapple and grapes, should also be avoided. Fertility stretching exercises *funin kikō* 不妊気功, which is a combination of breathing and stretching exercises, may also be prescribed. For further information, see "Alternative Healing."

Japanese Tips for Fertility

■ Be aware that the electric *kotatsu* (a low table with an attached heating unit), as well as hot baths may alter the blood circulation in the lower body and kill or slow sperm.

■ Take vitamin C for healthier eggs, and vitamins E and B-12 for healthy sperm production.

■ Exercise regularly to increase blood circulation to the pelvis.

■ Avoid tight underwear and trousers, which cut off circulation to the lower half of the body (applies to both men and women).

■ Practice good posture for total body health and for keeping the pelvic organs in the correct and normal positions.

■ Take frequent exercise breaks to increase circulation to the lower half of body during long car trips.

Ovulation Prediction Tests　*hairanbi kensa-yaku* 排卵日検査薬

These are sold in boxes of five or seven. These tests monitor the surge in hormones which precedes ovulation. A woman will be most fertile during the two to three days after the surge takes place.

Check One LH (by Arax)

1. Urinate thoroughly on the absorbent tip for 5 seconds. 2. Re-cap the tip while holding it pointing downward. Then place it on a flat surface so that you can see the windows. 3. The two windows will show a blue line in a transient process. Wait eight full minutes before reading the results. 4. If both windows still show blue lines, this is a positive result, and you can expect ovulation within twenty four to thirty-six hours.

Dotest LH (by Rotto)

1. Urinate on and thoroughly wet the test pad. 2. Replace cap and wait 15 minutes or more to read the results. 3. A clear line in the positive *yō* 陽 window indicates that ovulation will occur within thirty-six hours.

Where to Go for Help

It is usual in Japan for the wife to start at a gynecology clinic (*fujin-ka* 婦人科) and for the husband to be referred to a urology clinic (*hinyōki-ka* 泌尿器科), for their first examinations. Some gynecologists, however, will also perform the initial sperm tests. The next step is to be referred to an infertility specialist.

Infertility specialties (*funin gairai* 不妊外来) are still comparatively rare but can be found at university hospitals. Call beforehand to check the days on which clinics are held.

Infertility Clinics

Odawara Women's Clinic
小田原ウイメンズ クリニック
4-4-7 Ebisu, Shibuya-ku, Tokyo
03-3473-1031
OBS/GYN/Menopause/Assisted Conception
Refers patients for delivery.

Hara Infertility Clinic
原インファティリティー クリニック
1-7-8 Sendagaya, Shibuya-ku, Tokyo
03-3470-4211

Sanno Clinic
山王クリニック
8-5-35 Akasaka, Minato-ku, Tokyo
03-3402-3151
(Dr. Inoue)

Narita Hospital
1-20-30 Oosu, Naka-ku, Nagoya
052-221-1595/052-221-6039

International Medical Crossing Office
(see page 133)

Kanda 2nd Clinic (see page 134)

Toho Women's Clinic (see page 130)

Tojo Women's Clinic (see page 130)

Higashi-Fuchu Hospital (see page 130)
(Specialist comes from St. Luke's International Hospital)

Jikei Medical University Hospital
(see page 343) (Dr. Ochiai)

Toranomon Hospital (see page 344)

Keio University Hospital (see page 343)

Shisei-kai Second Hospital (see page 343)
(Many women doctors, some speak English.)

Toho University Omori Hospital (see page 344)

Mie University Hospital (see page 347)

Kobe University Hospital (see page 348)

Support Groups

You may be able to find an ongoing infertility support group by checking with TELL (see the endpapers). Or start your own group. Ask your specialist if you can post a notice in a prominent spot in the waiting room.

Resolve
1310 Broadway, Somerville, MA 02144-1731
USA
1-617-623-0744

http://www.resolve.org
A referral, support, and advocacy group also providing booklets, newsletters, and telephone support for problems of infertility.

Impotence *inpotensu* インポテンス

Male problems of the reproductive and urethral tract (including impotence) are treated at urology clinics *hinyōki-ka* 泌尿器科. Don't be surprised if the stressful life-style in Japan causes problems where none were present before. Of course the new impotence drug Viagra has not been approved by the government. However, once the cause is identified, treatment is available in Japan. Behavioral pattern changes *kōdō ryōhō* 行動療法, self-training (self-control) methods *jiritsu kunren hō* 自律訓練法, medication, and/or silicon penile implants *puresutēshisu* プレステーシス are used in Japan.

The urology departments of the following hospitals have impotence specialists. If these are outside your area, try calling a university hospital.

Menopause   *kōnenki*   更年期

"I was disgusted when I went to a well-known hospital in Tokyo for treatment of several very uncomfortable menopausal symptoms. All the doctor did was to give me a prescription for tranquilizers, without even telling me what they were. I then tried a hospital that I had seen written up in an English newspaper. Since they treat the heart as well as menopause (I have a family history of heart disease), I find that it's a good hospital for me."

In Japan, menopause is considered to be a natural period in a Japanese woman's life—one of the several seasons that her life encompasses—rather than a condition requiring treatment. Japanese women tend to ignore, or to take in their stride, physical and/or mental changes during this time, such as hot flashes, sweating, dryness of the vagina, heart palpitations, and chills in the hands and feet. Only ten to fifteen percent of menopausal women report the symptoms to be unmanageable, compared to twenty-five percent of American women. So if you should seek treatment for menopause in Japan, don't be surprised if a pep talk is the only treatment you are offered.

Self-help treatment is stressed. Believing that menopause is a normal stage of life that will soon pass is the first step in self-treatment. The menopausal woman is encouraged to take part in new activities and to get proper exercise. A balanced diet high in calcium and moderate exercise daily are usually offered as the treatment for both physical and mental symptoms.

Medical intervention can come in two forms. Oriental medications (see page 277) are very popular and widely used. Visit a *kanpō* practitioner, or a Western-style doctor with knowledge of *kanpō* to get appropriate medication. Many nonprescription *kanpō* medications for menopause are also available at the drugstore. Hormone Replacement Therapy (HRT) is used conservatively, and may be prescribed for short periods if symptoms are extremely severe. But HRT is gaining in popularity, and Japanese women are becoming more outspoken in their requests for treatment. The choice of medications seems more limited than in other countries. Medications including Premarin, Estraderm TTS Patch (the only estrogen patch available), Primodian Depot, and some others are available by renewable, one-month prescription. Long-term use is usually avoided, due to the possibility of side effects. Some Japanese gynecologists prescribe Estriel (estriol), a form of estrogen not used in many other countries. Its gentler action and fewer side effects seem more suitable for long-term use.

Resources

Toho Women's Clinic (see page 130)

International Medical Crossing Office (see page 133)

Kanda 2nd Clinic (see page 134)

Odawara Women's Clinic (see page 108)

Tokyo Medical and Surgical Clinic (see page 33) (Dr. Bliah)

Koyama Takao Clinic
6-14-2 Ginza, Chiyoda-ku, Tokyo
03-3545-4300
(Dr. Takao Koyama)
Pioneer in HRT in Japan.

Women's Adult Disease Clinic
Josei Seijinbyo Clinic
女性成人病クリニック
6-11-14 Ginza, Chiyoda-ku, Tokyo
03-3573-1008 (Eng.; call ahead)
Gynecologist Masako Horiguchi and internist Dr. Fuyoko Murasaki.

Kita-kanto Cardiovascular Hospital (see page 34)

Keio University Hospital, Menopause (Konenki) Clinic (see page 343)
Menopause clinics in many large hospitals, particularly university hospitals.

Sexually Transmitted Diseases (STDs) *seibyō* 性病

Until very recently, sexually transmitted diseases—and the HIV virus in particular—were believed to be problems that afflicted only foreigners and prostitutes, and not the Japanese themselves. The fact that in some cases Japanese men were bringing the diseases back from trips abroad did not seem to enter into the discussion.

The incidence of most STDs in Japan has been decreasing for some time. The number of HIV and AIDS patients, on the other hand, is very small in comparison with other first-world countries, but is rising. A dramatic increase has been seen, however, in two STDs in both men and women: genital herpes (for which there is no cure) and chlamydia-caused urethritis.

The seeming rise in the incidence of chlamydia infection (nongonococcal urethritis) is especially notable among teenagers, who are becoming sexually active increasingly early. Inadequate sex education in junior and senior high schools, a public health policy that does not encourage pelvic exams for women until they reach the age of thirty (see page 92), and the fact that a sufferer may have no symptoms all suggest that this trend will continue.

Treatment and Prevention

If you have reason to suspect that you may have an STD—whether or not you have any symptoms—go to an STD specialty clinic (*seibyō-ka* 性病科) to be examined and treated. For men, an alternative to the STD clinic is a urology clinic (*hinyōki-ka* 泌尿器科) or a dermatology/urology clinic (*hifu/hinyōki-ka* 皮膚泌尿器科), while a gynecology clinic (*fujin-ka* 婦人科) is an alternative for women. If possible, take or send your sex partner, too. If you are diagnosed with an STD, it is important to continue treatments until the doctor says that you are cured. This may mean going back for another examination to make sure that all traces of the disease are gone when you have finished your medication.

By law, the doctor must report each new case of an STD to the Public Health Department, which keeps track of communicable diseases. No names are used. The doctor will not report to the parents of an infected teenager. However, one public health nurse has pointed out that it may be difficult to keep this information private from the family if a teen has to borrow the family health insurance card for the doctor's visit.

Those described below are just a few of the more than 20 known STDs. It is very possible to have more than one sexually transmitted disease at the same time.

Chancroid, Soft Chancre *nanseigekan* 軟性下かん
Prevalence in Japan: Common in Southeast Asia and Africa. Rare in Japan, only 6 reported cases in 1996. Prostitution plays a role and occasional outbreaks around ports or military bases are reported.
Treatment and Notes: Antibiotics orally or by intramuscular injection. After therapy starts, healing takes about 9 days. Usually responds well to treatment.

Genital Herpes *inbu herupesu* 陰部ヘルペス
Prevalence in Japan: Over 1,000 new cases reported in 1992, versus 500,000 cases anually in the U.S.
Treatment and Notes: There is no known cure. Treatment is palliative and involves pain relievers, antibiotics, the use of medications to accelerate healing of the ulcers (Zovirax [acyclovir]), and frequent warm baths. The timing and severity of flareups varies.

Genital Warts *sei ibo* 性いぼ, *senkei konjirōma* 尖圭コンジローマ
Prevalence in Japan: Over 1,000 new cases reported annually, about the same rate as genital herpes.
Treatment and Notes: Removed by electrical cauterization or liquid nitrogen, *not* an over-the-counter wart removal medication.

Gonorrhea (Gonococcal urethritis) *rin byō* 淋病
Prevalence in Japan: 2,201 new cases were reported in Japan in 1996. Disease peaked in 1984 and has been on decrease since then. Penicillin-resistant gonorrhea is a problem worldwide, especially in Southeast Asia where about 40–50% of cases are penicillin-resistant. Antibiotics other than penicillin can be used.
Treatment and Notes: 1. Have smear taken. 2. Wait 3–7 days for results. 3. If positive, take antibiotic for several days. Antibiotic may be by injection and/or by pills in a single dose or over several days. May be asked not to bathe during first 1 or 2 days of treatment, or not to drink alcohol while taking antibiotic. 4. After completion of treatment have another smear examined to see if cured. (Frequently no symptoms at all. If left untreated, can cause sterility.)

Nonspecific Urethritis (NSU), Urine Infection *hitokui-sei nyōdōen* 非特異性尿道炎

Nongonococcal Urethritis *hirinkin-sei nyōdōen* 非淋菌性尿道炎

Prevalence in Japan: Recently overtook gonorrhea as the most common STD in Japan.
Treatment and Notes: Up to 14 days of antibiotics (for example, Erythromycin) as treatment for the underlying *chlamydia* infection, usually followed by a second examination to make sure the infection has been completely cured.

Pubic Lice, Crabs *kejirami* 毛虱

Prevalence in Japan: No statistics kept.
Treatment and Notes: Quickest treatment: shave! Or use Sumisurin Powder (see page 260). Can be caught from dirty bedding, etc.

Syphilis *baidoku* 梅毒

Prevalence in Japan: Declining. 565 new cases reported in 1996. Highest incidence among the 20–30 age group.
Treatment and Notes: First and second stages: highly contagious, but quickly cured by antibiotic (penicillin) injections or pills. Third stage: *No cure* once brain and blood vessels have been damaged.

AIDS (see pages 206–208)

Viral Hepatitis B and C (see page 199)

Food for Thought: The number two cause of *preventable* infertility today is STDs. In almost all cases STDs are life-style diseases. Healthy life-style choices and honesty between partners can keep you healthy. In Japan, too, sex is great but disease is not!

Resources

Call AMDA (see the endpapers) or an information service in your area (see "Regional Resources") for the medical institution nearest you that offers STD screenings. Or call your local public health department (in Japanese).

See also prenatal testing (page 135).

Having a Baby

"My second child was born in a clinic. I arrived at 2:00 A.M. and we were put into a room with two beds. My husband slept on one bed, while I labored on and around the other. Breakfast for two came at 7:00, and lunch at noon. By 2:00 in the afternoon my husband was chatting with the midwives who were massaging my back. Eventually I was fully dilated, and with some help I waddled to the next room and climbed onto the delivery table. The obstetrician appeared, but remained in the background while the midwives instructed me in pushing, and guided our son out into the world. No episiotomy and no tears. We stayed together for two hours. My son was then taken to the central nursery and I hobbled to a tatami room where two futons were waiting for me and the baby. The midwife told me that she would bring my son when he stopped spitting up amniotic fluid, maybe twelve hours later. After insisting, I was finally allowed to take my baby to my room, but the midwives couldn't understand why I didn't want to rest. I was delighted. I loved my stay there, and breast-feeding was so easy with my son on the futon next to me."

Childbirth Traditions

Taking a look at some of the traditional customs and beliefs concerning childbirth in Japan gives some fascinating insights into many of today's practices, which, at first sight, often seem totally foreign and incomprehensible.

The oft-cited reluctance to allow men to take part in the birth process can be partially understood by a glance at old traditions surrounding childbirth. In many parts of Japan, birth took place not at home, but at a one-room hut located at the edge of the community and used as a communal birthing place. This hut was usually furnished with an altar to the god of birth, a birthing bed of straw and rags, a thick rope hanging from the ceiling for the woman to grasp as she squatted to push her baby out, and a few simple tools for cutting the umbilical cord and bathing the baby. There may also have been amulets or a burning fire to ward off the evil spirits. If the community had no birthing hut, birth took place in an isolated part of the woman's house, or even on the ground outdoors. Usually, only a female relative, the godmother, and the *toriage-baasan* (lay midwife) attended the birth. Sometimes a Buddhist priest would be present to pray for an easy birth (*anzan*) or to use his physical strength or knowledge of Chinese medicine if the birth proved difficult. In most districts, the father of the child, if present, remained outside, perhaps performing rituals intended to hurry the birth to a safe and happy conclusion. His other role was to carry away the placenta after the birth to be buried near the outhouse on an auspicious day, in order to protect the child from future dangers. As late as the mid-1940s, birthing huts were still in use in parts of rural Japan. Even today, amulets and charms are still sold at shrines where pregnant women pray for an easy birth.

Childbirth took place in isolation because the birthing woman was said to be infected by *kegare* (sins, impurities) and her blood was regarded as unclean. Since *kegare* were considered contagious, anything which came in contact with the birthing woman was believed to be contaminated. *Kegare* were believed to travel through food and fire, so close relatives would prepare food for the new mother in a separate pot over a separate fire to prevent contamination. During the period of *kegare* (thirty-five days for the mother, thirty-two days for newborn girls, and thirty-one days for baby boys in the Edo period, 1603–1868), the woman and her newborn were confined to the birth hut or to an isolated room in the house. This may help explain why Japanese today readily accept the isolation of mothers and babies during the first month after birth. Nowadays they are encouraged to stay indoors in order to protect themselves, rather than the rest of society.

When the confinement was over, newborn babies were taken to the shrine by their grandmothers for purification. This custom still remains, although the baby's parents now join them. The mother would go through a separate ritual, preferably bathing in the sea, but alternatively taking a bath or simply sprinkling salt on herself. This view of the woman as something unclean and sinful contributed to her low status in society and the silencing of her voice. It partially explains the traditional passivity of Japanese women and why the women's movement in Japan has had such a long distance to travel.

Other restrictions were also placed on women during pregnancy and after the birth. According to the *Ishin-ho* (A.D. 984), the oldest extant Japanese medical text, the fetus was thought to be affected by what the pregnant woman ate, saw, or felt. For example, eating sweets might interfere with fetal bone formation, while hot and spicy foods might adversely affect the baby's temperament. Looking at rabbits might give the baby a harelip, while looking at "noble men" and "beautiful women" could help the fetus develop physically attractive characteristics. If a mother was obedient, polite, and mild-mannered, then her fetus would develop similar traits. In short, the woman could influence or "educate" her fetus through her behavior; this concept, which is termed *taikyō*, has recently experienced a resurge of interest. As time went on, the list of taboos and directives increased—sexual intercourse was forbidden during pregnancy, since it was believed to "exhaust the fetal *ki* [*qi* or *prana*] and the fetal blood," and women were cautioned against leaving the bed, and against washing in cold water or shampooing too soon after the birth.

Even today you will hear some of these taboos and directives, usually slightly adapted, which have been handed down over the years from mother to daughter, and from midwife to midwife. However, of all the traditional directives for pregnancy, the one most widely practiced and still suggested by the medical profession today is the wearing of an abdominal binder, the *hara-obi*, also known as *fukutai* or *iwata obi*.

The custom of binding the pregnant abdomen with this four-foot cotton sash dates back at least to the tenth century, since it is mentioned in *The Tale of Genji*. The reasons for binding the abdomen have changed through the ages, and vary in different parts of Japan. At one point, it was believed that the sash would prevent blood from "rising up to the liver" to cause a variety of problems ranging from hysteria to cold feet. Today, it is worn mainly for warmth and support of the abdominal muscles. Some midwives also use it to try to prevent the fetus from reassuming a breech position once the baby has turned.

Pregnant women begin to bind the abdomen during the fifth lunar month of pregnancy, which was believed to mark the beginning of the life of the fetus. On a lucky day of the same month (usually on the day of the dog, as dogs are believed to chase away evil spirits and are also associated with easy birth), pregnant women visit a shrine or temple dedicated to childbirth to pray for an easy birth and to buy her first *hara-obi*. A stop at the Suitengu Shrine in Tokyo or the Nakayama Temple in Osaka on the day of the dog will generally confirm that this custom continues today. Called *obi-iwai* or *chakutai-no-gi*, this ceremonial blessing can also take place at any nearby shrine; the *obi* can also be bought at any maternity shop or department store. Originally the *obi* was presented by the expectant mother's own family or by her *obi-oya*, a couple blessed with many children and called upon to be the first to bind her abdomen. Today, women usually buy the *obi* themselves or with their husbands, and are shown how to use it during a prenatal visit. Some women wear the *obi* only on this day, otherwise substituting a maternity girdle.

Until the early 1900s, most babies in Japan were delivered by lay midwives, whose task it was to deliver babies from the "land of the gods" into the world of humans. It was believed that, until the age of seven, children were still "children of the gods," belonging to both the heavens and the earth. However, with the new influence of Western (German) medicine, the lay midwives (*toriage-baasan*) were gradually replaced by midwives (*sanba*) with official training. In addition, many of the old customs were lost—traditionally, women had squatted while they pushed their baby out and then were kept seated after the birth to "let the blood run out," but Western medicine demanded that they lie down. Western practices also changed the dietary recommendations for pregnant women by including more protein and other nutrients. The midwife had the very difficult job of forcing the women they assisted to comply with all these new ways, but by 1940 statistics indicate that Western medicine was having a positive effect. Mortality rates for both mother and baby had fallen drastically, and throughout Japan the midwife had gained a respected status in the community, not only for the role she played during childbirth but also as a counselor on all kinds of family matters.

In 1950, more than 95 percent of births still took place at home. However, under the influence of the American occupation and with crowded living conditions, maternity health centers, hospitals, and obstetric clinics became more popular, and by 1965 nearly 85 percent of births took place in institutions; by 1991 the figure was virtually 100 percent. The occupation also influenced the training of midwives, who are now known as nurse-midwives, or *josanpu*. Only a very few midwives set up independent clinics; instead, most seek employment in hospitals or obstetric clinics working alongside obstetricians.

Childbirth practices in Japan today are a mixture of Western and oriental medicine and customs. If you are planning to have a baby during your stay, how can you prepare, and what can you expect?

Before Conception

English books (see page 119) can guide you in this important part of preparation. Women considering pregnancy are advised to take vitamin supplements (especially folic acid, vitamin B12, vitamin D, and vitamin E); eat a diet rich in calcium, protein, and iron; and abstain from cigarettes and alcohol. For information on nutrition, see the chapter on this subject. For smoking cessation, see page 241.

Infertility (see pages 105–108)
Pregnancy Tests (see page 102)

Registration of the Pregnancy

Once your pregnancy has been confirmed by a medical professional, if you are a resident of Japan, you must register the pregnancy at your local government office. Most offices do not ask your nationality or visa status, but only have you fill out a form giving the name of the doctor who confirmed the pregnancy and the name and address of his/her affiliated medical institution.

Mother and Child Health Handbook

The office will give you a handbook known as the *boshi kenkō techō* 母子健康手帳, in which will be recorded not only the course of your pregnancy and the birth, but also your baby's growth and immunizations through age six, when elementary schools begin to administer checkups and immunizations. You are expected to take it with you on each prenatal visit, to the birth, and every time you take your child to a pediatrician or for immunizations. The Tokyo government has put out a free, bilingual English-Japanese edition for residents of Tokyo, the *Mother and Child Health Handbook*. Another bilingual edition, titled *Maternal and Child Health Handbook*, can be purchased for a small fee at some clinics or hospitals catering to the foreign community, or ordered from Mothers' and Children's Health Organization (Boshi Hoken Jigyodan 母子保健事業団) 5-53-1 Jingumae, Shibuya-ku, Tokyo, 03-3499-3111. This organization also has bilingual editions in Tagalog, Spanish, Portuguese, Korean, Chinese, Thai, and Indonesian. Even if you buy this book, get the Japanese *boshi techō* from your local government office too.

The Japanese version includes a packet containing local information and immunization schedules in addition to coupons for free tests and immunizations at designated facilities. The coupons may vary according to area, but in most areas, two of the coupons, titled *ninshin kenkō shinsa jushin-hyō* 妊娠健康診査受診票, are for health checkups, one early and one late in pregnancy, including a urinalysis (protein and sugar) and blood tests for anemia, hepatitis B, and syphilis. The packet also contains a request form for a Guthrie test *senten-sei taisha ijō kensa mōshikomi-sho* 先天性代謝異常等検査申込書 (see page 141) and a Notification of Birth postcard (*shussan tsūchi-hyō* 出生通知表) to be filled in and sent back once the baby arrives. The card announces (not registers) the birth, and has space where you can request a free postnatal home visit (page 144). For mothers over age thirty-five, there may be a coupon for a free ultrasound during or after the twenty-eighth week of pregnancy. Some areas include coupons for the baby: immunizations, health checks, and a neuroblastoma exam at six months. Others send postcards about these after the birth, or announce them in local bulletins.

Birth Planning

Religious beliefs, cultural traditions, social attitudes, and many other factors influence the way women give birth. Developing realistic expectations, preparing yourself physically and mentally, and determining where and how you will want to give birth should set you in the direction of a safe and satisfying experience.

Finding Information About Birth

English books on childbirth can be ordered from the Foreign Buyers' Club (see the endpapers) or over the Internet. The following resources have annotated lists.

Capers Bookstore
P.O. Box 567, Nundah, QLD 4012 Australia
61-07-266-9573, fax 61-07-260-5009
capers@gil.com.au
Mail-order books on childbirth; send for catalog.

International Childbirth Education Association
P.O. Box 20048, Minn. MN 55420-0048 U.S.
1-612-854-8660, fax 1-612-854-8772
1-800-624-4934
Mail-order books and videos on childbirth; send for catalog.
http://www.icea.org

Maternity and Parenting Magazines
P. And, Balloon, and *Maternity* (all three are in Japanese, but contain many pictures of Japanese birth, etc.)
Mothering
P.O. Box 532, Mount Morris, IL 61054 U.S.

Today's Parent
955 Meyerside Dr., Missauga, Ont.
L5T 1P9 Canada
http://www.todaysparent.com

TWINS Magazine
5350 South Roslyn Street, Suite 400
Englewood, CO 80111 U.S.
http://www.twinsmagazine.com

Birthing exhibits are held every year on November 3, Good Birth Day *Ii Osan no Hi,* in Tokyo and sometimes other locations in Japan. Half the contributors are birth-related professionals and half are mothers—mostly members of various parenting groups. There is usually an English corner. For the location, call the Japan Association for Childbirth Education (JACE) 045-625-3560, also fax (in English).

Prenatal Education Classes *sanzen kyōiku* 産前教育
Most women benefit tremendously from attending classes provided by childbirth and breast-feeding preparation groups.

Tokyo Childbirth Education Association
(TCEA) Director: Elena de Karplus, C.C.E.
6-32-14 B Todoroki, Setagaya-ku, Tokyo
03-5760-3764; also 1-914-725-0150 (New York)
http://www.birthintokyo.com
Team of childbirth educators, midwives, nurses, and physiotherapists offer classes in English at locations around Tokyo and Yokohama. Includes Birthing in Tokyo, Prenatal Exercises, Baby Basics. Also labor assistance; telephone counseling; newsletter.

La Leche League Japan
Becky Oxley
2-30-15 Nishiogi-Kita, Suginami-ku, Tokyo
03-3394-4359
http://www.lalecheleague.org (LLL Int'l)
Miriam Eguchi 078-752-6654 (Kobe)
Carol Matsubara 078-581-3669 (Kobe)
Prepares pregnant women for breast-feeding and parenting and continues with support after

birth through telephone consultation, periodic meetings, lending-library, and sometimes breast pump rentals. Contact for information on local groups, in English and Japanese.

Maternity Room
151-4 Yamate-cho, Naka-ku, Yokohama
045-625-3560, also fax (J. or Eng.)
http://www.dali-lover.co.jp/ce/index.html
(home page in Japanese)
Active birth classes in Japanese by Ritsuko Toda, childbirth educator trained in the U.K. Also director of JACE.

Maternity Class
3-34-1-406 Kyuden, Setagaya-ku, Tokyo
03-3308-3345 (J. only)
http://www.dianet.or.jp/babycom/ (J. only)
Maternity coordinator Sakae Kikuchi offers active birth classes in Takadanobaba. In Japanese. She is also a good source of information.

Nagoya Foreign Mother's Group
Mikokoro Center 3 Fl., 3-6-43 Marunouchi
Naka-ku, Nagoya, Aiichi-ken
052-802-7047, also fax
http://www2.gol.com/users/rule/mothers
Run by English-speaking midwife Misako Iwa-
moto, who can also help with communication
difficulties with caregiver. Group meets bimonthly to share information on birth preparation,
doctors, hospitals, breast-feeding, childcare, etc.

Kansai Childbirth Education Organization
Birth preparation classes in the Kobe/Osaka
area. Includes Lamaze breathing techniques,
postpartum and newborn care, and breast-
feeding. Call Community House Information Center, 078-857-6540, for the current number.

Kyoto Birth Network
075-881-6385
Information and classes on birth preparation.

Tokyo Twins Group
Catherine Watters Sasanuma
03-3485-8557 cwstyo@gol.com
Monthly gatherings in Tokyo area to share ideas
on preparing for and raising twins. Also, answers inquiries from other parts of Japan.

Public Health Center Mothering Classes
Hokenjo no Haha Oya Gakkyu
保健所の母親学級 (J. only)
Midwives, public health nurses, and doctors
teach prenatal and parenting classes at public
health centers. Geared to Japanese women,
they supplement classes at individual facilities
and may not totally prepare you for birth. They
can, however, put you in touch with other expectant mothers and services in your area. You're
welcome to bring someone to help with communication. Videos on birth.

Safety

Birth in Japan is generally safe. The perinatal and infant mortality rates are reported to be
the lowest in the world (as of 1995, 7.0 and 4.2 respectively per 1,000 live births). These
favorable statistics are attributed not only to medical competence at the birth, but also to
access to good prenatal care, and to Japan's status as a relatively wealthy country with
universal health insurance and a population which is hygiene-conscious.

Although Japanese birth professionals in general have faith in natural birth, most are
also very capable of handling other kinds of birth as well. With the exception of certain
experimental techniques, virtually all obstetric procedures in use in Western countries are
available in Japan. With the falling birthrate, most obstetricians continually update their
practices to keep up with the competition. However, not all places of birth have the
capacity for all procedures. Some don't have the facilities or staff to handle obstetric emergencies, perform cesarean births, or take care of premature or very sick babies. The once
relatively high maternal mortality rate (9.6 per 100,000 live births in 1988, as compared to
8.4 for the U.S. and 5.9 for the U.K. the same year) was often attributed by Japanese caregivers to the lack of access to emergency care at some birthing facilities. Efforts to improve
prenatal care and reduce the incidence of toxemia had lowered this rate to 6.1 by 1994.

Cost
Insurance Coverage
Since normal pregnancy and birth is not considered an illness, Japanese public health
insurance does not cover the cost of normal maternity and obstetric care. Instead, a

monetary "gift" is awarded after the birth. Public insurance, however, covers the cost of medical care for pregnancy and birth complications, including cesareans (see pages 72–73 and 76–77 in "Health Insurance").

Fees

Typically, each prenatal visit costs between ¥4,000 and ¥20,000, depending on the facility and how many tests are performed. At some facilities ultrasound is routine and included in the basic fee. Others charge up to ¥5,000 extra. Some tests (such as amniocentesis, which can be as much as ¥100,000), can raise the cost considerably. You can reduce the cost of prenatal visits by using the coupons included with your *boshi techō*. The average cost of a normal delivery and five- to seven-day postpartum stay is currently ¥350,000–¥500,000, but a private room can add on another ¥10,000–¥40,000 a day. Deluxe facilities may charge ¥800,000–¥1,000,000 or more. Midwife clinics and national institutions are often more reasonable than other facilities.

Gift-giving Customs

In addition to the fees charged, it is customary (though not obligatory) to give caregivers a gift after the birth. Usual gifts for the nurses and midwives are a box of cakes or handkerchiefs (about ¥3,000); the doctor is usually given gift coupons, scarves, or whiskey. For the doctor; a gift equivalent to ¥10,000 is most common for normal birth (double for cesareans). Some foreign women have substituted homemade cookies as their gift to the nurses, and given items from their own country to the doctor. See also page 43.

If you choose to follow Japanese custom, another expense will be the cost of the *uchi-iwai*. This is the present which the new mother gives in appreciation to everyone who gave her baby gifts. The usual practice is to return something which costs approximately one-third of whatever was received, or one-half if the gift cost ¥10,000 or more. Typical return gifts are: coffee, potpourri, beer coupons, or a telephone card with the baby's name on it.

Maternity Leave and Benefits for the Working Mother

Mothering in Japan is still considered to be a full-time occupation. Although more women work outside the home than before, labor laws regarding benefits for pregnant women and new mothers lag behind those in many other countries. With the declining birthrate, the Japanese government is now trying to change these laws, to encourage women to reproduce.

The national labor laws apply to all women workers, regardless of nationality or whether they work full- or part-time (see page 61).

Government Assistance

Other benefits are also available to low-income mothers, working mothers, and those with toxemia, diabetes, anemia, obstetric hemorrhage, heart disease, and certain other conditions. Financial aid can also be requested for babies born prematurely or with certain potential disabilities or chronic diseases. See page 62 for more details.

Father's Participation *otto tachiai bunben* 夫立ち合い分娩

In Japan, fathers are not always permitted at the birth, and only 20–30 percent of Japanese fathers attend. At some facilities, fathers are not allowed in the labor room if other women are sharing it, but may be permitted into the delivery room. At others, the delivery room may be off-limits. In cases in which the mother is not Japanese, the father is often welcome to help with communication, especially if problems arise.

Some hospitals do not permit fathers to hold their babies during the postpartum stay. To avoid possible exposure to outside germs, babies are kept in a central nursery where they can be viewed during visiting hours only through a window. Even if the baby is allowed to room-in with the mother, hospital regulations may require returning the baby to the central nursery during visiting hours.

Birth Assistants

Japan does not have a system of independent professional birth assistants whom you can hire to assist you at a hospital birth. Most hospitals have regulations against independent hiring of this sort. However, if you have communication problems, or if your husband is unable to attend the birth, some hospitals will allow you to bring a friend or relative who can interpret for you and assist you.

Natural Birth *shizen bunben* 自然分娩

Non-medicated birth is still the norm in Japan, and the majority of women give birth without the aid of pharmaceutical pain relief. In nearly all birthing facilities, midwives assist the mother and deliver the baby, with the obstetrician, if one is present, taking more of an advisory role, unless medical intervention is needed.

This, however, does not mean that births are totally natural. With the exception of midwife clinics, even at facilities promoting natural birth, some medical procedures are customary, including ultrasound at prenatal visits, continuous electronic fetal monitoring during second stage and, especially for first-time mothers, episiotomies (with local anesthetic) during delivery. To prevent postpartum hemorrhage, the use of medication such as oxytocin or ergometrine to contract the uterus is also routine. After the birth, antibiotics and sometimes stool softeners are prescribed to prevent postpartum infection and constipation.

Traditionally, the Japanese expectant mother was expected to endure the pain of labor, helped only by her midwife's massage and encouraging words. Today, most women take prenatal classes to learn relaxation, breathing, and other techniques similar to those of natural childbirth methods in the West. Caregivers are likely to be familiar with the

Japanese version of the Lamaze method. Breathing patterns vary and may differ somewhat from those taught elsewhere, but can easily be learned in prenatal classes, or even at the birth under a midwife's direction. The British concept of active birth, which encourages the woman to keep mobile during labor and gives her freedom of position at the birth, is also practiced in some facilities. Other imported methods and techniques for birth or birth preparation include sophlologie, reflexology, aerobics, maternity swimming, aromatherapy, image training, and waterbirth. Some caregivers specialize; others are familiar with nearly all of these, including the oriental techniques below, and use a combination or leave the choice to the mother, in the "free-style" approach.

Traditional oriental techniques and others recently invented in Japan are also used, even in some hospitals and Ob/Gyn clinics. The Tokyo Metropolitan Police Hospital has introduced the REIB (Relaxation, Exercise, Imagination, Breathing) Method *ribu-hō* リーブ法 based on qigong that teaches the mother to relax both body and mind through exercise and abdominal breathing, and to facilitate the pregnancy and birth by visualizing and relating to her unborn baby. The method has spread elsewhere and videos are also available. At other facilities, doctors use massage, *kanpō*, moxibustion, acupuncture, qigong, and *seitai* (see "Alternative Healing").

The most natural of births are conducted by midwives in independent practice, either at home or at midwife clinics. Most are familiar with the Japanese versions of Lamaze and active birth. Some also make use of aromatherapy, imagery, yoga, acupressure, moxibustion, qigong, and *kanpō*. Midwives in Japan are limited in the medical procedures they can perform—they mainly check blood pressure, weight, the height of the fundus, and the circumference of the uterus; do urine tests and check the fetal heartbeat; give enemas; deliver the baby, and cut the umbilical cord. In an emergency situation, under the direction of a doctor, midwives can perform other medical procedures. Independent midwives are well trained in labor support and techniques to protect the perineum. If tears do occur during the birth, repair is done with clamps.

Anesthetized Birth masui bunben 麻酔分娩

The number of Japanese women using pharmaceutical pain relief for normal childbirth, (other than a local anesthetic for episiotomy repair), is much lower than in the West. Methods vary, but can include analgesics such as meperidine (demerol/pethidine), and spinal and epidural anesthesia; and/or what is called "balanced" or "cocktail" anesthesia, a combination of small doses of sedatives, painkillers, and anesthesia as needed to maximize the pain relief and minimize the side effects. The "walking epidural," which is a combination of spinal and epidural anesthesia and uses a lower-dose "cocktail" than regular epidurals, is not commonly used in Japan. Use of and availability of pharmaceutical pain relief varies, especially among smaller clinics. Some hospitals and clinics are noted for anesthetized birth; at others it may be available but seldom used, and, due to shortage of staff, reliable continuous monitoring is sometimes unavailable. To guarantee sufficient staff to monitor the anesthesia, some practitioners routinely control the timing of these births through planned induction. Dosages tend to be smaller than in the U.S. or U.K. If the anesthesia prevents the mother from pushing her baby out, vacuum extractions are more common than the forceps delivery customary in the U.S.

Induced Birth *jintsū yūhatsu* 陣痛誘発

For several years the rate of elective induction for convenience was rising in Japan, along with controversy over the relative safety of this kind of birth. Proponents of elective induction claim birth is safer, as well as more humane to the caregivers, if it is controlled so as not to occur during the night or on weekends, when staffing is low and emergency care less accessible. This is particularly the case at some small Ob/Gyn clinics and at facilities conducting anesthetized birth. Others contend that the possible dangers and increased discomfort of induced or augmented labor outweigh these or other potential benefits. These hazards include premature birth or rupture of the uterus, especially if the procedure is badly timed or handled improperly. The most recent statistics show that campaigns against unnecessary inductions have considerably lowered the rate.

Induction may start with stripping of the membranes (loosening the membranes near the cervix with the fingers), perhaps at a prenatal visit. If labor does not begin within a few days, you will usually be hospitalized and laminaria (dried seaweed) sticks inserted overnight and again in the morning to absorb liquid and expand and soften the cervix. Next, you will be given a prostaglandin and/or pitocin hormonal intravenous drip to stimulate the contractions. At this point, artificial rupture of the membranes is also a possibility. If natural labor is imminent, gentler means of induction, such as castor oil, may be used.

Cesareans *teiō-sekkai* 帝王切開

In Japan, cesarean birth is not usually considered an option which women can "choose," as it is in some countries. Although the cesarean rate in the U.S. is relatively high, at twenty percent, the rate here is about eleven percent. Most Japanese obstetricians believe in women's ability to give birth vaginally and are reluctant to perform cesareans. Caregivers pay particular attention to the mother's weight during pregnancy, telling her that she will increase her chance of a cesarean if she gains over seven to ten kilograms. Recent years have seen a slight rise in the cesarean rate, perhaps due to a corresponding decline in induced births, but other factors are contributing as well. More doctors are routinely delivering breech births by cesarean, and with older first-time mothers, the number of complicated births, including twin births, is rising.

Note that an obstetrician must have the woman's consent in writing to proceed with a cesarean. Epidurals and spinals are now customary; general anesthesia may be used for emergencies. The "classical" (vertical) incision is still practiced, but the lower abdominal (horizontal) "bikini cut" is becoming more common. Pharmaceutical pain relief after the birth is sometimes limited, although you can request it. A new trend is to continue the epidural in a low dosage for a couple of days after the birth. Hospital stays are comparatively long: 6–10 days, as opposed to 2–5 days in the U.S.

Postpartum Stay *sanjoku-ki nyūin* 産褥期入院

After a normal birth Japanese women usually stay in the hospital for 5–7 days, as opposed to 1–3 days in the U.S. and the U.K. This system is popular since the mothers can rest and adjust to the new baby with the help of professional caregivers. The long stay and recuperation at home (now 3–4 weeks) are believed to contribute to the lower incidence of uterine disease and hysterectomies among older Japanese women.

Rooming-in is not as widespread in Japan as in the West. In spite of the general promotion of breast-feeding, separation of mother and baby continues, reportedly due to limited staff, a lack of space, fear of infection, and the belief that new mothers need rest. Many facilities however do promote, or at least allow, varying degrees of rooming-in. At midwife clinics, mothers and babies remain together throughout their stay, and in some hospitals and Ob/Gyn clinics 24-hour or day-time rooming-in is possible, usually after an initial separation of 8–36 hours, depending on space, hospital policy, and/or the condition of the mother and baby. Some hospitals will only allow rooming-in in private rooms.

However, the benefits of rooming-in are slowly becoming better known in Japan, in response to the WHO/UNICEF recommendations for the promotion of breast-feeding. Attention was first drawn when Okayama National Hospital was awarded the WHO title of "Baby-friendly Hospital" in 1991. The WHO/UNICEF requirements include that breast-feeding be initiated within thirty minutes of birth, that there be no separation of mother and baby unless medically indicated, that mother and baby can stay in the same room (twenty-four hours a day), that the baby be fed nothing but breast milk unless medically indicated, and that the baby be fed on demand. In 1992, St. Mary's Hospital in Kurume, Fukuoka-ken, was granted the same award. Other hospitals, including the Nagasaki University Medical School Hospital and the Tottori Kenritsu Chuo Hospital, have now adopted the WHO recommendations.

Written Birth Plans バースプラン

Some women write birth plans describing alternatives they would like and present them to their caregivers, either to check the acceptability at that facility or to confirm agreements already reached. Written plans can be useful, especially if time is limited and communication difficult. Keep in mind, however, that while some Japanese caregivers may be responsive to your plan and appreciate your desire to share in the decisions surrounding your childbirth experience, others may be offended and consider your approach aggressive and distrustful. Japanese caregivers are accustomed to dealing with Japanese women, who tend to leave the management of birth completely up to them. Although the Japanese maternity media is now encouraging women to assume more responsibility, many women remain passive and select their place of birth chiefly on the basis of convenience and reputation. In addition, Japan is a country where following rules is the norm, and requests for individual exceptions can be considered selfish. Keep in mind also that no matter what birthing situation you choose, you need to be flexible. Birth is never totally predictable, and your plans may need revision as you go along.

Choosing a Place for the Birth

Research this topic early in your pregnancy. Some caregivers require a non-refundable deposit for the delivery midway through the pregnancy, and some will not accept women after a certain month.

Ask friends for recommendations or contact one of the parenting groups on pages 119–20. The AMDA Centers (see endpapers) have an extensive list of childbirth facilities accepting English-speakers, especially in the Tokyo and Kansai areas. If you live in Kansai also get *Medical Access: A Foreigner's Guide to Health Care in Kobe* (see page 27). The Internet web sites of the parenting groups also give some information. Unfortunately, Japanese medical institutions do not offer the public classes introducing their birthing practices, but if you can read Japanese, several guides are available at bookstores (see "References and Further Reading").

Suggested facilities are listed in the following pages after the discussion of each type of birthplace. All these facilities have been recommended by non-Japanese women who have given birth there. Note that the level of English proficiency varies.

You may not find the perfect situation, but many Japanese caregivers are understanding of differences in cultural attitudes and medical practices surrounding birth, and will try to incorporate your wishes. You may be able to negotiate alternatives that are closer in line with your views of birth—for example, obtaining a freer birthing position, greater contact with your baby, or a shorter postpartum stay.

Questions to Ask when Choosing a Place for the Birth

■ Check policies on inductions and other interventions: "natural birth" may be interpreted in different ways.

■ If you want the baby's father to be at the birth, find out beforehand not only if he can be present but to what extent he will be able to participate.

■ If you think you'll need access to pharmaceutical pain relief, look for a facility accustomed to using it. Find out how many women who give birth there actually use it, what methods are used when, and if possible, ask a few women who used it how well the pain relief worked. However, don't generalize on the basis of one person's experience.

■ Check how long the postpartum stay will be.

■ Check to what extent rooming-in is permitted and if the father may be with the baby.

■ Discuss also the procedures for cesareans. Ask what kind of anesthesia and incision are used, and what pain relief is available postpartum.

■ If you have or suspect any complications, be sure you are in a facility which can accommodate your needs—remember the obstetric emergencies are not totally predictable. Even if you are a good candidate for a normal birth and want to give birth in a small clinic, be sure it has sufficient staff and good emergency backup.

Where to Give Birth

About thirty percent of Japanese women still follow the custom of *satogaeri bunben* 里帰り分娩, in which the mother-to-be returns to her own family for the birth, spending the month or so before and after the birth at her family home.

If you decide to go home, plan ahead. Some airlines forbid flying after the thirty-fourth week of pregnancy and many require an obstetrician's written approval (in triplicate) during the ninth month. In addition, finding a doctor and facility willing to accommodate you in the final stages is not always easy. Your newborn will need a passport (and visa) to return. If the baby is entitled to Japanese citizenship, you must register the birth at a Japanese embassy or consulate within fourteen days. Check on what you'll need for all these procedures before you go. Also, be sure that your health insurance will cover any complications you or your baby may have while you are there.

(The following statistics are for all births in Japan in 1995, from the Ministry of Health and Welfare publication *Maternal and Child Health Statistics of Japan, 1996.*)

HOME BIRTH (less than 0.1 percent of births) *katei bunben* 家庭分娩

"If I'd found a place I liked nearby which would let me keep my baby with me from birth, I might not have had a home birth. I was checked by an obstetrician right through the last week. He offered to be on call if I needed him at the birth. Our midwife agreed to everything in our birth plan, which we'd had translated into Japanese. We spent the first part of labor talking with the midwives and my children. I took a bath when I was around 6 cm and was fully dilated an hour later. The children were in awe as I pushed their new sister out. We celebrated with champagne and called it a night. The midwife returned over the next few days to check on both of us. On the fifth day, we went to our family doctor and my obstetrician to be checked further."

Home birth may be a possibility if you are young and healthy, and are seeking a familiar and natural environment for birth. Home births are usually attended by a midwife in independent practice. She will recommend you see an obstetrician regularly for prenatal visits to confirm that everything remains normal, and will also check you herself, usually once during early pregnancy, and then periodically starting in about the seventh or eighth month. It's up to you to arrange for medical backup at a nearby facility. As a rule, two midwives attend the birth. During the week or two after the birth, the midwife will return daily or every other day to check on you and the baby, and to give the baby a bath.

However, very few Japanese women choose to give birth at home, probably because most question its safety. If you do decide on a home birth, you may have difficulty finding a willing, capable midwife (or doctor) and acceptable emergency medical backup, especially since Japan does not have the support found in parts of Europe, such as flying squads (vehicles with emergency staff and equipment that park outside the home during the birth or can be there within minutes).

Midwife Seiko Kamiya
神谷整子助産婦
3-35-8 Koishikawa, Bunkyo-ku, Tokyo
03-3812-0707 and fax

Aquariel
(Midwife Michiko Sugata)
57-8 Enshoji-cho, Okazaki, Sakyo-ku, Kyoto-shi
075-752-1634 (Eng.)

MIDWIFE CLINICS (0.9 percent of births) *josan'in* 助産院

"Our son was born in a midwife clinic on the tatami with the aid of a beanbag chair and a wooden birthing stool. The communal feeling in the delivery room was very supportive—everyone joined in with the breathing as we chanted fu-un *to help push him out. I had no anesthetics, episiotomy, or intervention of any sort. My husband cut the cord and held our son while the midwives prepared futons for me, my husband, and the baby. The next day the baby and I moved into a room with a Japanese woman and her new baby. We stayed there for the next four nights. The entire experience was even more wonderful than I could have imagined."*

Because most midwife clinics belong to elderly independent midwives who have been in private practice since before WWII, the number of midwife clinics has been steadily declining. But very recently the trend has reversed as an increasing number of younger midwives have begun leaving hospitals and setting up their own practices or joining others. These midwives have formed organizations such as the Japanese Midwives' Organized Network (JIMON). With over 250 members (some independent, others hospital-employed), this group is gradually changing the face of Japanese midwifery today. For information on midwives in your area, you are welcome to contact the following organizations.

JIMON
(Japanese Midwives' Organized Network)
fax 03-3414-3207
e-mail: jimonnet@ca2.so-net.or.jp
(J. or Eng.)

Japanese Midwives Association
Nihon Josanpu Kai
日本助産婦会
03-3262-9910 (J. only), fax 03-3262-8933 (in Eng.)

Facilities at midwife clinics vary, but they usually provide a flexible, family-like atmosphere. In addition to the head midwife, an assistant midwife, and household help, staff including specialists in breast massage may be available. Prenatal visits are conducted by the head midwife, with the exception of two or three checkups done with the *shokutaku-i* (part-time obstetrician), who forms part of the medical backup for the birth. Emergencies, which are rare if prenatal care and screening has been good, are sent to the nearest emergency facility. Postpartum stay is from five to seven days.

Midwife Clinics (some also do home births)

Fukuoka Josan'in
福岡助産院 (Midwife Teruko Fukuoka)
4-32-9 Higashi-Mukojima, Sumida-ku, Tokyo
03-3611-7563 (Eng.)

Fun Josan'in
黄助産院 (Midwife Fujiko Sugiyama)
1-25-9 Narita-Nishi, Suginami-ku, Tokyo
03-3313-5658 (Eng.)

Aqua Birth House
アクワ バースハウス
(Midwife Setsuko Yamada)
4-16-21 Sakuragaoka, Setagaya-ku, Tokyo
03-3427-1314 (Eng.)

Inada Josan'in
稲田助産院 (Midwife Yoshie Fujii)
2-4-7 Sugekitaura, Tama-ku, Kawasaki-shi
044-945-5560

Childbearing House Mirai
ベビーヘルシー美蕾 (Midwife Fusako Sei)
500-1 Minami-Ota, Ina-machi

Tsukuba-gun, Ibaraki-ken
02975-8-3708 (Eng., Indo.)

Ayumi Josan'in
あゆみ助産院 (Midwife Kazuko Sako)
999-2 Yamamura-cho, Fukakusa
Fushimi-ku, Kyoto-shi
075-643-2163

Namase Josan'in
生瀬助産院 (Midwife Hatsu Namase)
24 Takahashi-cho, Kinugasa, Kita-ku, Kyoto-shi
075-461-3408 (Eng.)

Mana Josan-jo
マナ助産所 (Midwife Ikuko Nagahara)
2-10-8 Hiyodoridai, Kita-ku, Kobe-shi
078-742-3474 (Eng.)

Mori Josan-jo
毛利助産所 (Midwife Taneko Mori)
4-13-3 Mikage Ishi-machi
Higashi-Nada-ku, Kobe-shi
078-841-2040 (Eng.)

OB/GYN CLINICS (44.4 percent of births) *sanfujin-ka i'in* 産婦人科医院

"My first child was born in a U.S. hospital. When I became pregnant with my second child, I felt that I didn't want to give birth in a large hospital, yet I wanted to be sure that pain relief would be available. After some research, I found that one of the Ob/Gyn clinics in our neighborhood specializes in anesthetized birth. Although it was my second child, I had a very long, hard labor and eventually did end up with an epidural, which by the way was fine, in spite of all the stories I'd heard about the inefficacy of Japanese pain relief.

I was exhausted after the birth, and so pleased to be in a place where someone else could look after my baby while I rested—I stayed the full week."

A clinic (a medical facility with less than twenty beds) is a popular choice of birthplace. Often family businesses headed by one or two family members who are obstetricians, or an obstetrician-and-midwife couple, clinics often have a homey atmosphere; others are luxurious, with hotel-like accommodations and even French gourmet cooking. Typically, the clinic has a small delivery room which may also be used for outpatient gynecological or obstetric procedures, as well as for cesarean birth. Most also have a central nursery for the newborn babies.

Methods of birth vary. Some clinics specialize in high-tech, anesthetized deliveries, while others promote natural birth. Without the red tape found in large hospitals, these clinics can be innovative and creative. Some have attached swimming pools for maternity swimming or studios for maternity aerobics.

One clinic in Okazaki-shi, Aichi-ken, the Yoshimura Byoin, takes an unconventional approach to natural childbirth. In the belief that a traditional life-style is important for nurturing the natural instinct for an easy, safe birth that modern women seem to have lost, an Edo-period farmhouse has been prepared on the grounds of the clinic. Here mothers-to-be can prepare for birth in an ideal setting by chopping wood and performing other traditional housekeeping chores.

Clinics can be wonderful, but they are not without their limitations. In many, the obstetrician is assisted only by nurses, in spite of recommendations that at least one midwife be available to cover situations that could arise when the obstetrician is away or busy. Not all clinics have up-to-date equipment or the staff or facilities to administer anesthetics or perform cesareans. When a staff is small, it can sometimes be necessary to control the timing of the birth, so at clinics artificial labor induction, and speeding of the rate of labor, once it has begun, are common.

Ob/Gyn Clinics

Toho Women's Clinic
Toho Fujin Kurinikku
東峰婦人クリニック (Dr. Hisami Matsumine)
5-3-10 Kiba, Koto-ku, Tokyo
03-3630-0322 (Pub. Ins., Eng.)
Emphasis on natural birth; infertility specialty.

Sanno Clinic
(Minato-ku, Tokyo; see page 108)

Tokyo Maternity Clinic
Tokyo Mataniti Kurinikku
(Dr. Yoichiro Yanagida)
東京マタニティー・クリニック
1-20-8 Sendagaya, Shibuya-ku, Tokyo
03-3403-1861 (Eng.)

Shohei Clinic
Shohei Fujin-ka
昇平婦人科 (Dr. Shohei Hayashida)
3-14-8 Amanuma, Suginami-ku, Tokyo
03-3393-5171 (Pub. Ins., Eng.)

Higashi-Fuchu Hospital
Higashi-Fuchu Byoin
東府中病院 (Dr. Shin Juzoji)
2-7-20 Wakamatsu-cho, Fuchu-shi, Tokyo
0423-64-0151 (Pub. Ins., Eng.)

Totsuka MT Clinic
Totsuka MT Kurinikku
戸塚ＭＴクリニック (Dr. Hirobumi Chikuni)
3970 Totsuka-cho, Totsuka-ku, Yokohama-shi
045-862-0050 (Pub. Ins., Eng.)
Natural birth, maternity swimming, aerobics, yoga; pediatrics.

Isezaki Women's Clinic
(Naka-ku, Yokohama-shi; see page 83)

Tojo Women's Clinic
Tojo Uimenzu Kurinikku
東條ウイメンズクリニック (Dr. Ryutaro Tojo)
2-23-7 Maruyamadai, Konan-ku, Yokohama-shi
045-843-1121 (Pub. Ins., Eng.)

Nishikawa Clinic
Nishikawa I'in
西川医院 (Dr. Masahiro Nishikawa)
2-16-10 Tennoji-cho, Kita-Abeno-ku, Osaka-shi
06-714-5218 (Pub. Ins., Eng.)

Iitoh Women's Clinic
Iitoh Sanfujin-ka
飯藤産婦人科 (Dr. Yuriko Hashimoto)
5-6-6 Izumi-cho, Suita-shi, Osaka-fu
06-388-0141 (Pub. Ins., Eng.)

Iwasa Ladies Clinic
(Dr. Yoshihiko Iwasa)
9-22 Korien-cho, Hirakata-shi, Osaka-fu
0720-31-1666 (Pub. Ins., Eng.)

Ueda Hospital
Ueda Byoin 上田病院 (Dr. Rokuro Ueda)
1-1-4 Kunika-dori, Chuo-ku, Kobe-shi
078-241-3305 (Pub. Ins., Eng.)
Also pediatrics; appointment required.

Matsuoka Women's Clinic
Matsuoka Fujin-ka Kurinikku

松岡産婦人科クリニック
(Dr. Kenji Matsuoka)
1-6-18 Midori-cho, Kita-ku, Kobe-shi
078-582-0003 (Pub. Ins., Eng.)

Hisa Ob/Gyn Clinic
Hisa Sanfujin-ka
久産婦人科 (Dr. Yasuo Hisa)
23-1 Juroku-sen, Tawaramoto-cho, Ishiki-gun
Nara-ken
0744-33-3110 (Pub. Ins., Eng.)
Natural birth, waterbirth.

HOSPITAL BIRTH (54.5 percent of births) *byōin shussan* 病院出産
The majority of foreign women in Japan give birth in hospitals (medical facilities with twenty beds or more). For childbirth, this can be further categorized into the following:

General Hospitals *sōgō byōin* 総合病院

"Because I suffer from epilepsy, I decided to choose a general hospital. I still wanted my husband to be present and to have as natural a birth as possible. We started out at a university hospital, which had said my husband could be present at the birth. But when we discovered at eight months that "at the birth" meant not in the labor room as we had expected, but in the delivery room, we decided to switch to another hospital. I had a natural birth and although I never needed extra medical care, I felt comfortable knowing that it was easily accessible."

If you have, develop, or suspect complications, your best choice may be the obstetric department of a general hospital which also has departments handling other fields of medicine. If the hospital you choose has an NICU, your baby can also receive any intensive care necessary.

Another reason for choosing a general hospital would be communication—some are used to taking care of non-Japanese, and staff may be familiar with different birthing customs. Pharmaceutical pain relief is also available, and if you want a natural birth, most large hospitals' rates for cesarean and other interventions are relatively low.

The greatest disadvantage of a large institution is the systematization of the care and the difficulty in accommodating individual wishes. An obstetrician at one such facility likened the care at his hospital to a conveyor belt. Further, appointment systems are rare, so at prenatal visits you may wait two or three hours for a five-minute consultation. Continuity of care can also be a problem. By timing your appointments on days when the doctor you want to see is on duty, you will have a greater chance of seeing the same obstetrician for all your prenatal visits, though there may be no guarantee he/she will be present at the birth. At some hospitals, certain doctors will accept requests to have them attend the delivery.

Privacy can also be a problem. Prenatal checks can be an assembly line of women waiting half-naked for the doctor; labor rooms may accommodate five or more women, with only a skimpy curtain, if that, between one person and another. Sometimes six women (and their babies) share a postpartum room. If the hospital is a teaching hospital, even your delivery may be a public affair. Private rooms are few, and priority may be given to those with serious complications.

All the following general hospitals accept Japanese public insurance and have English-speaking obstetricians:

Jikei Medical University Hospital
(Minato-ku, Tokyo; see page 343)
03-3433-1111

Japanese Red Cross Medical Center
(Shibuya-ku, Tokyo; see page 343)
03-3400-1311
Complete rooming-in, LDR; emergencies.

Seibo International Catholic Hospital
(Shinjuku-ku, Tokyo; see page 343)
03-3951-1111

St. Luke's International Hospital
(Chuo-ku, Tokyo; see page 344)
03-3541-5151
Private LDR's and postpartum rooms.

Tokyo Adventist Hospital
(Suginami-ku, Tokyo; see page 344)
03-3392-6151
Emphasis on anesthetized birth; vegetarian.

Tokyo Women's Medical University Hospital
(Shinjuku-ku, Tokyo; see page 344)
03-3353-8111
Maternal and child health center.

Kitazato University Hospital
(Sagamihara-shi, Kanagawa-ken; see page 344)

0427-78-8111
Emergencies; emphasis on anesthetized birth.

Shonan Kamakura General Hospital
(Kamakura-shi, Kanagawa-ken; see page 345)
Coordinates with Bluff Clinic (see page 34)

Kobe Adventist Hospital
(Kita-ku, Kobe-shi; see page 348)
078-981-0161

Konan Hospital
(Nada-ku, Kobe-shi; see page 348)
078-851-2161

Kobe Kaisei Hospital
(Nada-ku, Kobe-shi; see page 348)
078-871-5201

Rokko Island Hospital
(Higashi-Nada-ku, Kobe-shi; see page 348)

Yodogawa Christian Hospital
(Yodogawa-ku, Osaka-shi; see page 348)
06-322-2250

Japan Baptist Hospital
(Sakyo-ku, Kyoto-shi; see page 347)
075-781-5191

Maternal and Child Health Specialty Hospitals *san'in* 産院

"We really couldn't afford to have a baby. I thought about a midwife clinic, but it was my first experience, and I wanted more medical backup. Public maternity hospitals appealed, because they are inexpensive and because most of the care is provided by midwives, yet with medical backup. Everything went fine, but I sometimes felt I was on an assembly line. The

worst was the prenatal internal exams—five of us lying on beds in little cubicles separated by curtains, half naked, with our legs spread apart. The doctor would go from one person to the next, hardly uttering a word. The strangest part of the exam was the curtain which separated the upper part of my body from the lower and me from the doctor. The birth wasn't as bad, but I got the doctor to let me leave with my baby after three days."

The advantage of specialist maternity hospitals is that they are specifically designed to accommodate both mother and baby. If complications arise, both an obstetrician and a pediatrician should always be on duty and can be at the birth. As specialists in this field, if the facility is well funded, practices should be current and equipment up-to-date. If the hospital is large, however, it has the same disadvantages of general hospitals. Note also that not all facilities are able to care for very premature babies. The following are private maternal and child health specialty hospitals:

Aiiku Hospital
Aiikukai Byoin 愛育会病院
5-6-8 Minami-Azabu, Minato-ku, Tokyo
03-3473-8321 (Pub. Ins., Eng.)
Emphasis on natural birth.

St. Barnabas Hospital
Sei Barunaba Byoin
聖バルナバ病院
1-3-32 Saikudani, Tennoji-ku, Osaka-shi
06-779-1600 (Pub. Ins., Eng.)

COMBINATION SYSTEM

Although prenatal care and delivery usually take place in the same facility in Japan, a few obstetricians, mainly those catering to the foreign community, conduct prenatal care at outside outpatient clinics and have delivery rights or referral connections at a hospital. Prenatal visits are usually on an appointment basis; communication is relatively good and the atmosphere comfortable and reassuring. Note that not all the clinic or hospital staff will speak English, although some usually do and others somehow manage and are relatively familiar with Western ways. The obstetrician will usually appear at the beginning of labor, and then be on call for complications, reappearing for the birth. The midwives will monitor labor, give assistance, and alert the obstetrician when the birth is imminent or if any abnormalities are detected. The fees for this system, however, can be considerably higher, and Japanese public insurance may not apply to complications.

Obstetricians Offering Prenatal Care at Outpatient Clinic and Delivery at Hospital

Tokyo Medical and Surgical Clinic
(Minato-ku, Tokyo; see page 33)
03-3436-3028 (Eng., Fr., Sp.)
Dr. Joshua Suzuki
Dr. Takumi Yanaihara
Dr. Hideki Sakamoto (also at Nihon University Hospital, Itabashi)
Dr. Claudine Bliah (see next page)

Deliveries at Seibo Hospital (see page 343) or Sanno Clinic (see page 108).

International Medical Crossing Office
(Dr. Ryoko Dozono)
4-2-49-401 Minami-Azabu, Minato-ku, Tokyo
03-3443-4823 (Eng.)
Prenatal and postnatal care. For delivery, referred

elsewhere. (Also general gynecological check-ups, acupuncture, family planning, counseling for teenagers. Medical coordination for both men and women.)

Kanda 2nd Clinic (Dr. Sayoko Makabe)
Umeda Bldg. 2 Fl., 3-20-14 Nishi-Azabu
Minato-ku, Tokyo
03-3402-0654 (Pub., Ins., Eng.)
Delivery at Aiiku Hospital (see page 133)

Dr. Claudine Bliah

03-3400-9942 (Eng., Fr.)
Prenatal care at Tokyo Medical and Surgical Clinic, referral to obstetrician there from mid-pregnancy. Also, at Aiiku Hospital, and referrals to obstetricians there for birth.

Bluff Clinic
(Naka-ku, Yokohama-shi; see page 34)
Delivery at Shonan Kamakura General Hospital (see page 345); obstetrician comes to the clinic twice a month.

During Pregnancy *ninshin* 妊娠

While most Japanese advice to pregnant women is similar to that given in the West, more attention is often given to the idea of avoiding stress and cold. For example, you may be told that driving during the last month of pregnancy is too stressful; riding a bicycle is too bumpy; wearing a mini-skirt is too cold, at least without thick tights; and washing the bathtub is too dangerous. Some of the advice you'll hear may sound outdated, but some may also make sense, considering the Japanese life-style.

Reading about pregnancy and birth will help you understand the tests you will undergo and prepare you for the coming event.

Prenatal Care *sanzen keā* 産前ケアー

Although in the West we usually speak of 40 weeks or 9 months of pregnancy, in Japan, pregnancy is said to last 10 months: the first month is 0 (the week of your last period)–3 weeks; the second month 4–7 weeks; the third 8–11 weeks; and so on, ending with the tenth month (36–39 weeks). For your ease in talking with caregivers in Japan, this system is used in this chapter.

Since prenatal care follows the guidelines of both the Ministry of Health and Welfare and local governments, similarities are found throughout Japan. The following tests performed at prenatal visits are general guidelines followed in Tokyo.

Prenatal visits
Once every 4 weeks until the 28th week, once every 2 weeks until the 35th week, and once a week from the 36th week.

Check at every visit:
■ Urine *nyōkensa* 尿検査 for protein and sugar.
■ Blood pressure *ketsuatsu sokutei* 血圧測定.
■ Weight *taijūsokutei* 体重測定.
■ Swelling *mukumi* むくみ; edema *fushu* 浮腫.
■ Abdominal circumference *fukui sokutei* 腹囲測定.
■ Height of the fundus of the uterus *shikyūtei chōsokutei* 子宮底長測定.

■ Fetal heartbeat, usually by doppler ultrasound *doppurā kensa* ドップラー検査 (from the third month).

Additional procedures and tests
■ Questions on medical history, life-style, etc. *Monshin* 問診 (first visit).
■ Internal exam *naishin* 内診; many facilities use a vaginal ultrasound probe *keichitsu chō-onpa kensa* 経腟超音波検査 (first visit; and weekly in the tenth month).
■ Measurement of pelvis (once during the pregnancy).

■ Blood tests *ketsueki kensa* 血液検査 to check for anemia (twice: early and late in pregnancy), blood type (ABO, RH), syphilis. hepatitis B, rubella (if suspicion of exposure in early pregnancy), toxiplasmosis (if suspicion of exposure). If you test positive for hepatitis B, your baby is entitled to free vaccinations against the virus from a designated facility after the birth.

■ External exam *gaishin* 外診 to check fetal size, position (every visit from the fifth month).

■ Breast and nipple exam *nyūbō to nyūtō kensa* 乳房と乳頭検査 (sixth month).

■ Dental exam (at dental clinic).

Supplementary tests

The following tests and procedures, although not included in the general guidelines for Tokyo, are routine at many facilities:

■ Abdominal ultrasound scan *keifuku chō-onpa kensa* 経腹超音波検査 from 10 weeks; frequency varies according to condition of mother and baby and obstetrician's practice—some two or three times (in early, mid-, and late pregnancy), others every visit; usually performed by an obstetrician, and not an ultrasound specialist.

■ Swab test to check for vaginal infections *chitsuen kensa* 腟炎検査 such as candida, group B streptococcus (seventh month).

■ Blood tests to check for the bleeding disease, idiopathic thrombocytopenic purpura (ITP) (third, ninth, and tenth months); nutritional deficiencies (fourth, seventh, ninth, and tenth months); liver disease (GOT, GPT) (fourth month); human T-cell leukemia-lymphoma virus (HTLV-1), which is endemic in Japan (seventh month); and hepatitis C.

■ Counting of fetal movement (ninth month, if indicated).

■ Non-stress test (tenth month).

■ Urine test to check placental functioning (for those who go past their due dates; at some clinics, routine for all women in the tenth month).

■ HIV/AIDS test *eizu kensa* エイズ検査 Routine at about 70 percent of hospitals (third month).

■ Ultrasound via vaginal probe for more accurate view and measurements is sometimes performed in the early months.

Optional tests

■ Pap smear *shikyū gan kensa* 子宮癌検査 (first visit).

■ Amniocentesis *yōsui kensa* 羊水検査 (at 16–18 weeks or as indicated).

RH Incompatibility *RH futekigō* RH不適合

Although Caucasians from northern Europe have a very high incidence of RH incompatibility, among Japanese the incidence is below ten percent. Most Japanese caregivers are not accustomed to handling this incompatibility, so if you are RH-negative and the father is positive, find a caregiver with recent experience of this condition, perhaps at an international facility or a large teaching hospital.

Testing for Fetal Disorders *taiji no kensa* 胎児の検査

Genetic testing in Japan is usually for those with family histories of congenital disorders *senten ijō* 先天異常. It is not recommended as routinely for expectant mothers over the age of thirty-five as it is in the U.S. Your doctor should be able to refer you to a testing center, however, at your request. Amniocentesis, which detects such disorders as Down syndrome and spina bifida, is performed at certain institutions around the country. The alpha-feto protein test (AFPT) screening is available at some hospitals. Chorionic villus sampling (CVS) is not presently used, because it can potentially do harm to the fetus. Discuss your situation with your doctor who will refer you if you are to be tested.

Screening for Tay-Sachs disease, sickle-cell anemia, and thalassemia is not generally available in Japan. If your ethnic origin (Eastern European [Tay-Sachs], black [sickle cell], or Mediterranean [thalassemia]) makes you a possible candidate for these conditions, discuss testing with your doctor, who will arrange for the test or give you a referral. The Toronomon Hospital in Tokyo (see page 344) is well known for its prenatal genetic testing and has a special outpatient clinic for this (*iden gairai* 遺伝外来) which you can use even without an introduction from your doctor. In Kansai, you may be referred to the Kobe University Hospital, Osaka Boshi Center, or other—especially university—hospitals in the area.

Resources

Tokyo Metropolitan Maternal and Child Health Services Center
03-3941-8818 (see page 58)
Information and referrals Mon.–Fri. 5:00–9:00 P.M.

The National Institute of Neurological Disorders and Stroke
31 Center Dr., MSC 2540, Bldg. 31, Rm. 8A16,
Bethesda, MD 20892-2540 U.S.
1-301-496-5751, 1-800-352-9424
http://www.ninds.nih.gov/
Information on screening for Tay-Sachs disease.

Japan Family Planning Association Genetic Counseling Center
Nihon Kazoku Keikaku Kyokai Iden Sodan Senta
日本家族計画協会遺伝相談センター
Hoken Kaikan Shinkan, 1-10 Tamachi, Ichigaya
Shinjuku-ku, Tokyo
03-3267-2600
Information on genetic testing.

For more resources, see page 163.

Morning Sickness tsuwari つわり

As with other conditions, Japanese caregivers are often more ready to hospitalize women who suffer from severe morning sickness.

Weight Gain taijū no zōka 体重の増加

Recommended weight gain during pregnancy is 8–10 kg in Japan, as opposed to 12–16 kg, depending on the size of the mother, in the U.S. Japanese caregivers tend to be very strict about weight control during pregnancy, because of their emphasis on natural birth and association of excessive weight gain with toxemia, diabetes, difficult deliveries, and more cesareans. Western caregivers are less strict about weight gain and are more adamant in warning women not to *lose* weight during pregnancy. If you are concerned about your caregiver's warnings on weight gain, consider his reasoning and perhaps get a second opinion, here or in your own country.

Childbirth textbooks for Japanese women give detailed advice on low-fat, low-sugar and low-salt diets for pregnancy and strict weight-gain schedules. Most suggest: a 500–800 g increase per month through the fifth month, and 1–2 kg per month after that, depending on how much was gained in the early stage of pregnancy. Women who gain 3–4 kg in any one month are advised to restrict fats and sugars and to exercise more. Some practitioners recommend a cesarean if total gain is more than 15 kg. With the change in the average size of the Japanese, however, one would expect these recommendations to become more flexible.

Nutrition eiyō 栄養

Japanese dietary recommendations naturally center around Japanese foods. Because of the high salt content in Japanese foods (the average daily intake is 11.7 g but can easily rise to 20 g), you'll notice a heavy emphasis on low salt intake. Women are told to allow themselves no more than 10 g per day (1 g = 1/5 tsp. of salt or 1 tsp. *shoyu*), and to avoid salty foods, such as *ramen* broth, Japanese pickles, *tonkatsu* sauce, and other sauces. They are told to avoid excess fat and sugar, and to be wary of highly-processed foods containing these and chemical additives, such as ready-made curry roux and bottled salad dressings.

Tokyo Government Dietary Advice for Mothers-to-be

Non-pregnant daily diet: 1,800 calories
(1 unit = 80 calories)

1 serving of milk or milk product (e.g., 200 ml milk); 1 egg.

60–80 g of lean meat; 60–80 g of lean fish; 60–80 g more of either meat or fish.

1 serving of soybeans or soybean products (e.g., 1/3 block tofu or 1 tbsp. *miso*).

100 g green or yellow vegetables (e.g., spinach, carrots); 200 g combination of pale vegetables (e.g., cabbage, *daikon*) and seaweed.

1 serving of fruit (e.g., 1 large *mikan* or 1/2 apple).

5 small bowls of rice or 5 thick slices of bread (loaf cut into 6 slices); 1 serving of potato (e.g., white potato 50 g).

2 servings of fat (e.g., 1 tbsp. margarine and 2 tsp. vegetable oil); 2 tbsp. sugar.

Early-pregnancy diet: 1,950 calories
To the "nonpregnant daily diet" add 1 glass of milk.
Increase meat serving by 20 g (if possible liver; increase fish serving by 10 g small fish (includes bones).
For vegetables, eat *hijiki* seaweed often.

Late-pregnancy diet: 2,150 calories
To the "early-pregnancy diet" add 10 g liver; 30 g green vegetables; 1 bowl of rice; 1 tsp. salad oil.

Breast-feeding diet: 2,500 calories
To the "late-pregnancy diet" add 1 1/3 glasses of milk; 1/2 bowl of rice and 2 tsp. vegetable oil.

Vitamin and Mineral Supplements

Prenatal vitamin, iron, and calcium supplements are not routinely recommended in Japan. Women are expected to get these from a healthy diet. Iron supplements are prescribed if deficiencies are detected (one in three women is said to develop anemia during pregnancy).

Exercise undō 運動

Japanese caregivers recommend very light exercise during the first four months and the last month of pregnancy. Maternity aerobics, swimming, and yoga classes are popular in Japan, and accept women from the fifth month of pregnancy. A midwife is often present at the classes for consultation and for minor checks such as blood pressure or weight gain. Many foreign women also enjoy these classes and benefit greatly from them. Some, however, criticize the underwater breath-holding practiced at maternity swimming classes, since it deprives both mother and baby of necessary oxygen.

For suggestions on prenatal exercise, ask your childbirth preparation teacher, ask at your local public health center or private fitness club, or try any of the following:

Maternity Yoga and Aerobics

The Yoga Circle
Minato-ku, Tokyo (see page 287)

Japan Maternity Yoga Association
Nihon Mataniti Yoga Kyokai
日本マタニティ・ヨーガ協会
Tokyo-to Josanpu Kaikan 5 Fl.
1-8-21 Fujimidai, Chiyoda-ku, Tokyo
03-3979-4688 (J. only)
Classes offered here and around Japan.

Japan Maternity Aerobics Association
Nihon mataniti-bikusu Kyokai
日本マタニティビクス協会
c/o High Hat Studio, Tanaka Bldg. 6 Fl.
5-25-1 Okusawa, Setagaya-ku, Tokyo
03-3725-0071 (J. only)
Classes from the fifth month offered here and around Japan.

Maternity Swimming

Children's Castle
Kodomo no Shiro
子供の城
5-53-1 Jingumae, Shibuya-ku, Tokyo
03-3797-5667 (J. only)

Nice Sports Tokyo
4-27-10 Higashi-Ikebukuro, Toshima-ku, Tokyo
03-3986-2233 (J. only)

Oahu Club Kiyoicho
TBR Bldg. 1 Fl., 5-7 Kojimachi, Chiyoda-ku, Tokyo
03-3234-1180 (J. only)

Tamagawa Swimming School
たまがわスイミングスクール
1-1455 Sanno-cho Kamimaruko, Nakahara-ku
Kawasaki-shi
044-422-5222 (J. only)

Massage and Other Therapies

To relieve the strains and stresses of pregnancy, Japanese women sometimes visit therapists for massage, shiatsu, acupuncture, aromatherapy and moxibustion. Midwives are generally familiar with these forms of treatment; try asking a midwife affiliated with the place where you will give birth, or contact one of the organizations on pages 119–20, for the name of a therapist in your area who is accustomed to treating pregnant women.

Miscarriage ryūzan 流産

Although complete bedrest is also suggested in the West for threatened miscarriage *seppaku ryūzan* 切迫流産 resulting from problems with the uterus, caregivers in Japan are more likely to suggest close medical observation in the hospital, possibly because Japanese insurance will cover this care.

If you do miscarry, Japanese obstetricians often use transvaginal ultrasound to check if a curretage (either suction *kyūin* 吸引 or sharp *sōha* 掻爬) is necessary to clean the uterus or if the miscarriage has been total. If you are scheduled to have the procedure, discuss anesthesia with your doctor beforehand. It is usually general anesthesia by intravenous drip, but some doctors use just a local cervical or paracervical block.

Japanese caregivers tend not to counsel women who have lost babies early on. You may want to contact an infertility specialist for genetic and other tests, especially for repeated problems (see page 135). The Prenatal and Infant Death Support Group (see page 331) has helped many to deal with their grief and to obtain published materials in both English and Japanese.

Admission to the Hospital/Clinic *nyūin* 入院

As you'll probably give birth at the facility where you received prenatal care, registration is usually just a matter of showing your patient ID card and then answering questions about the course of labor so far. You may also be asked to fill out a form or be questioned on what kind of food you want, etc.

What to Bring for a Five- to Seven-Day Stay (Typical advice; see also page 43)

Sold at the maternity/infant departments of most department stores:

■ 2 or 3 nursing bras *junyū-yō burajā* 授乳用ブラジャー.
Large sizes may be hard to find; try Isetan Department Store in Tokyo, or mail order from your country.

■ 2 abdominal binders *fukutai* 腹帯 or postpartum girdles/waist nipper 産後用ウエストニッパ.

■ 1-2 *koshimaki* 腰巻, a cotton flannel cloth (for winter) or bath towel (summer) to wrap around lower body, usually fastening with magic tape; keeps you warm after birth and protects your nightgown from getting soiled.

■ 6–7 postpartum pants *sanjoku-yō shōtsu* 産褥用ショーツ to hold pads in place.

■ 1 pack breast pads *bonyū paddo* 母乳パッド

■ 5–6 gauze handkerchiefs for wiping baby's mouth, etc.

■ 1 pack of large size sanitary napkins, special for birth *o-san-yō napukin* お産用ナプキン.

■ 2–3 cotton *T-jitai* T-字帯, a cotton G-string used instead of underpants to hold the pads in place.

Sold at most pharmacies:

■ sterile cotton with antiseptic *shōdoku men* 消毒綿 (to wipe perineum).

Also:

■ 2–3 nightgowns (cotton, front opening); 1 bathrobe; slippers; cup; chopsticks; spoon/fork; towels; toiletries (soap in container); shower cap; coins for laundry and vending machines; personal seal; *boshi techō* (including coupons); health insurance certificate; hospitalization certificate; telephone card; clock; plastic bags; tissues, clothes for the baby to wear going home.

Labor *jintsū* 陣痛

Practices vary. At births with an independent midwife, you can expect a very minimum of medical intervention—periodic doppler or trumpet monitoring, perhaps an enema. After being admitted to an Ob/Gyn clinic or a hospital, unless you've requested otherwise, you'll probably be given an enema and possibly a partial shave, then be put into a labor room until you're ready for delivery. External fetal monitoring may be intermittent or constant, depending on hospital/clinic policy, your condition, and the condition of your baby. Most caregivers today will encourage you to be upright and to move around periodically during labor. Intravenous glucose drips are not routine at all facilities, but many routinely insert a needle so that a vein will be ready in case of an emergency. Eating during labor is rarely prohibited, although most women have little appetite and stick to fluids and foods that are easy to digest. Some facilities permit showers during labor, but this is still rare.

Delivery *bunben* 分娩

At many hospitals or Ob/Gyn clinics, women are hooked up to an IV when they enter the delivery room, for possible emergency use. Although Japanese women traditionally squatted for birth, you'll probably be confined to the dorsal, semi-reclining, or seated position, though caregivers are increasingly more flexible about positioning. Instructions for pushing the baby out vary, ranging from forceful straining and prolonged breath-holding to gentle pushing and breathing the baby out. About 80–90 percent of first-time mothers have episiotomies, but some caregivers have much lower rates. As your baby is born, his/her breathing passages will probably be suctioned out vigorously. There is no custom in Japan of the father's cutting the cord. The cord will be cut and clamped by one of the caregivers and your baby put onto an infant warmer, if available, where the midwives will measure and check him/her. Although in some Western countries this practice has been abandoned, an antibiotic will be put in the baby's eyes to prevent infection. Some practitioners will, on request, deliver the baby onto the mother's abdomen and then give him/her to the mother to be put to the breast. If your facility still follows the Japanese tradition of *ubuyu*, the first bath after birth, your baby will be bathed as soon as he/she has been measured and determined healthy, about thirty minutes to an hour after the birth, and then wrapped up and handed to you for inspection. At some facilities, the baby is left with the mother to feed and to enjoy the two-hour stay in the recovery room together. More often, unfortunately, he/she is taken to the central nursery until the first breast-feeding several hours (or days) later.

Umbilical Cord *heso no o* へその緒, *saitai* 臍帯

In Japan the umbilical stub, which remains attached to the baby after the cutting of the cord, is kept for good luck after it dries and falls off. Don't be surprised if you are presented with a special box for it when you leave the hospital.

Premature Birth *sōzan* 早産

You are required to notify your public health center if your baby's birth weight was below 2,500 grams. If the doctor thinks it necessary, your baby will be hospitalized in a designated hospital and the care completely paid for by your insurer and the government. Remember that you can generally expect excellent care in Japanese neonatal intensive care units. Mothers are encouraged to express their breast milk and deliver it daily to their hospitalized baby. If you find you are being denied access to your baby without apparent reason, talk to your baby's doctor. Some mothers have been able to negotiate more participation in their baby's care.

Postpartum Care *sango keā* 産後ケアー, *sanjoku-ki keā* 産褥期ケアー

Although in the U.S. a sitz bath is commonly recommended to help soothe and heal the wound left by the episiotomy, in Japan baths are typically discouraged. Many facilities provide a toilet with a bidet. Most Japanese women don't use pain medication for the associated pain, though it is possible to ask for pain killers—usually a rectal suppository which will not affect breast milk. In Japan, postpartum recommendations for the new mother place a great emphasis on rest, keeping warm, and returning gradually to normal life. To prevent colds, you'll probably be told not to shower or shampoo until the third day or more after the birth (the eighth day if you've had a cesarean). For the same reason—and also to avoid infection—you'll probably be advised against taking a bath for three weeks after the birth, until the lochia has nearly stopped. The reason for this directive could also be because family members use the same bath water in Japan. In addition, you may be told not to read, to avoid straining your eyes during the first three weeks after birth.

Care of the Newborn *shinsei-ji no keā* 新生児のケアー
During the postpartum stay, most facilities provide instruction for new mothers in baby care and breast-feeding. Since the classes use visual aids, attending these classes can be interesting even if you don't understand Japanese.

Circumcision *katsurei* 割礼, *hōkei rinsetsu-jutsu* 包茎輪切術
Japanese babies are not circumcised, so Japanese caregivers are not accustomed to counseling on this procedure or performing it. Even in U.S. hospitals, circumcision is no longer a routine medical procedure, and the decision is left to the parents. You can find discussion on circumcision in most U.S. childbirth texts. Some Japanese obstetricians, usually those who have studied in the U.S., are familiar with infant circumcision, and will perform it on request. Urologists can usually perform the operation as well, but are not used to operating on little babies. Some doctors have required that the baby be kept in the central nursery for observation for up to twenty-four hours after the operation.

Sleeping Position *nekashi-kata* 寝かし方
Your baby will most likely be positioned on his/her back, in keeping with Japanese tradition. Several years ago the U.S. custom of putting babies to sleep on their stomachs was adopted by some facilities. However, recent research on Sudden Infant Death Syndrome indicates that putting babies to sleep on their back during the first six months is safer for most babies. In view of this, most have returned to the traditional Japanese practice.

Tests on the Newborn *shinsei-ji no kensa* 新生児の検査
At some point between the fifth and seventh days, babies are given the Guthrie inhibition assay test, a blood test to screen for hypothyroidism and inborn errors of metabolism including phenylketonuria (PKU), maple syrup urine disease, some forms of homocystinuria, and galactosemia. Most facilities routinely perform this test on all babies, but if the place where you give birth does not, or if you leave before the fifth day, you can have the test performed at a designated local clinic. A request form for this test is in-

cluded in the *boshi techō* packet (see page 118). The form should be sent to the facility you choose, preferably before the birth. Note that the test is free only at designated facilities. During the postpartum stay, your baby will also be checked for jaundice and treated if necessary. Blood typing is not routine but can be requested. Within a few days of the birth the obstetrician (a staff pediatrician at some facilities) will check your baby for any other abnormalities.

Vitamin K

During the postpartum stay, babies are routinely given a vitamin K syrup to prevent hemorrhaging, once 24 hours after the birth and again at discharge, 5–7 days after the birth. A third dose is given at the checkup at one month.

Bathing the Baby akachan no o-furo 赤ちゃんのお風呂

Although in the West babies are usually kept out of water until the umbilical stump falls off, in Japan your baby is likely to have the first bath within hours of birth. A nurse or midwife will also probably bathe your baby daily during your postpartum stay. Details vary, but the usual practice is to keep the baby dressed or wrapped in a cotton cloth while the midwife washes, rinses, and dries the face using a separate basin of warm water and gauze washcloth. Next, she submerges the baby, cotton cloth and all, up to the neck in water about forty degrees centigrade, and washes the hair and body with soap while the baby clutches the cloth, now floating freely in the water, to feel secure. She'll then hold the baby out of the water over the tub and pour clean, warm water over the body to rinse off the soapy water. After the bath, she'll clean the area around the umbilicus with a cotton bud dipped in alcohol to prevent infection.

If you want to learn the Japanese method of bathing a baby, attend the baby care classes offered during your postpartum stay or attend a class at your local public health center. The midwife from the public health center who visits you after the birth should also be able to show you how to bathe your baby this way in your own home.

For the first three weeks it is the custom for someone other than the new mother, usually the baby's grandmother or father, to bathe the baby. This explains why you'll see fathers attending bath demonstrations at the hospital or prenatal classes, even if they are missing at the birth! After the first month, babies use the big, family bath, usually held by the father, after being washed outside the tub in the usual Japanese fashion.

Breast-feeding bonyū junyū 母乳授乳, bonyū ikuji 母乳育児

A combination of tradition, U.S. postwar teachings, and recent Japanese innovations, you'll find some breast-feeding management in Japan quite different from that current in the West, and different from that presently recommended by the World Health Organization (see page 125). After the twentieth week of pregnancy, unless you are experiencing uterine contractions, most Japanese caregivers recommend nipple rolling and pulling, along with the application of olive oil or cold cream, to toughen the nipples. About 12–24 hours after the birth, midwives will routinely perform breast massage to encourage the flow of breast milk. There are several schools of thought on this procedure. The Oketani Method promotes a rigorous massage by professionals and restricts the mother's diet in various ways. Others encourage self-massage before or after the birth, and only recommend professional massage if problems arise.

With the exception of midwife clinics and facilities following the recommendations from WHO, breast-feeding in Japanese hospitals usually begins 8–24 hours or more after the birth. The first three days, until the "real milk" comes in, are considered a practice time, and breast-feeding is scheduled every 3–4 hours, supplemented with bottles of glucose water or formula. Although it is known that the colostrum, the "beginning milk," contains antibodies and other nutrients helpful to the baby, emphasis is more on letting the mother rest and become exposed gradually to the baby's sucking. This limited stimulation from the baby may partially explain the popularity of breast massage in Japan. In the West, to build up the mother's milk supply, the current recommended practice is not to give breast-fed babies bottles during the first three to four weeks, unless there is a medical reason. If supplementation is necessary, it is often given by a small medicine spoon, or a cup, to prevent nipple confusion.

Breast-feeding Resources

Viva Mamma

ビバマンマ (Midwife Kaoru Yanagisawa)
03-3643-0081
(Kiba, Tokyo; next-door to Toho Women's Clinic [see page 130])

La Leche League
(See page 119)

■ **Hiroko Hongo, MSW, IBCLC**
International Board Certified Lactation Consultant at Keikyu Department Store (045-848-1111) 5 Fl. Parenting Corner *ikuji sōdan-shitsu* in Kami-Ooka, Yokohama. Tues. 11:00 A.M.–4:00 P.M. Confirm hours with Maternity Dept. (*maternity uriba*) before visiting. Free of charge.

Bottle-feeding *jinkō eiyō* 人口栄養

Japanese women are all expected to breast-feed their babies, so you'll rarely be asked if you prefer to bottle-feed. But, since supplementation is extremely common, you'll find all kinds of formulas *miruku* ミルク and equipment. The midwives will teach you how to prepare formula during your postpartum stay. See page 305 about special formulas.

Returning Home

The security felt during the postpartum stay can break down when you return to your own home, and it's easy to feel isolated and insecure. If you have older children, getting rest can seem impossible. Don't hesitate to pick up the phone and call a friend or the childbirth or breast-feeding preparation groups for help and information.

In Japan, you are expected to stay in bed during the first two weeks after birth, and, in the third week, to be in and out of bed. During the fourth week, you'll be told you can gradually start to do light laundry, cook, tidy rooms, and bathe your baby and take him/her outside. From the fifth week on, with the permission of your doctor, you'll be advised that you can resume your regular life-style.

Home Help, Baby-sitting *hōmu herupā* ホームヘルパー, *bebī shittā* ベビーシッター

Several services in Japan will take care of older children while you are away for the birth and/or help you when you arrive home. Ask at childbirth preparation classes or La Leche meetings.

Resources

Poppins Service
(Minato-ku, Tokyo)
03-3447-2100 (Eng.)
http://www.poppins.co.jp

Baby Life Center
03-3485-0630, fax 03-3469-7387 (Tokyo area, including Chiba, Saitama, Kanagawa)
Ministry of Labor-approved company offers baby-sitting 24-hours a day; also light housework, postpartum care; very reasonable.

San Mark Mothering Center
03-3209-7612 (Eng.)
(Tokyo area, Sapporo, Sendai, Shizuoka, Nagoya, Kyoto, Osaka, Hiroshima, Fukuoka)
Professional total care of mother and baby; baby bath; breast massage; postpartum care. Rates reasonable.

Goonies
06-311-2911, fax 06-311-2912 (parts of Osaka, Nara, Kobe, and Kyoto)
Open all year; baby-sitting 24-hours a day while mother is in hospital; postpartum care. Rates reasonable, but minimum of three hours.

Home Visits *sango hōmon* 産後訪問

Sometimes foreign midwives or doulas will make home visits. If they aren't licensed to work in Japan, they cannot give medical advice, but they will be happy to visit your home to answer other questions about breast-feeding, baby care, and postpartum recovery. Call any of the childbirth education groups on pages 119–20.

Japanese midwives specializing in breast-feeding and breast massage can also be of help. Some have clinics; others pay home visits. For a referral ask at the facility where you gave birth, or try one of the midwives' organizations on page 128.

By sending in the postcard included with your *boshi techō*, you can also request a free visit from a public health nurse or midwife during the week or two after you return home. She will check both you and the baby, offer advice, answer questions, and come again if you request.

Postpartum Hostels

Jiairyo 慈愛寮
Shinjuku-ku, Tokyo
Apply through Tokyo Metropolitan Women's Counseling Center (To no Josei Sodan Senta 都の女性相談センター 03-5261-3110) or your local welfare office (in Japanese). Serves as a temporary dorm for single mothers or battered pregnant women from the eighth month until the baby is six months old.

Yachiyo Midwife Clinic
Yachiyo Josanin
八千代助産院
1-8-21 Fujimi-cho, Chiyoda-ku, Tokyo

03-3261-0626
Will house and take care of mothers and their
newborns for one month after the birth, even if
the birth was elsewhere.

Baby Equipment bebī yōhin ベビー用品

You can often save money by renting baby equipment. The groups on pages 119–20 also advertise secondhand items from time to time. For detailed information on baby needs in Japan, check out *Japan for Kids* (see "References and Further Readings").

Baby Equipment Rental Companies

Aiiku Baby 愛育ベビー
0120-350-540 (Tokyo/Yokohama)

Futabado 双葉堂
0120-17-2810 (Kyoto)

Osaka Baby Center 大阪ベビーセンター
0120-123747 (toll-free; Osaka)
0120-152655 (toll-free; Kobe)

Pediatricians shōni-ka'i 小児科医

Generally, the obstetrician, midwives, and a hospital pediatrician examine your newborn during your hospital stay and if problems arise during the first month of life. It is up to you to locate a pediatrician, preferably before the birth, who will become your child's primary caregiver after that. See page 157 for a list of pediatric clinics.

Registration of the Birth shussei todoke 出生届

The hospital or clinic will give you a birth certificate, which you must use to register your baby. Note that you may need a version in your language as well for registration at your embassy. There is no custom of foot printing. The deadline for naming babies is fourteen days after birth. All babies born in Japan must be registered within fourteen days of the birth at the local government office where they live or where they were born. You will need the Japanese birth certificate, the *boshi techō*, your national health certificate (members only), and both parents' alien registration cards. If you are enrolled in a National Health Insurance plan, you should also bring your health insurance certificate. You'll be issued two copies of a Japanese-language certificate of registration.

Check with your embassy about the procedures for birth registration and passport application for your own country. Usually the embassy requires the certificate of registration, the translation of the hospital birth certificate, photos of the baby, the passports of both parents, and a certified or original copy of your marriage certificate.

Unless your baby has Japanese citizenship, you must bring the certificate of registration to the alien registration section of your local government office for alien registration within sixty days of birth. Apply for a visa at the immigration office within thirty days of birth; you'll need the baby's passport, both parents' alien registration cards, and the registration certificate. Within fourteen days of receiving the visa, bring the baby's passport and registration certificate to your local government office for registration.

If your baby has Japanese citizenship, be sure to register him in the family register and get a Japanese passport. It is illegal for him to leave the country without it.

Postnatal Checkups *sango kenshin* 産後健診
One month after the birth, both you and your baby will return for a checkup to the place where your baby was born. If you have any problems before that time, you can always call the midwives or doctors there.

Emergency Birth
Even if you have a car, keep a list of taxi companies' phone numbers, and learn how to direct them in Japanese to your home. Know the layout of your hospital and where the emergency/night entrance is.

Ambulances may not be used for normal birth, but can be called for obstetrical emergencies like heavy bleeding. Although you may ask the crew to take you to your selected hospital, in an emergency, for the sake of you and the baby, you'll want quick attention. See the front endpapers for phrases to use when calling an ambulance.

Kyūkyūsha onegai shimasu.	Ambulance, please.
Akachan ga sugu ni umare sō desu.	My baby is about to be born.

Childbirth Terms
(See also the Glossary.)

General

female doctor *joi* 女医
home birth *katei bunben* 家庭分娩
midwife clinic *josan'in* 助産院
midwife, nurse-midwife *josanpu* 助産婦
obstetrician *sanka-i* 産科医
part-time doctor *shokutaku-i* 嘱託医
waterbirth *suichū shussan* 水中出産

Pregnancy *ninshin* 妊娠

abortion *(jinkō ninshin) chūzetsu* （人工妊娠）中絶
acupressure *shiatsu* 指圧
acupuncture *hari* 鍼
amniocentesis *yōsui kensa* 羊水検査
bleeding *shukketsu* 出血
blood type *ketsueki-gata* 血液型
due date, expected date of delivery *bunben yotei-bi* 分娩予定日
ectopic pregnancy *shikyū-gai ninshin* 子宮外妊娠

engagement (fetal head) *kotei (jitō)* 固定（児頭）
fetal heartbeat *taiji shin'on* 胎児心音
fetus *taiji* 胎児
heartburn *muneyake* 胸やけ
high blood pressure *kō-ketsuatsu* 高血圧
inverted nipple *kanbotsu nyūtō* 陥没乳頭
iron-deficiency anemia *tetsu ketsubō-sei hinketsu* 鉄欠乏性貧血
last menstrual period *saishū gekkei* 最終月経
low-salt diet *teien-shoku* 低塩食
miscarriage *ryūzan* 流産
morning-after pill *yokuasa no hinin-zai* 翌朝の避妊剤
morning sickness *tsuwari* つわり
moxibustion *o-kyū* お灸
nausea *hakike* 吐き気
ovarian cyst *ransō nōshu* 卵巣のう腫
overweight *futorisugi* 太りすぎ
pelvic exam, internal exam *naishin* 内診
pelvis *kotsuban* 骨盤

post-term pregnancy *kaki ninshin* 過期妊娠

pregnancy test *ninshin hannō* 妊娠反応

pregnant *ninshin shite iru* 妊娠している

pregnant woman *ninpu* 妊婦

prenatal *sanzen* 産前

raped *gōkan sareta* 強姦された

threatened miscarriage *seppaku ryūzan* 切迫
流産

toxemia *ninshin chūdoku-shō* 妊娠中毒症

twins *futago* 双子

ultrasound scan, sonogram *chō onpa kenshin*
超音波検診

unmarried *mikon* 未婚

uterine fundus *shikyū-tei* 子宮底

uterine myoma *shikyū kinshu* 子宮筋腫

vagina *chitsu* 腟

vaginal discharge *taige, orimono* 帯下、
おりもの

Labor and Birth *jintsū to shussan* 陣痛と
出産

abnormality *ijō* 異常

afterbirth, placenta *taiban* 胎盤

amniotic fluid *yōsui* 羊水

analgesic *chintsū-zai* 鎮痛剤

anesthesia *masui* 麻酔

artificial rupture of the membranes *jinkō
hamaku* 人工破膜

(artificial) speeding of labor *jintsū sokushin*
陣痛促進

balanced anesthesia *baransu masui-hō*
バランス麻酔法

birth *shussan, osan* 出産、お産

birth canal *sandō* 産道

bloody show *shirushi* しるし（産徴）

breathing pattern *kokyūhō* 呼吸法

breech position *sakago* 逆子

castor oil *himashiyu* ひまし油

cesarean *teiō-sekkai* 帝王切開

continuous epidural anesthesia *jizoku kōmakugai masui* 持続硬膜外麻酔

contraction *shūshuku, itami* 収縮、いたみ

deep breath *shin-kokyū* 深呼吸

delivery *bunben* 分娩

delivery room *bunben-shitsu* 分娩室

dilate *hiraku* 開く

dilation *kaidai* 開大

effaced *tentai shita* 展退した

electronic fetal monitor *monitā, taiji kanshi
sōchi* モニター、胎児監視装置

enema *kanchō* 浣腸

episiotomy *ein sekkai* 会陰切開

father attending birth *otto tachiai bunben* 夫立
ち合い分娩

fetal distress *taiji kashi* 胎児仮死

forceps *kanshi* 鉗子

full dilation *zen-kaidai* 全開大

general anesthesia *zenshin masui* 全身麻酔

hyperventilation *ka-kanki* 過換気

inhalation anesthesia *kyūnyū masui* 吸入麻酔

induction of labor *jintsū yūhatsu* 陣痛誘発

labor *jintsū* 陣痛

labor room *jintsū-shitsu* 陣痛室

local anesthesia *kyokubu masui* 局部麻酔

massage *massāji* マッサージ

meconium staining *taiben senshoku* 胎便染色

nitrous oxide anesthesia *shōki masui* 笑気麻酔

normal delivery *seijō bunben* 正常分娩

nothing by mouth *zesshoku* 絶食

perineal tear *ein resshō* 会陰裂傷

perineum *ein-bu* 会陰部

physiological jaundice *seiri-teki ōdan* 生理的
黄疸

pitocin *pitōshin* ピトーシン

placenta *taiban* 胎盤

placenta previa *zenchi taiban* 前置胎盤

position during delivery *bunben tai-i* 分娩体
位

precipitous delivery *kyūzan* 急産

premature birth *sōzan* 早産

prolapsed cord *saitai dasshutsu* 臍帯脱出

push, to *ikimu* 息む

relax *rirakkusu* リラックス

shave *teimō* 剃毛

spinal anesthesia *sekizui masui* 脊髄麻酔

squat, to *shagamu* しゃがむ

stillbirth *shizan* 死産

suture *hōgō* 縫合

transition *ikō-ki* 移行期

umbilical cord *heso no o, saitai* へその緒、
臍帯

vacuum extraction *kyūin bunben* 吸引分娩

vaginal delivery *keichitsu bunben* 経腟分娩

1st (2nd, 3rd) stage *bunben dai ikki (niki, sanki)*
分娩第一（二、三）期

How frequent are your contractions? *itami wa
nanpun oki desu ka* 痛みは何分おきですか

My contractions are ten minutes apart *itami wa
juppun oki desu* 痛みは十分おきです

I had the bloody show *shirushi ga arimashita*
しるしがありました

My waters broke *hasui shimashita* 破水
しました

I want to push *ikimitai* 息みたい

Push now *ima ikinde* 今息んで

Don't push *ikimanaide* 息まないで

Breast-feeding bonyū junyū 母乳授乳

bottle *honyū-bin* 哺乳ビン

breast *oppai, nyūbō* おっぱい, 乳房

breast massage *nyūbō massāji* 乳房マッサ
ージ

breast pump *sakunyū-ki* 搾乳器

breast-feeding room *junyū-shitsu* 授乳室

breastmilk *bonyū* 母乳

colostrum *shonyū* 初乳

formula *miruku* ミルク

glucose water *tōsui* 糖水

mastitis *nyūsen'en* 乳腺炎

mixed feeding *kongō eiyō* 混合栄養

nipple *nyūtō, chikubi* 乳頭, 乳首

nipple shield *nyūtō ate* 乳頭あて

suck *su-u* 吸う

I want to breast-feed *o-chichi o agetai desu*
お乳を上げたいです

My nipples are sore *chikubi ga itai -desu*
乳首がいたいです

My breasts are full *o-chichi ga hatte imasu*
お乳が張っています

Postpartum sanjoku-ki 産褥期

afterpains *ko-jintsū* 後陣痛

baby *akachan* 赤ちゃん

birth certificate *shussei shōmei-sho* 出生証
明書

circumcision *katsurei, hōkei-rinsetsu-jutsu*
割礼, 包茎輪切術

home visit *sango hōmon* 産後訪問

jaundice *ōdan* 黄疸

lochia *orimono, oro* おりもの、悪露

meconium *taiben* 胎便

naval, umbilicus *heso* 臍

neonatal intensive care unit (NICU) *shinsei-ji
shūchū chiryō-shitsu NICU*, 新生児集中治
療室

newborn baby *shinsei-ji* 新生児

nursery *shinsei-ji-shitsu* 新生児室

postnatal *sango* 産後

rooming-in *boshi dōshitsu* 母子同室

vernix *taishi* 胎脂

Please bring my baby *akachan o tsurete kite
kudasai* 赤ちゃんを連れてきてください

May I hold my baby? *akachan o daite mo ii desu
ka?* 赤ちゃんをだいてもいいですか

May I see my baby? *akachan o mite mo ii desu
ka?* 赤ちゃんを見てもいいですか

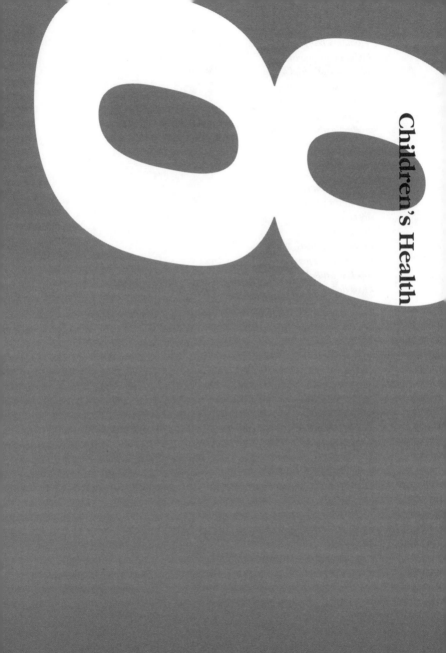

Children's Health

"I took my baby out of the house for the first time when she was three weeks old, in a front-facing baby carrier. It was an American-style product with support for the baby's neck, and so it could be used with a newborn. A middle-aged Japanese woman whom I had never met before stopped me on the street and asked me how old my daughter was. When I told her, she was shocked and asked what I was doing outside (I didn't know then that Japanese babies don't leave the house for the first month). Then she asked me why I was carrying my daughter in such a carrier, and said it looked like the baby was suffocating. Needless to say, it was upsetting to be accosted with this unsolicited advice, particularly from someone I didn't even know."

Cross-Cultural Troubleshooting

At times the hardest thing about being a parent in a foreign country is being bombarded with advice and suggestions about child-rearing practices that you don't understand, or that contradicts everything that you have been taught.

Every culture has its own thinking and traditions about child care. When comparing ideas from Japan and your own country, you don't have to decide that one is right and the other is wrong, just bear in mind that they are different and that they offer you new alternatives that you might not have thought about before. Your doctor or nurse may make a suggestion on some point of childrearing with which you cannot agree. It's probably best to listen politely. Later on, you may want to consider whether the advice is culturally based, or whether it's practical advice that happens to work well in the Japanese environment. For example, your own mother may be astounded to hear that you are bathing your baby in water heated to forty degrees centigrade, but in Japanese homes, where there is no central heating, this is a good way to warm up just before going to bed. If you don't think someone's advice is useful, ignore it if you wish; just don't try to convert anybody to your own way of thinking, since this may lead to hard feelings. Here are a few possible areas of contention and potential topics for gossip in your neigborhood:

Children Should Be Lightly Dressed

After a child reaches about four kilograms in weight he has enough body fat to regulate his own body temperature. Many in the Japanese medical community believe that in order to raise a child resistant to colds, etc., a baby should be dressed in one layer less than an adult.

Traditionally the Japanese feel that as long as the abdomen is well covered, a child will be able to maintain his body temperature. For this reason, special belly bands *haramaki* 腹巻き are sold to wear at night, so that even if a child throws off his covers, his stomach area won't get cold. Nurses often tell mothers not to put socks on their babies' feet while in the house, since wearing socks limits the baby's ability to directly sense and perceive the outside world. Some mothers, however, carry this to extremes and prefer not to use socks at all, even outside on winter days, in the belief that this helps the baby to regulate his own temperature.

School-age children are encouraged to become *kaze no ko* 風の子 or "children of the wind," dressing in shorts, skirts, and thin jackets even in winter. Some private kindergartens have taken this concept even further by creating year-round "shirtless" classes.

No Bath Until a Sick Child Is Fully Recovered

Since the water in Japanese baths is traditionally used for relaxing and is very warm, children who have a fever and a slight cold or cough are usually instructed not to bathe. The American practice of bathing a febrile child in lukewarm water to lower his temperature is rarely practiced here; instead, ice packs are wrapped in a towel and placed under the child's head and neck and under his arms.

Breast-feeding, Weaning, and Appropriate Weight Gain

"After the birth of my first child, a public health nurse made a home visit, and we ran into problems when we started talking about breast-feeding. I told her that I was following the suggestions of the La Leche League and giving my daughter only breast milk. She insisted that I had to give her water twice a day in a bottle. I disagreed. She later called my husband at work, was very concerned, and said that if we wouldn't agree she would have to make a return visit. My husband quickly lied and said that of course we would do it. I guess that I shouldn't have turned this into a philosophical battle, and should have just nodded my head in the first place."

Opinions may vary on any of these points. In Japan, mothers may be told to start soup at two months and solids when the child reaches about seven kilograms (nineteen pounds), usually at five or six months. Mothers are also encouraged to make their own home-made baby foods, or "weaning foods" *rinyū shoku* 離乳食 (see pages 305–306).

Remember that percentiles for growth charts are determined by the average Japanese child, and that charts for your own country may differ slightly. Perhaps surprisingly, though, the Japanese and the American charts are almost identical.

Early Toilet Training

Many doctors encourage parents to have their children sit on a potty chair from the age of eighteen months, at a specified time each day, while the parent makes a whooshing sound to encourage defecation. This training—which from a Western point of view is likely to have little effect until the child is good and ready to be trained—is supposed to continue so that by two years of age, the diapers are removed completely and the child is basically trained.

No Diagnosis of Infantile Colic

Americans usually say that a baby has colic when he has daily periods of loud crying, as if they were in abdominal pain, for no apparent reason. It's said to start at two to four weeks of age and end at three to four month. Japanese haven't identified this syndrome but they do use *yonaki* 夜泣き to describe uncontrollable crying at night for no known reason. There's also a traditional term *kan no mushi* かんの虫 that describes continual hard crying, which is resolved by going to a designated temple to pray.

"Skinship" and Sleeping

The word *sukinshippu* スキンシップ has been borrowed—or, rather, invented—from English to denote touching the skin to deepen a relationship or a feeling of love. It's usually used to describe the bonding process, when a mother and baby touch after birth, and so develop an emotional and physical attachment. It's also used now for the need to hug and touch your child, so that he or she feels your love, and is used in reference to older children too. Japanese mothers traditionally have not used kisses as a way to express their love, but have used other forms of physical closeness, like bathing together and carrying their babies everywhere on their backs with a special baby strap *obui himo* おぶいひも.

When it comes to sleeping, or putting the baby or child to bed, the need for skinship is often emphasized these days. Parents and children have traditionally slept together, but now the emphasis is different: mothers are encouraged to lay down beside their child, talk them to sleep, and share skinship with them (although caution should be used, since the number-one cause of accidental death among children under one is suffocation, usually in bed).

Doctors Take a Wait-and-See Attitude

"My second child was an early walker, and at one was already attempting to run. However, whenever he tried to, he'd step on his feet and fall flat on his face. I took Bobby for a well-child checkup at the maternity clinic where he was born and questioned the pediatrician, but she felt that his legs were not unduly out of alignment and that he would "grow out of it." This did not seem right to me, so I took him to the same internist who treated the rest of the family. He did not seem especially concerned either, but since I was worried he referred me to an orthopedic surgeon. The surgeon agreed that my son did need treatment to straighten his legs, and after wearing leg braces for a short time, he was soon running in the park."

In Japan, doctors often take the attitude that children will grow out of anything, including delayed speech or difficulties in walking, if given a little time. This may be true in some cases, but not always. Certain conditions need to be evaluated and treatment started early. Treatment delays may be compounded by long waits for hospital beds for elective surgery.

Maternal Guilt

"A friend's one-year-old son Yohei burned his hand on some hot soup that had been placed on a low table. When she rushed him to the nearest clinic, the first question the doctor asked her was whether her husband had been angry with her for the negligence that had allowed Yohei to be injured."

As mothers are expected to be perfect, problems with the child are often blamed on lapses in maternal care. It is not unusual for mothers to be made to feel guilty. For example, the mother of an asthmatic child may be assumed to be a poor housekeeper, and injuries suffered in normal playground activity are blamed on lack of parental supervision.

Although most of the examples given here focus on young children, you'll probably find that differences in thinking about parenting continue to arise throughout the course of your child's development. Try not to let different beliefs and customs come between you and your doctor, nurse, or other health care provider.

Be Prepared

In Japan you may be living far from grandparents and other extended family members, so you may feel isolated or unsure of the "right way" to do something. For handy references on children's health, growth, and development, that you will want to keep on your shelf, see "References and Further Reading."

Choosing a Pediatrician

In a foreign country, sudden bouts of fever or illness can be quite frightening, and you can be sure that these will probably happen at the worst possible time, such as late at night or during a holiday. Prepare ahead. Choose your child's doctor in advance, and plan what you'll do in an emergency.

Ideally, one pediatrician would take care of all your child's needs, but in reality you may need to look for more health providers. In Japan, pediatricians (or other doctors) are rarely available after hours, and they prefer that certain ailments be treated by other specialists, such as ENT physicians or dermatologists. Even if you need to use various clinics and hospitals, choosing one pediatrician to coordinate your child's care and assist you in finding the necessary resources is highly recommended (see page 25 for hints on how to choose a doctor and a hospital). Try asking your friends or neighbors for recommendations. Check out the doctor by visiting him for a minor ailment—nothing can beat the assurance that there is someone to turn to when your child gets sick. During your first visit, don't forget to ask whether the doctor is available after hours and in emergencies. Some doctors offer a phone-in consultation service for regular patients for a small fee. This may or may not be available after clinic hours. Also ask the doctor's advice on what to do in an emergency.

Some neighborhood internists will also treat children. Their location may make them convenient for minor problems, but since they're not pediatricians they may misinterpret symptoms. If you decide on a pediatrician in the outpatient department of a hospital, make a note of the days he comes in, since doctors often rotate.

If your child needs hospitalization, see "Choosing a Caregiver and Using the System." Note that visiting times and rules about staying overnight with a child will vary from one hospital to another. See page 62 for more on health care subsidies for children.

Notes on Treatment Differences

Common childhood diseases may sometimes be treated differently in Japan.

■ Ear infections (or otitis media) *chū ji en* 中耳炎 in children seems to be a problem worldwide. Many times ear infections can become a recurring concern. In Japan, ear problems are treated by ENT doctors rather than pediatricians; in fact, your doctor may never look into your child's ears. So as a parent you may have to be more on your toes, especially if your child has chronic problems. Children who suffer from chronic otitis media can have a fluid buildup behind the eardrum that is difficult to drain. Known in English as serous otitis media, or otitis media with effusion, *shinshutsusei chūji en* 浸出性中耳炎 can affect a child's hearing. For children under three, the standard treatment policy in Japan is medical. For older children, doctors will treat the condition for three months and if no improvement is seen, will perform such surgical treatment as inserting a tube to drain the ear. In the case of younger children, this is usually an inpatient procedure.

■ Childhood allergies like asthma and atopic dermatitis are very common in Japan, perhaps due to the environment. See pages 183–84 for information on the way these are usually treated.

■ Squint eye, or strabismis *shashi* 斜視, occurs when the eyes do not move in synch. If your child has an oriental eye shape with extra skin along the inner eye, it can sometimes be difficult to tell if the eyes are moving together or not. Eye exams can be done by an ophthalmologist *ganka-i* 眼科医 (see pages 94–95).

■ A febrile convulsion *nessei keiren* 熱性痙攣 can be very frightening for both parent and child. To prevent a recurrence, parents are instructed in Japan to keep a careful watch on their child's temperature and general condition. Ice packs and an oral fever medication are recommended for feverishness, and a suppository of diazepam (an anti-convulsion medication available by prescription) is given at that time, to prevent convulsions from recurring.

■ If a child has a cold and a fever, the cause is probably viral, but some Japanese medical texts recommend that a physician prescribe four days of antibiotics to prevent the child's condition from worsening.

■ As Japanese public health insurance and hospital policies discourage long-term antibiotic treatment, remember that pediatricians will only prescribe antibiotics for a short time, asking you to return frequently for follow-up visits—usually every two to three days—so that they can keep a close watch on the child and renew the prescription.

Communicable Diseases in Children

■ See pages 198–208 for details on many "catching" diseases.

■ Because of a new law that recently went into effect, making vaccinations elective, there may be an increase in the incidence of preventable diseases like whooping cough and measles among children in Japan.

■ Some diseases such as roseola *toppatsu sei hosshin* 突発性発疹 occur with such regularity that the majority of children under the age of one contract them (see pages 204–205).

■ Acute bronchiolitis *kyūsei saikikanshi-en* 急性細気管支炎 is very contagious and occurs frequently in Japan from winter through early spring in children ranging from six

Children's Health

weeks to two years old, and particularly often in children about six months old. Various viruses can cause it, but in Japan, the culprit in sixty percent of cases is the respiratory syncytial virus (RSV). Because one of the symptoms is wheezing, this is sometimes mistakenly diagnosed as the first episode of bronchial asthma *kikanshi zensoku* 気管支喘息. It is interesting to note that since male babies have smaller airways then females, they may be more susceptible to acute bronchiolitis.

■ Acute vomiting and diarrhea in Japan are usually viral. To replace lost fluids, sports drinks like Pocari Sweat or Gatorade can be given with a spoon. Medical electrolyte solutions like Aqualite アクアライト are also available in large drugstores.

■ Children love to play in sandboxes. In Japan, however, dogs and cats like to play there too, which poses dangers to children of roundworm infection. If a child ingests feces, they may develop this infection, also known as ascariasis. Sometimes there are few symptoms, with the only indication being white eggs in the child's stool. Tokyo and other cities are now constructing sandboxes with wire fencing to prevent animals from entering.

Tips for the Parent for an Outpatient Visit

■ If the child has a communicable disease, call ahead to ask when is the best time to register, etc.

■ If you're not used to the metric system, bring conversion tables for weight, height, and temperature so that you and the doctor can speak the same language. Note also that temperatures are usually taken under the arm in Japan, which gives a lower reading than temperatures taken in the mouth, rectum, or ear. So be sure to take your child's temperature under the arm at some point when he is not sick, so you have a gauge of what a normal temperature is for him.

■ Depending on the day and time, you may have a long wait before you actually see the doctor, so give your child some fever medicine before you go, so he won't suffer unduly—preferential treatment is rarely given to "sicker" children.

■ Medications prescribed in powdered form are very common. The paper envelopes are supposed to be ripped open and the powder swallowed in one gulp—something that is very difficult for small children to do. One idea is to dilute the medicine in a teaspoon of water and give it with an eyedropper. Make sure that you learn the name of the medicine from the pharmacist who prepares the packet. Sometimes more than one type will be mixed together, especially in the case of cold preparations, and there are no identifying numbers on the medicine itself (as there would be with pills or capsules).

Pediatric Clinics

For other English-speaking pediatricians, contact one of the AMDA centers (see the endpapers). Also see major children's hospitals (pages 164–65) and major general hospitals with pediatric departments (listed in "Regional Resources").

Suwa Michiko Pediatric Clinic
Nikko Royal Palace Rm. 103, 5-16-4 Hiroo
Shibuya-ku, Tokyo
03-3444-7070 (Pub. Ins., Eng.)
Canada- and U.S.-trained doctor.

Akaike Clinic
O.A.G. House 4Fl., 7-5-56 Akasaka,
Minato-ku, Tokyo
03-3584-1727 (Pub. Ins., Eng.)

**Tokyo University Hospital
(Dept. of Pediatrics)**
Tokyo Daigaku Igakubu Fuzoku Byoin (Shoni-ka)
(Bunkyo-ku, Tokyo; see page 344)
03-5800-8903 (Dr. Yoichi Sakakibara)
Fluent English; specializes in pediatric neurology
and development, but also does general pediatrics. Also assists in coordinating vaccination
schedules. Appointment necessary.

Dr. Norio Endo
2-24-13-305 Kami-Osaki, Shinagawa-ku, Tokyo
03-3492-6422 (Pub. Ins., Eng.)
Pediatrics and internal medicine.

Yamamoto Pediatric Clinic
Yamamoto Shoni-ka I'in 山本小児科医院
1-7-3 Hon-cho, Kokubunji-shi, Tokyo
042-325-3101 (Pub. Ins., Eng.)

Abe Clinic Abe I'in 阿部医院
2-5-7 Taira-cho, Meguro-ku, Tokyo
03-3717-2288 (Pub. Ins., Eng.)

Saito Pediatric Clinic
Saito Shoni Naika Kurinikku
5-13-10 Shimo-Hoya, Hoya-shi, Tokyo
0424-21-7201 (Pub. Ins., Eng.)
Pediatrics and internal medicine.

Shioda Clinic
Shioda I'in 塩田医院
6224-6 Izumi-cho, Izumi-ku, Yokohama-shi
045-804-6655 (Pub. Ins., Eng.)

Mukaiyama Clinic
Mukaiyama Shoni-ka I'in 向山小児科医院
22-1 Honmoku-Sannotani, Naka-ku

Yokohama-shi
045-623-7311 (Pub. Ins., Eng.)

Tame Pediatric Clinic
Tame Shoni-ka ため小児科
6-14 Yamanote 2-jo, 1-chome
Nishi-ku, Sapporo-shi
011-611-3718 (Pub. Ins., Eng.)

Takashita Pediatric Clinic
Takashita Shoni-ka I'in 高下小児科医院
Daiichi Bldg. 2Fl., Nishi 16-chome, Kita 4-jo
Chuo-ku, Sapporo-shi
011-631-6521 (Pub. Ins., Eng.)

Yamanaka Tatsuru Pediatric Clinic
Yamanaka Tatsuru Shoni-ka Byoin
山中たつる小児科病院
3-9 Minami, Nango-dori 11-chome, Shiroishi-ku
Sapporo-shi
011-866-5555 (Pub. Ins., Eng.)

Kyogoku Children's Clinic
Kyogoku Shoni-ka Kurinikku
京極小児科クリニック
8-13 Kusunoki-cho, Ashiya-shi, Hyogo-ken
0797-31-2735 (Pub. Ins., Eng.)

Kobayashi Medical Clinic
Kobayashi I'in 小林医院
3-31-4 Higashi-Kohama, Sumiyoshi-ku, Osaka-shi
06-671-3101 (Pub. Ins., Eng.)
Pediatrics, internal medicine, and dermatology.

Kimura Pediatric Clinic
Kimura Shoni-ka きむら小児科
11-41 Toyotsu-cho, Suita-shi, Osaka-fu
06-338-5050 (Eng.), fax 06-821-0885

Sono Clinic
Sono Naika Shoni-ka ソノ内科小児科
3-13-16 Nishi-Midorigaoka, Toyonaka-shi
Osaka-fu
06-848-0057 (Pub. Ins., Eng.)
Doctor has U.S. experience.

Yamawaki Pediatric Clinic
Yamawaki Shoni-ka 山脇小児科
5-16 Hon-dori, Naka-ku, Hiroshima-shi
082-247-0634 (Pub. Ins., some Eng.)

Well-Child Check *kenkō shindan* 健康診断

Well-child checks should be a chance to evaluate your child's development and discuss any problems or concerns with your doctor. The American Academy of Pediatrics recommends that your child be seen eight times during the first year of life, then at least yearly through puberty. Ideally, your primary pediatrician—who knows your child well—would also perform his growth and developmental screening, and many doctors in Japan will in fact do this. Some clinics and most hospitals also offer well-child visits, and usually schedule them so that well and ill children are not in the waiting room together. Compared with the usual "three-minute consultations" necessitated by the public health insurance system, doctors will usually take time to do a careful exam, answer questions, and offer guidance. However, these visits are not covered by insurance, since they are considered preventive, rather than a form of treatment.

In Japan well-child checks (the Japanese term for which is often shortened to *kenshin*), are traditionally conducted at public health centers. At the ages of three or four, six, nine, and eighteen months, and then again at three years, a pediatrician, public health nurse, and/or a dentist will perform the checks, and a nutritionist may also give a lecture—to the mother.

The checks frequently have an assembly-line feeling to them, and also may be difficult if you don't speak Japanese. However, these exams, like the vaccinations that are administered under Public Health Department mandates, are free of charge to community residents. Some checks are done at designated sites other than the public health centers.

The following should give you some idea of what to expect at the checkups given to children of various ages:

■ Age 3–4 months: Nutrition and weight gain checkup, advice on making your own baby food, consultation on skin allergies, TB skin test followed by BCG.

■ Age 6–7 months: Absorbent paper is mailed home for an early-detection urine test for neuroblastoma, a type of tumor in the adrenal glands above the kidneys.

■ Age 6 months and 9 months: Two more developmental screenings are usually offered free during the first year. These aren't usually held at the public health center, but at a central location; alternatively, you may be able to go to a doctor of your choice. Ask at your public health center.

■ Age 18 months: General physical checkup and an evaluation of language development. A dental check is also given at this time. Fluoride treatments may be started.

■ Age 3 years: Vision testing and language development are emphasized.

Vaccinations *yobō chūsha* 予防注射

If you look at the chart on pages 160–161 and compare the vaccination schedules for Japan, the U.S., the U.K., and the Philippines, you'll find that the vaccinations themselves are basically the same, and only the timing is different. Each country makes its schedule based on its own medical conditions. While in Japan, you'll have to decide if and when to vaccinate your child, and if you do, which schedule to follow.

You may want to consider whether you'll be here for a short- or long-term stay, where in Japan you'll be living, and whether your child will attend an international or a Japanese school. In Japan, the government schedule consists of six vaccines: polio *shōni mahi* 小児麻痺; DPT (also called the triple combined vaccine) *sanshu kongō* 三種混合, (including diptheria *jifuteria* ジフテリア, pertussis *hyaku nichi zeki* 百日咳, and tetanus *hashōfū* 破傷風); TB skin test *tsuberukurin hannō* ツベルクリン反応, given before the BCG vaccine, measles *hashika* 麻疹, rubella (German measles) *fūshin* 風疹, and Japanese encephalitis *nihon nōen* 日本脳炎. Chickenpox (varicella zoster) *mizubōsō* 水痘, mumps *otafukukaze* おたふくかぜ, and influenza *infuruenza* インフルエンザ vaccines are offered privately for a fee. Note that the Haemophilus influenza b (Hb) vaccine is not available except at a few foreigner-oriented clinics, and that the MMR vaccine is not available as a single vaccine in Japan.

On the chart, the numbers in parentheses indicate the age at which children can receive a vaccine from the public health department. If you don't vaccinate your child then for some reason, the vaccine can still be obtained free up to the upper age limit (also indicated on the chart), at a designated clinic.

The Japanese schedule tends to begin later, and seems more conservative, than the schedules of other countries. One reason for this is concern about possible side effects of vaccines. By law, the Japanese government will compensate children who suffer side effects from any vaccines that are included in the government schedule, usually by covering the cost of medical treatment.

With the revision of the Vaccination Law in 1994, vaccines are no longer compulsory, although they are still recommended. The Public Health Department still coordinates the program, but instead of group vaccinations at the public health center (except in the cases of polio and BCG vaccines), community pediatricians are now under contract to the government to administer the free vaccines.

When your child receives a vaccination in Japan, a questionnaire must be filled out, which varies with the specific vaccine. The BCG form will, for example, ask about skin troubles (皮膚のトラブル); the polio form about diarrhea (下痢); and the measles form about allergies to eggs (鶏卵). You will need to stamp the questionnaire with your personal seal to validate it, and also to report your child's morning temperature. After a vaccination, doctors recommend that children do not take a bath since it's assumed that they may have a fever or be in a weakened condition. Any vaccination your child receives will be recorded in your Mother and Child Health Handbook *boshi techō* (see page 118).

The timing of the vaccines, method of notification, and distribution of the questionnaire vary in different areas. Contact your local public health center for details about the system and names of doctors in your area who offer the free vaccines.

Vaccination Schedule Comparison Chart
(The figures in parentheses indicate the age at which the vaccine is given at public health centers.)

	Japan	USA	UK	Philippines
DPT	3 times at 3–8 week intervals between 3 months and 7.5 years; booster 12-18 months after initial series (varies in different areas)	2, 4, 6 months; 15–18 months; 4–6 years	2, 3, 4 months, Hb influenza given in combo injection	2, 3, 4 months; 18 months; 4–6 years; 14–16 years
DT	12 years	11–16 years	3–5 years	Included in DPT
Polio	Twice at 6-week intervals from 3 months to 7 years; (spring and fall at 6-month intervals between 3 months and 18 months)	2, 4, 6–18 months; 4–6 years	2, 3, 4 months, 3–5 years, 14–19 years	2, 3, 4 months; 18 months; 4–6 years; 14–16 years
MMR	Not available as one injection	12–15 months; 4–6 years	12–15 months; 3–5 years	15 months; 11–12 years
Rubella	1–7.5 years; 12–15 years; [1–3 years; also 6 years)]	Incorporated in MMR	Incorporated in MMR	Incorporated in MMR
Measles	1–7.5 years; (1–2 years; 6 years)	Incorporated in MMR	Incorporated in MMR	9 months
Mumps	Not in gov't schedule; available privately after 1 year	Incorporated in MMR	Incorporated in MMR	Not in gov't schedule

	Japan	U.S.	U.K.	Philippines
Chickenpox (Varicella Zoster)	Not in gov't schedule; available privately after 1 year	12–18 months	Not in gov't schedule	Not in gov't schedule
BCG	After a negative TB skin test BCG, 3 months to 4 years (3–12 months). Repeated at 6 and 13 years if necessary	Periodic TB skin test. BCG not recommended unless very high risk, as it may affect the results of the skin test	At birth if at risk, or after negative TB skin test at 10–13 years	Birth to 6 months
Hepatitis B	Given to newborn of carrier mother; 2 doses of HB immunoglobin at birth and 2 months; vaccine at 2, 3, 5 months	3 doses beginning at birth to 2 months	Given to newborn of carrier mother; 3 doses beginning at birth	6, 10, 14 weeks to newborn of carrier mother
Haemophilus (Hb) Influenza	Not available	Schedule differs depending on type; 3-4 doses during first 15 months	Incorporated in DPT	Available
Japanese Encephalitis	High risk 6 months–7.5 years; (2 doses at 3 years; booster at 4 years; then once every 4–5 years)	Available for overseas travel		Not in gov't schedule, but recommended
(source)	(Ministry of Health and Welfare, Japan; April 1998)	(Department of Health and Human Services, U.S.; April 1998)	(Department of Health and Social Services, U.K.; November 1996)	(Philippine Academy of Pediatrics; December 1996)

If you want to start before the suggested time, in accordance with your own country's schedule, you will find that vaccinations are given at specific times at large hospitals or at some clinics for a fee, or at the quarantine clinics. International clinics will have vaccines on demand. If in doubt, call the clinic or hospital beforehand to check the availability.

Notes on Familiar and Less Familiar Vaccines

A newly-formulated DPT vaccine was introduced in 1981, after the previous type had been discontinued, due to side effects. That year, the government began vaccinating children at twenty-four months of age, and the age is now gradually being lowered, although at six months it's still higher than in most countries. Each health district analyzes its own statistics and determines the opportune time to begin the series, so you will see the greatest variation nationwide in regard to the timing of this vaccine. Because polio does not exist in Japan, only two doses of the vaccine are given, which is thought to give ninety percent immunity. Health officials recommend that if you are traveling to other countries where you could be infected with polio, you should pay to have a third dose before leaving Japan. The MMR vaccine was given for a time, but then discontinued in 1993, because of reported side effects. This means that each component—measles, rubella (German measles) and mumps, has to be given separately. The first two are in the government's schedule, while mumps must be obtained privately. The influenza vaccine, which was removed from the government's schedule in 1994, is perhaps the most controversial in Japan, with proponents (who claim that the vaccine prevented deaths during the flu epidemic of 1997–98) and opponents (who cite side effects and questionable effectiveness) failing to reach a consensus. Although it is still available for a fee, the quantity which is produced has been greatly reduced, so it is possible that if there were a flu epidemic some year, supply might not meet demand.

The BCG vaccine is perhaps the most controversial outside Japan. After receiving this vaccine, your child will develop antibodies against TB, and so he will have a semi-positive reaction to a tuberculosis skin test (Tine test). Discuss with your doctor in your home country whether or not your child should have this inoculation. If you plan to live permanently in Japan, your decision may not be so difficult. The vaccine itself is given after a negative Tine test. The BCG vaccine is administered as a stamp (which looks like a grid) on the upper arm, in two spots. After two to three weeks there will be a local reaction, with tiny red blisters being formed. After a week, they should scab over and heal naturally. Do not bandage the area. If it looks infected, consult your doctor. The vaccine will not be administered if the child has any skin problems. It is said to provide fifty percent immunity to pulmonary TB and eighty percent immunity to tuberculosis meningitis. See pages 199 and 202–203 for details about tuberculosis.

The Japanese encephalitis vaccine is part of the government's schedule and usually given to kindergarten students. See pages 199 and 200–201 for details about the disease, to see if your activities warrant receiving it. The vaccine is usually given as an injection at three years, with the first and second doses given one to four weeks apart. A booster dose is given one year later, followed by shots every four to five years. There is a small possibility of an allergic reaction, so officials recommend that you remain at the clinic for thirty minutes after an injection. A very small percent of the vacunees report a low-grade fever, and redness, swelling, and dull pain at the site of injection.

Specialist Care

If your child has a chronic condition such as asthma, epilepsy or diabetes, or has symptoms that are difficult to diagnose, he probably needs specialist care. In the pediatric outpatient department of large hospitals, afternoons are usually dedicated to specialty clinics (these often require an appointment). Although many pediatricians in Japan specialize in neurology or gastroenterology, they do not use that title—for example, pediatric neurologist or pediatric gastroenterologist. The only designated specialty is pediatric surgeon.

Childhood Diseases that Are Uncommon in Japan

Some illnesses or conditions are genetically or ethnically determined. For this reason some diseases like cystic fibrosis (nōhōsei sen'ishō 嚢胞性線維症), Tay-Sachs Disease (ティーサックス病), and sickle-cell anemia (kamajō sekkekkyūbyō 鎌状赤血球症) are not found in Japan. To find a doctor here who is able to treat such a disease, it may be fastest to contact the national association in your own country, and ask them to suggest two or three doctors in Japan who have experience treating this or a similar type of condition. It would be best to do this before you arrive. If your child is born here, or arrives in infancy and then develops one of these diseases, it may be difficult to get an accurate diagnosis, since most hospitals will never have treated patients with these disorders.

If you have concerns about an inherited disorder, or if any such disorders run in your family, counseling may be available from your physician or (in Japanese) from the Japan Family Planning Association Genetic Counseling Center (see page 136), which also makes referrals to similar counseling centers around the country.

Cystic Fibrosis Trust
11 London Road, Bromley, Kent BR1 1BY U.K.
0181-464-7211, fax 0181-313-0472

Cystic Fibrosis Foundation
6931 Arlington Road, Bethesda, MD 20814 U.S.
1-301-951-4422 http://www.cff.org
Web site on home care, complications, helpful hints.

Sickle Cell Disease Association of America
200 Corporate Pointe #495
Culver City, CA 90230 U.S.
1-310-216-6363, fax 1-310-215-3722

March of Dimes Birth Defects Foundation
National Office
1275 Mamaroneck Ave., White Plains, NY 10605 U.S.
1-888-663-4637 http://www.noah.cuny.edu/pregnancy/march_of_dimes/birth_defects/taysachs.htm
Web page on Tay-Sachs–related facts, research, diagnosis.

Tay-Sachs and Allied Diseases Association
17 Sydney Road, Barkingside, Essex, Ilford U.K.

Emergency Situations

In a life-or-death emergency (shock, multiple injuries, etc.), call an ambulance and trust them to take you to the nearest appropriate hospital. If your child's condition is not life-threatening and you have time to make a phone call, a little knowledge of the system and preparedness (see pages 45–52) can ensure that your child will be treated at the hospital of your choice.

Note that most doctors and clinics aren't available after hours, and most smaller hospitals will not have a pediatrician on duty in their emergency room. One solution is to investigate the large hospitals (university, city, Red Cross, etc.) near your home ahead of time. Find out if they have a pediatrician on staff in the emergency room. If they do, take your child to the outpatient pediatric department during regular morning clinic hours as soon as he has the slightest problem. That way you'll have a registration number and the child's records will be on file. In an emergency, call the hospital and tell them your name and registration number and the child's problem, and ask permission to take your child there. They should agree.

As these larger hospitals are designated as emergency facilities, you're not supposed to use the emergency rooms if you do not arrive by ambulance. If, in addition to arriving by any means other than ambulance, you are not registered, the hospital may refuse to treat you.

Learn how to call an ambulance too, and know basic first aid. Since accidents are the number-one cause of death among toddlers, it's vitally important that you are prepared.

Major Children's Hospitals

The following are major children's hospitals; most require a letter of introduction from another doctor and an appointment. The major hospitals and university hospitals listed in "Regional Resources" also have well-equipped pediatric departments.

National Children's Hospital
Kokuritsu Shoni Byoin 国立小児病院
3-35-31 Taishido, Setagaya-ku, Tokyo
03-3414-8121

Tokyo Metropolitan Hachioji Children's Hospital
Tokyo Toritsu Hachioji Shoni Byoin
東京都立八王子小児病院
4-33-13 Dai-Machi, Hachioji-shi, Tokyo
0426-24-2255

Tokyo Metropolitan Kiyose Children's Hospital
Tokyo Toritsu Kiyose Shoni Byoin
東京都立清瀬小児病院
1-3-1 Umezono, Kiyose-shi, Tokyo
0424-91-0011

Kanagawa Children's Medical Center
Kanagawa Kenritsu Kodomo Iryo Senta
神奈川県立こども医療センター
2-138-4 Mutsukawa, Minami-ku, Yokohama-shi
045-711-2351

Saitama Children's Medical Center
Saitama Kenritsu Shoni Iryo Senta
埼玉県立小児科医療センター
2100 Magome-Ohaza, Iwatsuki-shi, Saitama-ken
0487-58-1811

Chiba Children's Hospital
Chiba-ken Kodomo Byoin
千葉県こども病院
579-1 Heta-cho, Midori-ku, Chiba-shi, Chiba-ken
043-292-2111

Hokkaido Children's Hospital and Medical Center
Hokkaido-ritsu Shoni Sogo Hoken Senta
北海道立小児総合保健センター
1-10-1 Zenibako, Otaru-shi, Hokkaido
0134-62-5511

Ibaraki Children's Hospital
Ibaraki Kenritsu Kodomo Byoin
茨城県立こども病院
3-3-1 Futabadai, Mito-shi, Ibaraki-ken
0292-54-1151

Shizuoka Children's Hospital
Shizuoka Kenritsu Kodomo Byoin
静岡県立こども病院
860 Urushiyama, Shizuoka-shi, Shizuoka-ken
0542-47-6251

Nagoya (Japanese) Red Cross First Hospital
Nagoya Daiichi Sekijuji Byoin
名古屋第一赤十字病院
3-35 Michishita-cho, Nakamura-ku, Nagoya-shi
052-481-5111

Nagano Children's Hospital
Nagano Kenritsu Kodomo Byoin
長野県立子供病院
3100 Toyoshina, Toyoshina-machi, Minami Azumi-gun, Nagano-ken
0263-73-6700

Hyogo Prefecture Kobe Children's Hospital
Hyogo Kenritsu Kodomo Byoin
兵庫県立こども病院
1-1-1 Takakura-machi, Suma-ku, Kobe-shi
078-732-6961

National Sanatorium Kagawa Children's Hospital
Kokuritsu Ryoyosho Kagawa Shoni Byoin
国立療養所香川小児病院
2603 Zentsuji-cho, Zentsuji-shi, Kagawa-ken
0877-62-0885

Fukuoka City Children's Hospital and Medical Center for Infectious Disease
Fukuoka Shiritsu Kodomo Byoin/Kansensho Senta
福岡市立こども病院／感染症センター
2-5-1 Tojin-cho, Chuo-ku, Fukuoka-shi
092-713-3111

Poisonings

Poisoning can pose a life-or-death situation. Identify the poisonous substance as quickly as possible, as well as the amount ingested and the period of time elapsed. See the front endpapers for poison control center numbers and post them by your telephone. When you call the center, give them information on any symptoms. Note that the medical advice that these centers can give you is limited to whether the situation is life-threatening and what first aid measures to take. If you think that the product ingested was Japanese, it may be better to phone the Japanese centers. If you cannot speak Japanese, find someone to call for you, or depend on ambulance personnel. Take the telephone numbers to the emergency hospital, as the doctor may want to call to confirm treatment.

If your child is conscious, the center may tell you to induce vomiting. Note that the emetic Ipecac syrup is not available in Japan. To make a child vomit without this syrup, give him some water, hold him over your knee, and press the back of his throat with a spoon. Prepare a bowl for the vomit, as the doctor may want to examine the contents. Also, if you know what the child took, bring a sample of it with you to the emergency room.

Infant and Small Children's Health

Safety

In Japan, accidents are the number-one cause of death among children aged one to four. If you are pregnant, childproof your house before your baby is born. Take a good look around your house or apartment to identify potential dangers. If you are living in a Japanese-style home some possible problems are that everything is low to the ground where it can easily be reached by a crawling infant, windows are usually the sliding type and easy to open, and bathtubs are deep.

Possible Causes of Injury in Japan

■ **Burns:** Low ironing boards, pushbutton thermos bottles ready for the next cup of tea, unregulated bathtub heaters, and portable space heaters.

■ **Poisoning:** Cigarette filters or butts; medicines left on low tables or shelves.

■ **Falls:** Cribs that don't meet safety standards for side height, narrow polished wood staircases without rails, unevenness of floor surfaces due to tatami matting, and air conditioning units set out on the veranda onto which a child can climb and then fall over the side of the railing.

■ **Drownings:** Deep bathtubs that have been filled but which aren't covered with a sturdy top, standing buckets of water, and open washing machines.

■ **Traffic Accidents:** Mothers riding a child or two on a bicycle, and small children walking along the side of the road in spots where there are no sidewalks.

Also check your own baby books to have a better all-around picture of safety measures needed to childproof your home.

Baby-sitting

In Japan, once the baby is born, mother and child are nearly always together. There are some possibilities for hiring a baby-sitter in the larger cities (some wards have lists of approved baby-sitters) but leaving the child with a relative stranger is not yet a common practice. When it's time for grocery shopping, some mothers leave the baby at home, trying to time their outings to coincide with the child's nap times. But there are sometimes reports of fires or accidents with this practice. Health officials suggest that you childproof your home so that accidents won't occur while you're away.

For parents who do have baby-sitters, another concern arises, which is the question of proper preparation for possible medical emergencies.

For the Baby-sitter

■ Leave all health records, including immunization records and health insurance information and cards, in one place.

■ Write and sign a general letter of permission for others to seek medical care for your child if it is needed. Indicate the name of the doctor or clinic where your child is usually treated.

■ Leave the sitter a family medical encyclopedia and any medicines which the child may need, along with directions for their use. Childproof your home by putting other medicines in a safe, inaccessible place.

■ Leave the name of an emergency contact person. If you are traveling, also leave a detailed itinerary of your travel plans, with hotel telephone numbers; at your child's school—especially with the school nurse—leave your babysitter's name and phone number, and your expected date of return.

Language Acquisition and Bilingualism

"My father is Japanese and my mother is American. I am now at college in the United States, but I've spent half my life in Japan. During school I went back and forth a few times between American and Japanese school systems. I did experience brief cases of ijime *during fifth and sixth grades, right after returning from a few years in the U.S., but by junior high school I no longer had the problem. When I went to an American high school in eleventh grade, I had difficulty at first with the different system, but ended up being happier. I did not go through any severe depression during these adjustments, and now I am definitely glad to be nearly bilingual and of course bicultural. I'm glad that my parents chose this for me, and if I had to do it all over I would do it all the same."*

It may be good to contemplate ahead of time how you will raise your child linguistically. Will your home be an English island? Do you plan to use Japanese too? What language would you like him to use to communicate with other family members? If you are raising him in a completely English environment, plan to bring books, videotapes, and music tapes or CDs from home so that he'll hear a variety of accents and new vocabulary. Ensure that he has English-speaking friends to play with. You may want to consider forming a play-group, or to enroll him in nursery school classes earlier than you would have otherwise.

If you're raising your child bilingually, it takes consistent effort to ensure that the child has opportunities to hear and use both languages. Many authors recommend that either a one-parent, one-language approach or a home language-school language division be used consistently. Don't forget to evaluate periodically how well your system is working. For good resources on raising bilingual children, see "References and Further Reading."

Resources

Two volunteer language study groups have been formed for bilingual English-Japanese children.

Children's English Circles
03-3444-2167, fax 03-3444-2204 (CWAJ)
Sponsored by the College Women's Association of Japan. For elementary school-age children returning from abroad. Children are expected to have begun the study of English while attending school in a foreign country.

International Children's Bunko Association
03-3496-8688
This organization welcomes bilingual children of elementary school age or above.

School-age Children's Health

Choosing a School

Choosing the appropriate school, either international or Japanese, for your child can be an important consideration in his or her well being. It's generally easier on the child if you stick to the same system. This isn't considering only language procurement but also that the teacher's expectations and appropriate classroom behavior is very distinct in two systems. If your child does switch from one system to another, it's possible that they will need extra tutoring or parental support until they catch up academically. Check in the reading list for accounts of two foreign families' experiences of sending their children to Japanese schools. You may want to consider the following kinds of points when making your decisions.

"We arrived from Poland two years ago. My daughter Lana initially spoke only Polish, but quickly became conversant in Japanese and enjoyed her first-grade class. When we moved to a new apartment the following year, she transferred to another school in a working-class neighborhood that rarely got transfer students, and never foreigners.

"From the beginning she could not adjust to the new atmosphere. Her classmates teased her and refused to play with her at recess. Although we had numerous conferences with the teachers, the situation didn't improve, and she began to refuse to go.

"We then transferred her to a government-designated school for Japanese children who had been educated overseas (kikoku shijo kyoiku ukeire suishin gakkō), and she quickly made friends."

"My four-year-old son is very shy and although he understands English, his mother tongue, well, he rarely speaks. Before I left for Japan, all my friends kept encouraging me to put him in a Japanese kindergarten, saying, 'Just think, with a little effort, he'll be bilingual,' but for my son who had a speech delay in addition his natural shyness, this wouldn't have been a good choice. Since an international school was available, we enrolled him there, and he is blossoming."

"I'm a Canadian with very little Japanese ability, with a Japanese husband and an eight-year-old daughter. My daughter is doing well in the local school, but since I can't help her with her homework, I've arranged for private lessons with a neighbor, to help her with her writing skills, and she goes to afternoon classes twice a week for math practice. Whenever we're called in for a conference with the teacher, my husband arranges to go on a Saturday when he's off from work, and although I don't understand very much, I always attend the large parent-teacher association meetings."

"My daughter has a hearing impairment, and at age six still needs reme-
dial classes to improve her speaking ability and comprehension. After
investigating numerous international schools, we found only one that
would enroll her."

"Our home language is Korean, and we had just spent six years in South
Africa when we were transferred to Tokyo last year. My older son com-
pleted sixth grade in an English-speaking school before arriving, but we
wanted him to learn Japanese, so we enrolled him in a public junior high
school. He attended the school for four months, but he made little progress
in the language, couldn't follow any of the classes, and was depressed
because he felt that he was losing his English. When we found out that he
would have to take an examination to enter high school after completing
ninth grade, we realized that we had placed him in an impossible situ-
ation, and had him transfer to an international school."

"Street Language" Versus "School Language"
Colin Baker, in his guide to bilingualism, writes about these two catagories of language
for second language learners. Street language refers to simple conversations that include
gestures and facial clues; it is used when playing or making social conversation. The
language of the classroom, on the other hand, after the first few years in elementary
school, has few gestures. The teacher's language and the material are more abstract, and
require a vocabulary that is more cognitively and academically demanding. Baker states
that it would take two years of immersion for a second-language learner to reach the
same level of proficiency as a monolingual in street language, but five to seven years to
reach the same level in classroom language.

The Problem of Bullying ijime いじめ
In Japan, particularly in the last twenty years, the problem of bullying has been a topic of
continuous debate among teachers, parents, students, and school board officials as to
what kind of students are likely to become bulliers or victims, why the entire problem
arises, and what can be done to stop it.

Junior high schools, in particular, provide an arena for bullying because of class sizes
that may include forty to fifty students (a number that is difficult to monitor), the stress of
the intense academic competition, and the perceived need for most Japanese to be part
of a group, with the accompanying mandate that anyone who is different does not belong.
Each year some victims seem to bear their pain in silence, without sharing their anguish
with parents or teachers, and then quietly commit suicide.

Since school is mandatory, author Sumio Hamada writes, it is not surprising that
bullying occurs there. Students can't choose their school or their classmates, and victims
may well feel that they are trapped in an untenable situation with no place to run. Bullying

involves identifying a victim as being different in some way. Bullied children may lack confidence, and to some extent even believe what bulliers say, which makes them feel still weaker and more defenseless.

In Japan particularly, *ijime* is a group activity, and the bulliers seem to feel that it reinforces the bonds between them and their friends. Some report that they use the activity as a form of stress relief, and say that they feel refreshed (*sukkiri shita*) afterwards.

Some teachers perpetuate the problem or even aggravate by saying that *ijime* is the victims' fault, and that bullied children need to make an effort to be more like everyone else. Japanese parents try to prevent any incidents by making sure that their children have the same kind of bookbags, pencils, haircuts, and clothes as their classmates.

There are various strategies for dealing with *ijime*, but perhaps the best is for parents and classroom teachers to discuss any problems immediately, since letting things go usually won't solve the problem, and may in fact cause the bullying to escalate. Hamada feels that the best form of prevention would be to encourage everyone to have self-pride and confidence, which are essential for self-defense, and that the Japanese society as a whole needs to strive to accept differences.

Resources

Bullying Hotline Ijime Sodan-shitsu
03-3493-2277 (J. only)
Mon.–Fri. 9:00 A.M.–8:00 P.M., Sat., Sun., hols.
9:00 A.M.–5:00 P.M.

Young Telephone Corner
Police hotline for any kind of worrisome problem.
03-3580-4970 (J. only)
Mon.–Fri. 8:30 A.M.–8:00 P.M. Sat., Sun., hols.
8:30 A.M.–5:15 P.M.

Health Care at International Schools

Most international schools have a school nurse, but most are not licensed in Japan, and so are designated as teachers. Nurses help provide health education, do simple health screening, and give simple first aid in emergencies.

International schools do not stipulate a particular vaccination program, because of the varying backgrounds of the students. Instead they rely on parents to maintain their own chosen schedule.

Requirements for returning to school after contracting a communicable disease vary from school to school, so check your school policy.

Health Care in the Japanese School System

A physical exam is administered at the school in the fall, for the five-year-olds who will enter school the following spring. After starting school, students receive annual health screenings, usually in April, which include a urine test, a stool test for pinworms, vision and hearing testing done by the school nurse, and quick reviews by a pediatrician, an ENT physician, and a dentist. If any problems are found, the parents are asked to take the child to their own doctor for further evaluation, and to report the findings back to the school. See "Health Checkups" for detailed information about and vocabulary useful for physical exams.

Vaccination was previously compulsory for entry into Japanese schools and booster shots were administered there after admission, but with the recent revision of the law, only a few vaccines such as the BCG are now offered at school, while the other shots are given by designated local doctors.

Children in certain grades undergo screening tests for colorblindness and scoliosis. Weight checks are done each month, and height checks three times a year, after which the school nutritionist provides counseling to any children who are considerably over- or underweight.

All the communicable diseases listed on pages 200–205 except hepatitis must be reported to the school: a doctor's certificate indicating that the child has recovered completely is required before he or she can return to school. These illnesses, together with measles, mumps, influenza, etc. are called required absences for communicable diseases *shusseki teishi no byōki* 出席停止の病気, and the school days missed are not counted as absences. If a child needs to be hospitalized for a long period, some hospitals will provide in-hospital schooling *innai gakkyū* 院内学級. If this service is not available, a private tutor may be hired, if appropriate.

Preventive Health Pointers from School Nurses in Japan

One recent survey indicated that although Japanese children are taller than they were thirty years ago, they also now suffer from more asthma, obesity, and dental and vision problems. School nurses stress the importance of the following in combatting these trends:

■ **Posture:** Good posture should be maintained both while standing and while sitting. All children's desks and chairs sold in Japan can be adjusted as a child grows, to maintain correct body alignment while studying.

■ **Eyesight:** In recent years, the number of children who require corrective lenses because their eyesight tests below 0.1 (20 x 20) has gradually increased. Computer game and TV time should be limited to one-hour intervals; parents should also require that children rest their eyes for a time after studying for one hour. Lighting is tested in the classrooms; at home, study rooms should have a brightness of at least 300 lux. In addition to the desk light, an overhead light should also be on while the child studies; the desk lamp should be three times as bright as the overhead light.

■ **Importance of Chewing Food:** The more times you chew, the more saliva is produced to help with digestion. This also helps rid the mouth of bacteria and strengthens the muscles, helping with jaw development, which in turn promotes good teeth alignment. A study has been done that compared the amount of time it took to eat dinner 200 years ago and today; two centuries ago it took 22 minutes, and people chewed 1,465 times, and at present it takes 11 minutes, and people chew only 620 times.

■ **Living Environment:** It is recommended that you should open the windows, especially in the morning, to let in fresh air. Appropriate room temperatures are 25–28 degrees centigrade in summer and 18–22 degrees in winter.

■ **Preventing Colds:** Since eighty percent of germs are passed from hand to mouth, also hand-washing and gargling, especially upon returning home from outside, can greatly reduce the risk of catching cold. Children are dressed lightly all year long, since this is thought to improve the body's resistance to disease.

■ **Low Body Temperature:** Research has been done which found that forty percent of the children studied had a low body temperature (below 36°C) upon waking in the morning. This is attributed to lack of proper sleep and exercise. Nurses often stress the need to establish an age-appropriate life-style rhythm of "early to bed, early to rise."

■ **Teeth:** Good brushing techniques are ex-

tremely important. Children should use a mirror every day to check their own teeth. Parents should also check children's brushing. Gingivitis is on the rise.

■ **Playing Outdoors:** Nowadays children are said to lack three things (san kan 三間); time to play (jikan 時間), open spaces (kūkan 空間) to play in, and friends (nakama 仲間) to play with. Outdoor play helps develop coordination and physical strength, and even improves eyesight by enabling children to adjust their vision to distant objects. Encourage, or shall we say *allow* your children to play outside several times a week.

Adolescent Health

In general, Japan is a relatively calm place to raise an adolescent. With the advanced transportation system, children can be quite independent, coming and going according to their own schedules; parents can also be freed from the duties of family chauffeur. Crime is low, and there are few illegal drugs about to tempt the unwary. But still, being aware of possible pitfalls may help you and your child avoid a few.

Japan is the "land of the vending machine," with more machines per person than any other country in the world. Almost everything is sold this way, including underwear, but most machines dispense soft drinks, beer, or cigarettes. Beer and cigarettes can cause problems for teenagers, because the law prohibiting the sale of alcohol or tobacco to anyone under the age of twenty is rarely enforced. One canned alcoholic beverage called chū-hai, made with grain alcohol (shōchū) and sweet juices, is very potent and can be very popular with adolescents. Another cause for concern is college students' practice of chugging drinks (ikkinomi), which can cause coma and even death (see Addictions, pages 241–44 for further information).

Other problems that are affecting Japanese youth in general, and that may affect your child at some point, are issues of sexual relations and the resulting dangers of sexually transmitted disease and unwanted pregnancy. According to a 1993 study by the Japanese Association for Sex Education, 57.3 percent of male and 43.3 percent of female college students are sexually active. The figure has doubled for male and quadrupled for female students over the last twenty years. Although the teenage pregnancy rate has more or less leveled off and is quite low when compared to Western countries, the rate of STDs, and especially chlamydia and genital herpes is rapidly increasing (see pages 110–12). There also seems to be a rising number of cases of eating disorders (see page 243).

While illicit drugs have not posed as great a problem among Japanese youth as in the West, drug use is becoming more common among young people, and the age at which problems begin is falling. The main reasons given for drug use among young people are no different from those cited elsewhere—loneliness, dysfunctional families, materialism, and peer pressure. Teenage drug users in Japan tend to start by sniffing paint thinner *shinna* シンナー. Other drugs that are abused are amphetamines *kakuseizai* 覚醒剤 (with the young person starting out with either stimulants to stay awake while studying for exams or with diet pills), and marijuana (or hemp) *taima* 大麻. Stopping drug use early is important because teenagers who start with thinners may move on to other more dangerous substances (see pages 242–44 for therapists who are experienced in treating substance abuse).

Young people up to the age of eighteen usually consult a pediatrician for regular illnesses, or possibly an internist. Since the problems inherent in the Japanese medical system—lack of privacy and very little time for consultation with the doctor—may be especially worrying to a teenager, you may have to look around to find a doctor that has an interest in really getting to know the teen and his or her problem, and who works in a setting that offers sufficient privacy. Many large hospitals have special adolescent clinics for teenagers *shishunki gairai* 思春期外来. Tokyo Women's University Hospital has a well-known adolescent outpatient clinic for girls. The urology department at Toho University Hospital Omori is known for its attention to the problems of adolescent boys.

Speech and Physical Delays

Children develop mental and physical skills in the same order—for example, they sit before they can walk—but the age when these skills are learned varies enormously. If you're concerned about your child's language development, evaluate how much language he is actually hearing, as well as how much he can understand of what is being said. It has been reported that about five percent of all children, whether bilingual or not, will have difficulties in learning to speak. In some cases, a natural delay can be compounded by a bilingual environment. Your child may require speech therapy (see page 175) if he has a natural speech delay, articulation problems, or loss of hearing due to a buildup of fluid in the ear.

Physical delays may be attributed to the lack of an appropriate play area where you child can gain confidence in his physical abilities and have ample opportunities to explore his world. Remember that a child must literally "walk before he can run," so try to provide him with a stimulating, fun physical environment. But sometimes there can be other reasons for a physical delay.

Preschool Evaluation and Therapy

Children develop at different paces, but if there are large discrepancies between your child's development and what is described in baby books, you may want to have him evaluated. First of all try to clarify the areas of your concern then seek appropriate care. Japanese pediatricians in general like to take a "wait-and-see" approach, but if you are really worried, keep looking until you find a doctor who will take your concerns seriously and address them.

Most medical university hospitals and all children's hospitals have developmental consultation clinics *hattatsu sōdan gairai* 発達相談外来. A CT scan and brain wave test (EEG) are usually recommended to start with, to make sure that the child has no medical problems. The doctor may then recommend some type of therapy (speech or play, etc.). But if your child speaks only English, it may be difficult to find a therapist. See the resources on page 175, or if you live outside the Kanto area, call the nearest international school to see what services are currently being offered by threrapists or tutors in your area.

If your child understands Japanese, check with your local public health center for services offered by your local government and by area hospitals. Many areas now have rehabilitation centers *shinshin shōgai sentā* 心身障害センター where speech and play therapy may be offered for preschool children. Within the social services department *fukushi-kyoku* 福祉局 of every local city government office, a children's consultation service *jidō sōdan-jo* 児童相談所 is staffed by professionals such as psychologists, neurologists, and social services personnel, who are ready to offer assistance on diverse issues like childrearing practices, delayed development, and welfare benefits. Financial subsidies are available for children with disabilities or chronic health problems (see page 62).

Learning Disabilities

Learning disabilities *gakushū shōgai* 学習障害 is a term usually applied to children who are intelligent but due to any of a number of conceptual or perceptual difficulties may have problems in the classroom.

Acceptance at international schools depends on the type and the severity of the problem. If your child is experiencing problems at school, testing should probably be done to identify the problem so therapy can be started. For Kanto residents, see one of the resources listed on page 175. If you live in another area, call TELL or another helpline (see the endpapers) for information. Your child's school may also be able to recommend a therapist or even provide treatment.

If your child has an attention deficit disorder, treatment may be difficult because medications such as Ritalin are not usually prescribed by Japanese pediatricians or neurologists. Since children with this type of problem can be disruptive to classes, schools may be unwilling to accommodate them.

In the Japanese school system, the concept of children having learning disabilities is relatively new: few teachers are familiar with the new research, little provision is made for testing or treatment, and no additional support outside the regular classroom is provided by the school. Psychologists administer a very simple IQ test in third grade, but otherwise do not visit the schools. The Wechsler Intelligence Test for Children, Revised (WISC-R), used widely in testing for learning disabilities, has been translated into Japanese, and can be administered at various education centers *kyōiku sentā* 教育センター

or university hospitals. However, even if a problem such as dyslexia can be identified, remedial treatment is rarely offered in the school system; it must instead be arranged for privately by the parent. One exception is speech therapy. Therapists treat articulation problems and speech delay in children at the school district's designated center, usually located in one of the area elementary schools. The number of visits per week is determined by the child's need. The only drawbacks are that the parent is responsible for transporting the child to the center, and that the sessions are usually held during school hours, meaning that the child must miss the regular classwork.

Counseling and Consultations in English

Tokyo International Learning Community
(TILC; see page 177)
Offers early childhood program including preschool classroom, speech, and language services, as well as occupational therapy. Also psychological and physical therapy. Learning disabilities group meets on Saturday mornings.

Speech and Language Disorder Referrals
03-3780-0030 rosenbrg@gol.com
Therapists who are members of the Association of Foreign Speech Pathologists can provide therapy in English for adults and children in the Kanto area.

Aoibashi Family Clinic
(Kamigyo-ku, Kyoto; see page 240)
Family education, counseling, and play therapy.

Shoko Sasaki, M.S.
(Shibuya-ku, Tokyo; see page 240)
School psychologist/family therapist. Psychoeducational evaluations, individual/family counseling for school-related problems and related issues, etc.

Institute of Psychoanalytic-Systems Psychotherapy
Highland Bldg. 3 Fl., 2-5-19 Higashiyama
Meguro-ku, Tokyo
03-3760-3631
Japan/U.S.-trained psychotherapists Prof. Hidefumi Kotani and Dr. Akiko Ohnogi. Adult and child individual, group, family, and couples psychotherapy. Also, play therapy and parenting education, as well as workshops and training for professionals.

Ron Shumsky, Psy.D.
(Minato-ku, Tokyo and Yokohama; see page 240)
Psychotherapy with children, adults and families. Psychoeducational evaluation/testing, including learning differences, dyslexia, and ADD/ADHD. School consultation.

Betsey Olsen, Ed.D.
(Musashino-shi, Tokyo; see page 240)
Individual and family counseling.

International School Support Services
5-12-2 Shimo-Meguro, Meguro-ku, Tokyo
03-3710-1331, fax 03- 3712-3386
http://www.cyber.ad.jp/tfn
Special education classes, tutoring for any subject, and consultation services for students with learning difficulties or who need preparation in English for entering international schools. Also, assistance in finding a suitable school or remedial classes.

Japanese Learning Disabilities Association
Zenkoku Gakushu Shogai Ji Renrakukai
全国学習障害児・者親の会連絡会
39-1 Nishi-Shinchi, Chita-shi, Aichi-ken
045-333-3232 (Mr. Yamada in J. or Eng.), also fax
Comprises 48 regional parents' support groups that encourage an exchange of information and strive for governmental legislation.

Special Needs in Education

The Japanese educational system for people with special needs starts as a preschool program under the Ministry of Health and Welfare, transfers to the Ministry of Education during school years, and reverts to the Ministry of Health and Welfare after the age of eighteen. Anyone who is a resident taxpayer may utilize the programs, although all instruction and therapy is in Japanese. School-age children who have special needs are either identified at the pre-entry physical (which includes a very simple IQ test), or by their parents after consultation with the local school board of education (*kyōiku i-inkai gakumu-ka* 教育委員会学務課), whose office is usually within the local government offices. Each school's principal has the right to decide whether to admit a handicapped child to the school.

Although programs for children with moderate or severe mental or physical handicaps are offered, there is very little provision for children with mild handicaps (such as learning disabilities). Children with moderate mental retardation are usually placed in a special class (*shinshin shōgai gakkyū* 心身障害学級) located in one of the local schools. Transportation is not provided. Classes are generally small, with two teachers per fifteen students. The curriculum and pace of teaching are adjusted to the children's needs.

Parents of intellectually capable but physically handicapped children often have difficulty finding a place in a regular school for their children because of the lack of elevators, etc. Transportation to a central school (*shitai yōgo gakkō* 肢体養護学校), which usually serves a wide area, is provided for children with physical disabilities. Children in these schools are grouped according to intellectual capacity.

Children with severe mental disabilities go to a central school (*seishin hakujaku yōgo gakkō* 精神薄弱養護学校) that usually serves a large area. The student-teacher ratio is five to one or less and life skills are emphasized; transportation is provided.

Special schools for the visually impaired (*mōgakkō* 盲学校) and hearing impaired (*rō-gakkō* ろう学校) are also provided. These are often residential schools, but part-time classes for students who are mainstreamed into the regular schools are also provided.

Perhaps unique to Japan are special residential schools for the physically weak (*byōjaku yōgo gakkō* 病弱養護学校). Established by boards of education in large cities, these schools provide a year of "country living" to children at parents' request. Children attending this type of school are those who have missed a lot of regular school through asthma or general sickliness, or those who are overweight. The program is offered to elementary school students from grade three to six; a small amount is charged per day for food. Parents are only allowed one visit per month, and children can only return to their homes during school vacations.

A few national and private schools for children with special needs are also available. Tokyo's Musashino-Higashi School for autistic children offers schooling for both regular and autistic children, with some joint classes provided.

Resources for Children With Special Needs

Support Groups for Parents of Children with Special Needs
Contact TILC for current president's number.

Tokyo International Learning Community (TILC)
6-3-50 Osawa, Mitaka-shi, Tokyo
0422-31-9611, fax 0422-31-9648
Using a multidisciplinary team approach, special education teachers and therapists work with families to develop individually-tailored education programs, including emphasis on academic and life skills for independence. Tuition fees are comparable to those of other international schools, but in cases of financial need, scholarships may be possible. A bus service is available to some students, and for those who are not able to actually attend, a home training program or a tutor may be arranged.

Japan Baby-sitting Service
506 Shuwa Residence, 3-3-16 Sendagaya
Shibuya-ku, Tokyo
03-3423-1251
Regular and temporary home baby-sitting service for children with special needs such as autism, Down syndrome, and cerebral palsy. Sitters can care for children up to the age of twelve. Medical service is not provided, and English ability is limited.

Japanese National Council of Toy Libraries
(Omocha no Toshokan Zenkoku Renrakukai)
2-6-7 Komagata, 7 Fl., Taito-ku, Tokyo
03-3845-8994 (J.), fax 03-3845-2203 (J., Eng.)
For nationwide list of 400 toy libraries established for children with physical and mental disabilities, but open to everyone.

Organizational Resources

John Tracy Clinic Correspondence
806 West Adams Blvd., Los Angeles, CA 90007 U.S.
1-213-748-5481
Free correspondence courses for preschool hearing impaired, and for deaf-blind children and their parents.

National Institute on Deafness and Other Communication Disorders Clearinghouse
P.O. Box 37777, Washington D.C. 20013 U.S.
1-301-496-7243 http://www.dhhs.gov
Information on disorders involving hearing, smell, taste, voice, speech and language; also directory of related associations.

National Information Center for Children and Youth with Handicaps
P.O. Box 1492 Washington, D.C. 20013 U.S.
1-202-884-8200, 1-800-695-0285
http://www.nichcy.org/
Info on parent support groups, etc., in the U.S.; also fact sheets on specific disabilities such as cerebral palsy, Down syndrome, and epilepsy.

National Institute of Child Health and Human Development (NICHD)
Bldg. 31 Rm. 2A32, Bethesda MD 20892-2350 U.S.
1-301-496-5133 http://www.nih.gov/nichd
Access to a wide range of information on diseases, such as sickle-cell anemia, autism, febrile seizures, etc. Pamphlets may be ordered by mail or accessed on the Internet. Also try using the search engine of the National Institutes of Health at http://search.info.nih.gov/

The National Organization for Rare Disorders, Inc.
P.O. Box 8923, New Fairfield, CT 06812-8293 U.S.
1-203-746-6518, fax 1-203-746-6481

American Academy of Pediatrics
141 Northwest Point Blvd., P.O. Box 927
Elk Grove Village, IL 60009-0927 U.S.
http://www.aap.org/
General information on child care, parenting, and resources.
at http://intl.pediatrics.org The AAP journal *Pediatrics* can access search medline using the National Library of Medicine.

Japanese Association for Autism
Nihon Jiheisho Kyokai 日本自閉症協会

2-2-8 Nishi-Waseda, Shinjuku-ku, Tokyo
03-3232-6478 (J. only)

Japanese Association for Parents of Children with Down Syndrome
1-10-7-203 Kita-Shinjuku, Shinjuku-ku, Tokyo
03-3369-3462 (J. only)

Parents Association of Hearing-Impaired Children, Japan
Nanchoji o Motsu Oya no Kai
難聴児を持つ親の会
3-15-4-118 Higashi-Nogawa, Komae-shi, Tokyo
03-3488-0414 (J. only)

Other Resources Found on the Internet

The Japan Down Syndrome Network in English
http://infofarm.cc.affrc.go.jp/~momotani/dowj1-e.html

National Down Syndrome Society (USA)
212-460-9330, fax 212-979-2873
http://www.ndss.org/

National Autistic Society (UK)
http://www.oneworld.org/autism_uk/

For inexpensive lodgings where families can stay during a child's hospitalization, see page 331.

Child Abuse

The Tokyo English Life Line (TELL; see the endpapers) offers telephone counseling to victims of child abuse, as well as to parents who fear that they may be, or may start, abusing their children. Long-term counseling is also available from various professionals (see pages 239–40). Another resource is the Adult Child of Alcoholics Support Group, which helps people who suffer from any kind of abuse. TELL will know the telephone number of the current contact person for the group.

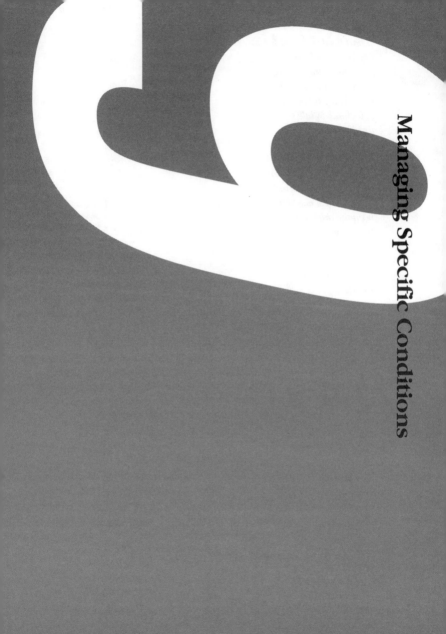

Managing Specific Conditions

"I had lived in Japan for five years and was packing up for a transfer overseas when I experienced my first episode of asthma. While sorting through all the closets and then sleeping on the floor amid stacks of boxes, I must have been exposed to a new kind of mold, or it could have been the added stress of the move."

"It was quite a shock when I was told I had diabetes. I had just turned forty when the doctor started questioning me about my health after the results of my annual physical showed a particularly high level of blood sugar. When I stopped to think about it, I realized that I had been under a lot of stress at work, I had gained about twenty pounds in the past few years, and my eyesight had weakened considerably. Fortunately, my condition quickly stabilized under the care of a specialist at a diabetes outpatient clinic at a nearby hospital."

Managing Specific Conditions

If you come to Japan while being treated for a chronic or serious condition, or are diagnosed with one during your stay, you will no doubt want to educate yourself about the ways that Japanese caregivers view and treat that condition. This chapter was included to try to point out some of the differences in treatment that you may encounter between your own country and Japan. We also try to give you some useful vocabulary and resources. It is beyond the scope of this book, however, to include complete and detailed descriptions of specific conditions or treatments. We encourage you to use your own family medical guide (see "References and Further Reading" for suggestions) and other reference to research information as fully as you can.

In Japan, the custom of wearing a medic alert wrist band or necklace has not been established. If you have a condition that could cause you to lose consciousness, you may want to carry a bilingual card in your wallet with an explanation of your medical condition.

Allergies

Allergies are a body's excessive reaction to common substances such as pollen, food, dust, or molds. Most allergies are an inherited tendency, and symptoms may vary from the runny nose and watery eyes of hay fever to the itchy rash of atopic dermatitis. Moving to Japan and coming in contact with new pollens, foods, stress, molds, or high concentrations of an allergen may cause allergic reactions in people who have never had problems before.

If you think that you have an allergy, see an internist at an allergy outpatient clinic, a dermatologist, or a pediatrician for testing. Tests done in Japan include checks of sensitivity to inhaled allergen *yūhatsu tesuto* 誘発テスト, skin tests *hifu tesuto* 皮膚テスト, blood tests for antibodies *kessei kōtai kensa* 血清抗体検査, and nasal smears *bijū tesuto* 鼻汁テスト. Once you know what you're allergic to, you may want to consider immunotherapy *men'eki ryōhō* 免疫療法. Hyposensitization treatments *genkansa ryōhō* 減感作療法 involve a series of allergy shots given over a period of two or more years to desensitize the body's reactions; opinions of their effectiveness vary widely.

House Dust and House Mites

In Japan, seventy percent of those who undergo allergy tests—including ninety percent of childhood asthmatics—are found to be allergic to house dust and the droppings of the tiny mite *dani* ダニ which live in house dust. These mites produce a large amount of droppings, and the only way that they can be killed is by high heat or the use of insecticides.

Doctors usually offer a long list of recommendations to prevent dust from collecting, such as daily dusting and vacuuming, the use of wooden flooring rather than carpets and of metal blinds instead of curtains, but these may not all be practical for you. Vacuuming the bedding (quilts or blankets, and futons or mattresses) weekly, and washing and then drying the sheets in a clothes dryer may help kill or remove the mites and droppings. Some models of vacuum cleaners kill dust mites by heat, and others by an insecticide in the dust collection bag; recent vacuum prototypes even use water. Japan's hot and humid summers provide ideal breeding conditions for dust mites, which make a beeline for closets where bedding and clothes are stored. Before using any goods that have been stored, remove dust and mites by airing, vacuuming or washing and drying them.

A mite-resistant fabric has also been developed in Japan. Look for the label marked *bō-dani kakō* 防ダニ加工 on furniture, bedding, stuffed animals, carpets, even pajamas. Anti-mite insecticides, such as carpet powder, tatami spray, and a fogging mist are available from *Earth Seiyaku* アース製薬.

Mold *kabi* かび

The heat and humidity of the rainy season and the damp caused by summer thunderstorms and typhoons provide ideal conditions for the spread of mold in your bathroom, closets, and shoe cupboards. Keep the mold under control with chlorine spray cleaners, moisture-collecting boxes, and dehumidifiers *joshitsuki* 除湿機.

Hay Fever *kafunshō* 花粉症

Japanese cedar trees, or *sugi*, were planted in large quantities after World War II to reforest the mountains. Dependent upon the wind for cross-pollination, cedars release massive amounts of pollen each spring, causing allergic reactions in over ten percent of the population. *Kafunshō* symptoms usually include a stuffed-up nose, itchy eyes, and frequent sneezing.

Pollen counts are higher on clear, windy days and between 6:00 A.M. and 3:00 P.M. Levels of cedar pollen seem to fluctuate yearly, with large amounts being released every three years. Researchers have suggested that increased pollen production may be related to dry hot weather the previous summer. In any case, listen for the pollen forecast *kafun jōhō* 花粉情報 broadcast during the weather report on television and radio.

If you are affected by pollen, try to stay inside as much as possible with the windows closed. Air filters *kūki seijōki* 空気清浄機 are sold by major electric appliance companies, with capacity measured by room size. Small ones can also be rented from baby supply companies. If you must go outside, try to avoid high pollen–count hours by going to work earlier and coming home a bit later. Wear a face mask and sunglasses or goggles to protect your eyes from pollen. When you come in from outside, brush your hair and clothes, wash your face, and gargle to prevent pollen from being released into the air inside the house. If possible, use a clothes dryer rather than hanging your wash outside; if you air your bedding outside, brush it well before bringing it in.

Other wind-borne pollens which cause symptoms on a smaller scale are *hinoki* (Japanese cypress) in spring, *kamogaya* (orchard grass) in summer and *butakusa* (ragweed), *yomogi* (mugwort), and *kanamugura* (humulus family) from late summer through fall.

ENT doctors or internists usually treat hay fever patients. In Japan, an antihistamine like Zaditen (ketotifen fumarate) may be prescribed three weeks before the start of the season, to help inhibit the allergic reaction. An aerosol medication such as Intal (cromolyn sodium) may also be prescribed. A wide variety of over-the-counter antihistamines and cold medications are available at pharmacies (see pages 257–59).

Atopic Dermatitis (Eczema) atopi アトピー

Atopic dermatitis is a noncontagious, itching allergic rash that occurs in all age groups. Although half of all affected infants seem to outgrow this allergy by eighteen months, for many children and adults it may become a chronic problem, amenable to treatment but prone to relapse. It usually occurs in the folds of the arms and legs, but may cover the entire body, particularly the face. For some reason it has become an increasing problem in Japan in recent years; doctors have suggested that new airtight housing materials, food additives, pollution, and stress are all contributing factors in the rising incidence.

Food allergies seem to be a major cause of this condition. In infants and children the top three allergens are said to be eggs, soybeans, and milk. Various low-allergen baby formulas *tei arugen miruku* 低アルゲンミルク such as Morinaga MA1 Atopi are sold in large drugstores. Doctors are undecided on whether to limit children's food, since complete elimination of such products as eggs could affect a child's growth and nutritional balance. Some doctors also recommend organically-grown produce and foods with no additives. Doctors usually prescribe corticosteroid ointments for short-term use and antihistamines to control itching.

For adult patients, *kanpō* preparations have become increasingly popular, used either alone or in combination with steroid ointments. Some examples of preparations are *jūmi haidoku tō* 十味敗毒湯 (containing the root of the Chinese bell flower, several varieties of parsley, and other ingredients), *shō fu san* 消風散 (containing gypsum, burdock root, and other herbs), and *byakkoka ninjin tō* 白虎加人参湯 (containing genmai, gypsum, ginseng, licorice, and other ingredients).

Other alternative therapies include salt water baths, ultraviolet light therapy, and garlic baths (see pages 289–90).

Asthma zensoku 喘息

For some asthma patients, a bout of mild wheezing can quickly develop into a life-threatening episode. If you are an asthmatic, plan ahead. Review the information on emergency care (see pages 45–52) and learn how to call an ambulance. Choose a hospital near your home in case you ever need it. Make a first visit to a doctor there; you will then have a patient identification number on file that will facilitate registration procedures in the event that you have an attack and need medical care.

The corticosteroid Vanceril/Becotide (beclo methasone dipropionate), the bronchodilator Ventolin (salbutamol hemisulfate), the antiasthmatic inhaler Intal (disodium cromoglycate), and the bronchodilator Theo-Dur (theophylline) are all available by prescription.

In Japan, stimulating the skin and acclimatizing it to lower temperatures by wearing lightweight clothing is said to improve various allergic conditions, especially asthma. Rubbing the chest and arms with a soft, dry towel (*kanpu masatsu*) or a cold, wet one (*reisui masatsu*), is said to train the skin to respond quickly to changes in temperature (however, this is not suggested for patients with eczema, since it would irritate the skin).

Children under eighteen who suffer from conditions like bronchial asthma or asthmatic bronchitis as a result of atmospheric pollution may be eligible for a partial subsidy of medical expenses (see page 62).

Others

Perennial rhinitis *tsūnensei arerugisei bi-en* 通年性アレルギー性鼻炎 usually causes the same symptoms as hay fever, but occurs year-round. Uticaria, or hives *jinmashin* じん麻疹, may be caused by an allergen, or may be a reaction to extremes in temperature (cleaning out your refrigerator, etc). *Kanpō* therapy can sometimes be effective in treating these conditions over a long period.

Japanese Products for Allergy Sufferers

■ Allergy Help-Clean Booth MC-1
An environmentally-controlled, enclosed booth of inflatable plastic one square meter in size. A quiet fan controls the air exchange. Can be placed on top of a bed or futon. Shuts out dust, pollen, and mites, so allergy sufferers can get a good night's sleep. Available from Toshin Products, Osaka.

■ Atopic Dermatitis Pajamas
"Atopitat Pajama"
Cotton pajamas with a natural antibiotic enmeshed in the cloth to help reduce itching from skin allergies, and with a pair of mittens to prevent new scratches. For children aged one through six. Japan Clinical Systems (Nihon Risho System), toll-free (0120) 77-2580.

Selected Hospitals and Clinics for the Treatment of Allergies

Japan Allergy Center
Nihon Arerugi Kenkyujo
日本アレルギー研究所
New Shinbashi Bldg. 3 Fl., 2-16-1 Shinbashi
Minato-ku, Tokyo
03-3591-5464 (by appointment only)

Yamada Skin Clinic
Yamada Hifu-ka
山田皮膚科
New Shinbashi Bldg. 3 Fl., 2-16-1 Shinbashi
Minato-ku, Tokyo
03-3580-7246 (Pub. Ins., Eng.)

National Children's Hospital
(Setagaya-ku, Tokyo; see page 164)

Allergy treatment for children.

Yokohama Children's Allergy Center
Yokohama Shoni Arerugi Senta
横浜小児アレルギーセンター
469 Futatsubashi-cho, Seya-ku, Yokohama-shi
045-365-3601 (by appointment)

National Sagamihara Hospital
Kokuritsu Sagamihara Byoin
国立相模原病院
18-1 Sakuradai, Sagamihara-shi, Kanagawa-ken
0427-42-8311
Allergy clinic; referral necessary.

See also the major hospitals listed in "Regional Resources.

Resource

National Institute of Allergy and Infectious Diseases
Bldg. 31 Rm. 7A32, 9000 Rockville Pike

Bethesda, MD 20892 U.S.
1-301-496-5717
Will answer questions on allergies, and send information.

Epilepsy *tenkan* てんかん

Epilepsy is caused by excessive electrical signals from one group of nerve cells in the brain which can overwhelm other areas and cause epileptic seizures (also caled fits or convulsions). Although epilepsy can't be cured, most seizures can be prevented with anticonvulsant drugs. All major antiepileptic medications are available in Japan by prescription, although the dosage may be lower than is usual in other countries. Since there are more than thirty types of seizures, specialist care is vital.

In Japan, children are usually treated by a pediatrician specializing in neurology. All national children's hospitals (see pages 164–65) have epilepsy outpatient clinics, and most university hospitals have a specialist. Adult patients will be treated by a neurologist or by a psychiatrist specializing in epilepsy. Epilepsy outpatient clinics are usually listed as *tenkan gairai* てんかん外来, *keiren gairai* けいれん外来 or *hossa gairai* 発作外来.

Epilepsy Treatment Centers
There are five national epilepsy treatment centers てんかんセンター, which are part of the pediatrics departments or neurology departments of the following hospitals:

National Sanitorium Kamaishi Hospital
Kokuritsu Ryoyojo Kamaishi Byoin
国立療養所釜石病院
4-7-1 Sadanai-cho, Kamaishi-shi, Iwate-ken
0193-23-7111

National Sanitorium Yamagata Hospital
Kokuritsu Ryoyojo Yamagata Byoin
国立療養所山形病院
126-2 Gyosai, Yamagata-shi, Yamagata-ken
0236-84-5566

National Sanitorium Shizuoka Higashi Hospital
Kokuritsu Shizuoka Higashi Byoin
国立療養所静岡東病院
886 Urushiyama, Shizuoka-shi, Shizuoka-ken
054-245-5446, fax 054-247-9781

National Sanitorium Nishi Niigata Chuo Hospital
Kokuritsu Nishi Niigata Chuo Byoin
国立療養所西新潟中央病院
1-14-1 Masago, Niigata-shi, Niigata-ken
025-265-3171

Utano National Hospital
Kokuritsu Utano Byoin
国立療養所宇多野病院
8 Ondoyama-cho, Narutaki, Ukyo-ku, Kyoto-shi
075-461-5121

Other Resources
Japan Epilepsy Association
Nihon Tenkan Kyokai 日本てんかん協会
Zenkoku Zaidan Bldg. 5 Fl., 2-2-8 Nishi-Waseda Shinjuku-ku, Tokyo
03-3202-5661; Mon.–Fri. 9:00 A.M.–6:00 P.M.
Contact for list of member doctors in Japanese, English, and French. Medical counseling by telephone is also available in Japanese by appointment.

Epilepsy Foundation of America
4351 Garden City Dr., Landover, MD 20785 U.S.
1-301-459-3700
Information and referrals.

Diabetes Mellitus *tōnyōbyō* 糖尿病

Diabetes mellitus occurs when the pancreas either stops producing insulin or does not produce enough, with the result that sugar and starch cannot be absorbed from the blood. It is classified into two syndromes: insulin-dependent, or juvenile onset, diabetes mellitus, and non-insulin–dependent, or adult onset, diabetes mellitus. The number of diabetics—especially those with the adult-onset type—is increasing, but early diagnosis and care can prevent complications. Since many people don't realize that they have a problem, tests for elevated blood sugar (hyperglycemia) and urine tests should both be a part of your annual physical checkup.

If you need care for diabetes in Japan it's suggested that you visit a specialist at a diabetes clinic *tōnyō senmon gairai* 糖尿専門外来 or an endocrinology and metabolism clinic *naibunpi taishaka* 内分泌代謝科 at a university hospital or specialty hospital (see below). Regular checkups will probably be necessary. Insulin, syringes, needles, and urine testing papers are all covered by health insurance; alcohol pads and blood testing strips are not. All medicines and supplies are prescribed for just one-month periods, which is inconvenient for those who must travel for any length of time.

Nutritional counseling for diabetics is done at the specialty hospitals, but different food preferences and body sizes may make the treatment of non-Japanese a challenge for the Japanese dietician. If you are a newly-diagnosed diabetic, make sure that you get help in understanding the dietary requirements of your condition, whether through books, one of the nutritionists listed on pages 310–11, or a quick trip home to receive counseling.

Oral antidiabetic medications such as Orinase and Rastinon (tolbutamide), and human isophane insulin such as Novolin or Humulin are available by prescription. Japanese doctors use the HbA1c test, which is part of the glycosylated hemoglobin assay, to test for diabetic control over a period of weeks. If a diabetic is completely faithful to his diet and takes medications as ordered, this HbA1c level should be six percent or less.

Suggested Hospitals for Treating Diabetes

Asahi Seimei Diabetes Research Center
Asahi Seimei Tonyo Kenkyujo (affiliated with Marunouchi Byoin)
朝日生命糖尿病研究所
Marunouchi Center Bldg., 1-6-1 Marunouchi, Chiyoda-ku, Tokyo
03-3201-6781/03-3213-0489 (call for appointment)

Tokyo Women's Medical University Diabetes Center
Tokyo Joshi Ika Daigaku Tonyobyo Senta, Dai-san Naika
東京女子医科大学糖尿病センタ第3内科
(Shinjuku-ku, Tokyo; see page 344)

National Kyoto Hospital Diabetes Center
Kokuritsu Kyoto Byoin Tonyobyo Senta
国立京都病院糖尿病センター
1-1 Fukakusa Mukai Hata-cho, Fushimi-ku
Kyoto-shi
075-641-9161

See also the major hospitals listed in "Regional Resources."

Resources

Japan Diabetic Society
Nihon Tonyobyo Kyokai 日本糖尿病協会
1-27-4 Hamamatsu-cho, Minato-ku, Tokyo

03-3437-1388; Mon.–Fri. 10:00 A.M.–5:00 P.M. Nationwide list of member doctors and affiliated hospitals. Nutritionist offers telephone counseling Wed. 1:30–4:00 P.M. (J. only).

Sakae さかえ
Sakae, a monthly Japanese magazine for diabetics, is available at bookstores nationwide.

National Diabetes Information Clearinghouse
Box NDIC, Bethesda, MD 20892 U.S.
301-654-3327; Mon.–Fri. 9:00 A.M.–5:00 P.M.

Many publications, plus a free quarterly newsletter on current diabetic therapy.
Juvenile Diabetes Foundation
432 Park Avenue S., New York, NY 10016 U.S.
1-800-500-2873/1-212-889-7575
http://www.jdfcure.com

American Diabetes Association
1660 Duke Street, Alexandria, VA 22314 U.S.
1-800-232-3472/1-703-549-1500, fax 1-703-549-6995
http://www.diabetes.org

Cancer

The very thought of cancer strikes fear in the hearts of many people, preventing them from seeking the advice of a physician when they most need it. Especially when you are far from home and your personal physician, it is easy to put off going for a checkup, deciding instead to wait for your next vacation. But needless to say, *cancer diagnosed in an early stage of growth is much more easily and effectively treated.* If you're experiencing any of the following seven warning signals, as outlined by the American Cancer Society, you should go for a checkup immediately: a change in bowel or bladder habits; a sore that does not heal; unusual bleeding or discharge; a thickening or lump in breast or elsewhere; indigestion or difficulty in swallowing; an obvious change in a wart or a mole; or a nagging cough or hoarseness.

If a diagnosis is made and treatment is needed, you can decide whether to have it done in Japan or in your own country. According to Japanese statistics, there are few doctors in Japan with a specialty in onocology. So at any facility other than the cancer specialty centers, which tend to take a team approach involving specialists in various fields, you would likely be treated by one doctor—either a surgeon or an internist—depending on the treatment chosen. The majority of cancers that afflict Japanese are tumors—such as stomach, lung, or liver—which respond well to surgery, so this is the primary form of treatment for seventy percent of patients. In the U.S., where many different types of cancer are diagnosed and medical costs are high, surgery is chosen by only fifty-five percent of patients.

In addition, chemotherapy *kagaku ryōhō* 化学療法 and radiotherapy *hōshasen chiryō* 放射線治療 are also used here. Chemotherapy with anti-cancer drugs *kōgan zai* 抗がん剤 is utilized to cure certain types of cancer like leukemia, decrease the size of a tumor, or reduce pain. One requirement for any anti-cancer drug's approval by the Japanese government is that it must reduce the size of the patient's tumor by half in at least twenty percent of cases. In 1997, the system of bedside or clinical trials with of experimental drugs or treatment *rinshō shiken* 臨床試験 was begun in Japan; this means that some medications or treatments not yet approved by the Ministry of Health may be used by doctors, but only with the informed consent of the patient as to the possible benefits and risks. If you are asked to participate in a drug trial, make sure that you consider carefully the risks and possible benefits before signing anything.

Since some anti-cancer drugs are oral and not only intravenous medications, it's important to know what you are being given, and to have one doctor coordinate all your medications so as to avoid dangerous reactions to incompatible drugs. Remember that each department keeps its own records, and that these are not usually available to be read by doctors from other departments.

Radiotherapy with either X-rays or implanted radioactive material is used in Japan. Also experimental therapy using proton rays *yōshisen chiryō* 陽子線治療 is being done at three locations, and the world's first heavy-ion medical accelerator *jūryū shisen chiryō* 重粒子線治療, which is used to treat certain types of throat, brain, and lung tumors, began operation in 1994. In Japan, where virtually everyone has health insurance and many cancers respond to surgery, the percentage of patients receiving radiotherapy is much lower than in other countries. This also means that it may be difficult to find doctors and technicians with experience in this type of treatment outside the specialty centers.

Another form of treatment, which loosely translates as heat therapy *onnetsu ryōhō* 温熱療法, is also done here. Cancer cells have been determined to be more sensitive to heat than normal cells. If a tumor is close to the surface, as is the case with skin, breast, or bladder cancer, heat applied in combination with chemo- and/or radiotherapy might be effective. There are two types. Localized therapy to the tumor with microwaves, ultrasound, or sometimes hot water is done once or twice a week in sixty-minute sessions. A probe is placed near the tumor to ensure that the area has been heated to forty-three degrees centigrade. For pain relief, a systemic therapy is also done under general anesthesia, in which the blood is pumped outside the body, heated to forty-two degrees centigrade, and then returned. This method seems to be effective. Immunotherapy known as *men'eki ryōhō* 免疫療法, which includes interferon therapy, etc., is also being done here.

There are statistics for death rates from cancer in Japan, but few reliable ones for the number of people treated and cured each year. Lung, stomach, and liver cancer are the top killers, and because stomach cancer was the number-one cause of death among Japanese for years, this country's diagnosis and treatment of the gastrointestinal tract is highly respected worldwide. Breast, colon, and prostate cancer may be slowly increasing with the Westernization of the Japanese diet, but they are still much lower than in most industrialized countries, so relatively few surgeons specialize in these types (for recommendations of doctors treating breast cancer, consult with patient support group Akebono Kai; see page 94).

As we've mentioned before, communication between doctors and cancer patients often leaves something to be desired in Japan, with the majority of patients not being informed of their diagnosis. In addition Japan still uses very little morphine for pain relief (although this has been changing in recent years), with both patients and doctors reluctant to use it, for fear of addiction; patients generally just bear their pain. Keep these points in mind, together with the fact that the most up-to-date treatment can likely be found at one of the following cancer centers or at a large university hospital when choosing a hospital and a tearm of doctors that meets your needs.

Some cancer centers require a letter of introduction from another medical facility. Testing for cancer can often be done without an introduction, particularly at the Adult-Onset Disease Centers *seijinbyō sentā* 成人病センター. More information on specific tests is given in "Health Checkups."

Selected Cancer Centers

There are at least fifteen other cancer hospitals nationwide. In addition, most of the major hospitals listed in "Regional Resources" also treat cancer.

Cancer Institute Hospital
Gan Kenkyukai Fuzoku Byoin Kenshin Senta
癌研究会附属病院検診センター
1-37-1 Kami-Ikebukuro, Toshima-ku, Tokyo
03-3918-0111

National Cancer Center Hospital
Kokuritsu Gan Senta Chuo Byoin
国立がんセンター中央病院
5-1-1 Tsukiji, Chuo-ku, Tokyo
03-3542-2511

Tokyo Metropolitan Komagome Hospital
(Bunkyo-ku, Tokyo; see page 344)

Saitama Cancer Center
Saitama Kenritsu Gan Senta
埼玉県立がんセンター
818 Komuro, Ina-machi, Kita-Adachi -gun
048-722-1111

Chiba Cancer Center
Chiba-ken Gan Senta
千葉県がんセンター
666-2 Nitona-cho, Chuo-ku, Chiba-shi
043-264-5431

Aichi Cancer Center
Aichi-ken Gan Senta
愛知県がんセンター
1-1 Kanokoden, Chikusa-ku, Nagoya-shi
052-762-6111

Osaka Medical Center for Cancer and Cardiovascular Diseases
Osaka Furitsu Seijinbyo Senta

大阪府立成人病センター
1-3-3 Nakamichi, Higashinari-ku, Osaka-shi
06-972-1181

National Kyushu Cancer Center
Kokuritsu Byoin Kyushu Gan Senta
国立病院九州がんセンター
3-1-1 Notame, Minami-ku, Fukuoka-shi
092-541-3231

Resources in English

Cancer Support Group
Call TELL (see the endpapers) for latest contact number for cancer support groups in Tokyo and elsewhere.

Cancer Information Service
National Cancer Institute, U.S.
1-410-955-8638; Mon.–Fri. 9:00 A.M.–5:00 P.M.
Information by phone.
http://cancernet.nci.nih.gov

Office of Cancer Communications
National Cancer Institute
Bldg. 31, Rm. 10A24, 9000 Rockville Pike
Bethesda, MD 20892 U.S.
Will provide information by mail.

International Union Against Cancer
Geneva, Switzerland
41-22-809-1811
Serves as an information clearinghouse on cancer organizations in other countries.

Thyroid Conditions

Hyperthyroidism *kōjōsen kinō kōshinshō* 甲状腺機能亢進症 is the excessive secretion of the thyroid hormone. It usually affects women (four times more often than men), and particularly those aged twenty to forty. Symptoms include agitation, heart palpitations, hand tremors while at rest, sweating, mood swings, and weight loss (despite a ravenous appetite) resulting from a high metabolism. Radioiodine therapy is the treatment most often chosen by adults in the U.S., but it is seldom used in Japan. Instead, an antithyroid medication *kō-kōjōsen yaku* 抗甲状腺薬 is prescribed, and the patient is monitored over a period of time.

Hypothyroidism *kōjōsen kinō-teika-shō* 甲状腺機能低下症 occurs most frequently in women aged forty to fifty; its symptoms are the opposite: a slowed metabolism, weight gain, tiredness, dry skin, etc. Forgetfulness is another symptom, and people sometimes mistake this condition for menopause. It is treated with hormone therapy.

Japanese specialists recommend that anyone with thyroid problems visit a thyroid specialty hospital or an endocrinology outpatient clinic *naibunpi taisha-ka* 内分泌代謝課 at the onset of their symptoms to be tested, to confirm the diagnosis, and to plan a treatment. Later the person's own internist can take over the treatment.

All the following thyroid specialty hospitals accept Japanese public insurance and have English speakers on staff.

Thyroid Specialty Hospitals

Itoh Hospital
Itoh Byoin 伊藤病院
4-3-6 Jingumae, Shibuya-ku, Tokyo
03-3402-7411 (Pub. Ins., Eng.)
Hospital director and other specialists with overseas experience.
Treats all types of thyroid conditions.

Noguchi Thyroid Clinic and Hospital Foundation
Noguchi Byoin 野口病院

6-33 Noguchi-Nakamachi, Beppu-shi, Oita-ken
0977-21-2151
http://www.coara.or.jp/~hkntc/ntceng.htm
Specializing in treatment and research on thyroid diseases. Has English home page. Accepts thyroid-related questions via e-mail.

Kuma Hospital
Kuma Byoin 隈病院
8-2-35 Shimo-yamate-dori, Chuo-ku, Kobe-shi
078-371-3721

Conditions of Middle Age

The following common conditions are often diagnosed at annual health checkups (see also page 87–91):

Hypertension *kō ketsuatsu* 高血圧

Hypertension, or high blood pressure, is almost always symptomless at first, but if left untreated can lead to stroke, heart failure, or kidney failure. In Japan, it is usually treated by an internist.

If life-style changes such as weight reduction, a low-salt diet and stress reduction are not effective, your doctor may prescribe medications. Since one in three Japanese men over the age of forty are said to be hypertensive, a wide variety of medications are available by prescription, including Tenormin (atenolol), Capoten (capitoril), Cardura (doxazosin mesilate), Adalat (nifedipine), and Inderal (propranolol hydrochloride), under various Japanese brand names. Note that despite their reputation for curative powers, hot springs are not the most relaxing of places for patients suffering from hypertension—going from a cold room into a bath heated to more than forty degrees centigrade can raise your blood pressure to critical levels in an instant.

High Cholesterol *kō koresuterōru ketsu shō* 高コレステロール血症

High cholesterol levels and high triglyceride levels *kō toriguriserido ketsu shō* 高トリグリセリド血症 (also called *chūsei shibō* 中性脂肪) can, if left untreated, cause coronary artery disease. Life-style changes such as weight reduction, a low-fat diet, and regular exercise may help; your doctor may also prescribe medication. For high cholesterol, the following medications are available by prescription under various Japanese brand names: Questran (cholestyramine), Lorelco (probucol), Zocar (simvastatin), and pravastatin sodium. For a high triglyceride level, the little-known medications bezafibrate, clinofibrate, and niceritrol may be prescribed.

Gout *tsūfū* 痛風

Gout usually attacks without warning, creating an intense pain in the joints. Avoid foods high in purines, such as liver, sardines, bonito, large shrimp, and dried squid. Drinking two liters of water a day to protect the kidneys is usually advised, as is weight reduction. Note that drinking alcohol and taking aspirin should be avoided, since these slow the excretion of uric acid from the body. Sufferers should be under the care of a doctor, because this chronic condition can be completely controlled with medication.

In Japan, internists or orthopedic surgeons usually treat gout. Available by doctor's prescription are the following medicines: ibuprofen and indometacin for inflammation and pain, and the medications colchicine, probenecid, and Zyloric (allopurinol).

Specialist Hospitals for Treating Conditions of Middle Age

Most of the following will also perform the *ningen dokku* health checkup.

(See also the list of major hospitals in "Regional Resources.")

Institute of Geriatrics Tokyo Women's Medical University
Tokyo Joshi Ika Daigaku Seijin Igaku Senta
東京女子医科大学成人医学センター
Toho Seimei Honsha Bldg. 21 Fl.

2-15-1 Shibuya, Shibuya-ku, Tokyo
03-3499-1911

The Institute for Adult Disease Asahi Life Foundation
Asahi Seimei Seijinbyo Kenkyu Byoin
朝日生命成人病研究附属病院
1-9-14 Nishi-Shinjuku, Shinjuku-ku, Tokyo
03-3343-2151

Osaka Medical Center for Cancer and Cardiovascular Diseases
Osaka Furitsu Seijinbyo Senta

大阪府立成人病センター
1-3-3 Nakamichi, Higashinari-ku, Osaka-shi
06-972-1181

Resources in English

National Heart, Lung, and Blood Institute
Box 30105, Bethesda, MD 20824 U.S.
1-301-251-1222; Mon.–Fri. 9:00 A.M.–5:00 P.M.
http://nhibi.nih.gov
Information on high cholesterol, high blood pressure, and cardiovascular disease.

National Institute of Arthritis Musculo-Skeletal and Skin Disease
Box AMS, 9000 Rockville Pike, Bethesda, MD 20892 U.S.
1-301-495-4484
http://www.nih.gov/niams/healthinfo
General information on osteoarthritis, gout, and rheumatoid arthritis.

American Self-Help Clearinghouse
St. Clare's Riverside Medical Center, Denville

NJ 07834 U.S.
1-973-625-7101
http://www.cmhc.com/selfhelp/
Send SASE for list of American support groups.

National Institute of Neurological Disorders and Strokes
Bldg. 31, Room 8A06, 9000 Rockville Pike
Bethesda, MD 20892 U.S.
fax 1-301-496-5751
http://www.nih.gov/ninds/
For information on coping with migraine headaches.

National Institute of Diabetes, Digestive and Kidney Disease
Bldg. 31, Room 9A04, 9000 Rockville Pike
Bethesda, MD 20892 U.S.
1-301-654-4415; Mon.–Fri. 9:00 A.M.–5:00 P.M.
http://www.niddk.nih.gov
Information on peptic ulcers, ulcerative colitis, gallstones, and hepatitis.

Death from Overwork *karōshi* 過労死

One unique condition now accepted as a direct cause of death among the Japanese is overwork. Known as *karōshi*, it may happen when someone works so many hours that their normal pace of life is disrupted and their mounting fatigue aggravates a preexisting condition such as high blood pressure. People who die from *karōshi* usually suffer a heart attack or stroke. Since the Labor Ministry has recognized this condition as being work-related, the death itself does not have to occur at the job site, and the surviving family members can claim compensation under the Workmen's Accident Compensation Law (see pages 59–60).

Warning signals of high risk for *karōshi* seem to fall into three categories:

■ **Health:** Has your health status changed in the last year or so? Has your weight, blood pressure, fatigue, forgetfulness, bad temper, headaches, or chest pain increased or seemed worse than usual?
■ **Lifestyle:** Do you go home only to sleep? Rarely see your family awake? Eat irregularly and often skip meals entirely? Smoke more than thirty cigarettes a day? Never exercise? Drink five or more cups of coffee a day?
■ **Work:** Do you work at least ten hours a day and most weekends and holidays? Have your responsibilities increased lately? Have you made some major errors at work lately that have added to your level of stress?

Long hours of overtime work can exhaust foreigners, too. Check out the information on relaxation and stress management in "Living in Japan" and "Alternative Healing."

Osteoarthritis *henkeisei kansetsushō* 変形性関節症

Living in Japan the Japanese way—with little furniture to support the back, sitting or kneeling on the floor at low tables to eat, and sleeping on futons that at times seem not much softer than the hard floor—puts plenty of extra stress on your joints. This added wear and tear, combined with the usual aging process that causes cartilage in your joints to flake and crack, may mean that your painful stiff joints are an indication of osteoarthritis. Common places to have this condition are osteoarthritis of the neck (cervical spondylosis) *keibusekitsuishō* 頸部脊椎症, the spine (lower back) *henkeisei yōtsuishō* 変形性腰椎症, the hip *henkeisei kokansetsushō* 変形性股関節症, and the knee *henkeisei shitsukansetsushō* 変形性膝関節症.

Self-help measures include taking simple painkillers like aspirin or ibuprofen, applying heat, wearing a supporter on the affected area, getting regular exercise to maintain your muscles, and losing weight, if necessary, to lessen the strain. If you have knee or hip problems, you should use a cane and should not be kneeling on the floor. In Japan, osteroarthritis is so common that many neighborhood clinics, even internal medicine clinics, have equipment for exercise therapy and heat that many people use daily. Warm baths in general are good for pain relief.

With knee and hip osteoarthritis, joint replacement surgery *jinkō kansetsu chikanjutsu* 人工関節置換術 may be necessary. Although materials have improved considerably in recent years, there is still some chance of failure, so Japanese doctors will probably prefer to wait as long as possible before doing this treatment.

Foot Care

"My Japanese mother-in-law was of a generation that thought feet were dirty things that should be kept hidden away. She would have been embarrassed to show her own feet even to a doctor, which was probably why she never had her enormous bunions treated. She always kept them covered by socks, tabi, slippers or shoes. In fact, she always seemed shocked that I would walk around displaying my bare feet."

Podiatry, or foot care, is not a recognized medical specialty in Japan. For foot problems you may see an orthopedic surgeon (*seikei geka*) for bone and joint conditions or a dermatologist (*hifu-ka*) for skin problems including infections, ingrown toenails, bunions, calluses, etc. There are also at least two foreign foot care specialists here and may be of help to you.

Josselyne Gourret
03-3495-6160 or (home) tel/fax 03-3495-6170
Also at the Tokyo Medical and Surgical Clinic, see page 33.
Qualified French podiatrist.

Eduard Herbst
078-382-2101, fax 078-382-2150 at K.K. Alice (shoe store) in Kobe
Qualified Austrian medical foot care specialist; can treat ingrown nails, corns, etc. and can make orthopedic shoes. Shoes for everyone but especially helpful for people with feet that are hard to fit, large, wide, etc.

Osteoporosis *kotsusoshōshō* 骨粗鬆症

A loss of calcium from the bones leading to humped backs, "settling" of the spine, and bone fractures happens to everyone with aging. Although both sexes can suffer from this often painful condition, it happens more quickly to women because of the rapid decrease in their estrogen levels during menopause, and so Japanese health care planners have placed more emphasis on prevention and treatment for women. At present, up to twenty percent of bedridden Japanese have osteoporosis, and since there has been little success in therapy aimed at restoring lost bone mass, early prevention is now being emphasized.

One recent study has shown that women living in Okinawa have the strongest bones of any Japanese women, probably because they eat a balanced diet which is high in calcium and which includes a lot of pork, fish (both high in vitamin D) and mineral-rich seaweed. The warm climate, too, allows them to be active outdoors year-round and this exposure to the sun helps form vitamin D in the body, aiding in the absorption of calcium. Moving to Okinawa may not be practical, but similar benefits can be gained from doing weight-bearing exercise, eating a diet high in calcium and vitamin D, and quitting smoking.

"Besides eating foods that have a lot of calcium, my sixty-year-old neighbor wears a pedometer on her waistband every day and checks it every night. Her public health nurse has encouraged her to walk ten thousand steps every day. However, she found that most days her total was between six and seven thousand, and that if she stays inside all day, it measures only about three thousand. She's always trying to increase the total number."

Japanese doctors may prescribe Hormone Replacement Therapy (HRT) during menopause in an effort to prevent osteoporosis, but they usually only do so for short periods because of fears of long-term side effects. Again physicians are divided on this issue. HRT therapy for osteoporosis prevention is not covered under Japanese public health insurance, but it can be used for treatment of an existing condition. For example, low-dosage Estriol is being prescribed for longer periods to treat osteoporosis in the elderly.

See also Bone check, page 97; Menopause, page 109; and Calcium, page 302.

Sports Injuries

Sports medicine is a fairly new medical specialty in Japan, and the country still has very few sports physicians (*supōtsu-i* スポーツ医). Although a majority of sports physicians specialize in orthopedic surgery, sports clinics are sometimes staffed by internists or pediatricians.

You do not have to participate regularly in sports to use a sports clinic. Remember that one large area of concern at sports clinics is the healthy, uninjured athlete who wants to stay healthy while building his strength and stamina. However, this kind of preventive treatment is not covered by national or employees' health insurance plans.

If you are a student, the school's health insurance policy will probably cover injuries that occur during school sporting activities. Schools and sports teams often have a sports doctor or hospital that they use regularly, and so can be a useful resource when looking for a sports doctor.

If you suffer a sports injury and are unsure where to go, call the outpatient department of a university or other large hospital to check if they have a sports orthopedic surgery department *supōtsu seikeigeka* スポーツ整形外科, a sports clinic *supōtsu kurinikku* スポーツクリニック or a sports outpatient department *supōtsu gairai* スポーツ外来. If no sports specialty is listed, go to the orthopedic surgery department *seikei geka* 整形外科. The advantage of going to a large hospital is that there will also be various other specialists on staff to care for any other problems you might have.

Information to Give at the Sports Clinic

■ Your sports history: sports specialty and level, practice routine (days and hours), exactly where you were hurt, when and how, what type of surface you were on when the injury occurred, whether you were using any preventive taping or bandaging, what types of treatment you have undergone before, and what types of health practitioner you have used before, etc.
■ Your own and your family's pertinent health history.
■ If applicable, a history of your menstrual health since you began taking part in sports.

After your initial treatment by an orthopedic surgeon, you may be referred to a physical therapist or an alternative treatment therapist for rehabilitation. If you have been treated initially at a large hospital and continue to have follow-up care at the same hospital, you may find that outpatient rehabilitation is done only in the morning. To avoid missing school or work, find a smaller orthopedic clinic that is more likely to have outpatient hours in the late afternoon and early evening.

Sports Clinics

Below is a list of hospitals and clinics staffed by either medical practitioners or alternative treatment practitioners. Alternative therapies such as *sekkotsu*, shiatsu, and acupuncture have also proved helpful in the treatment of sports injuries, particularly for massage and rehabilitation, following the primary diagnosis by a sports physician or orthopedic surgeon. Phone in advance for an appointment.

See also the hospitals listed in "Regional Resources."

Kanto Rosai Hospital Sports Clinic
Kanto Rosai Byoin Supotsu Kurinikku
関東労災病院スポーツクリニック
2035 Kizuki-Sumiyoshi, Nakahara-ku, Kawasaki-shi, Kanagawa-ken
044-411-3131 (Pub. Ins., Eng.)

Tokyo Koseinenkin Hospital Sports Clinic
Tokyo Koseinenkin Byoin Supotsu Kurinikku
東京厚生年金病院スポーツクリニック
5-1 Tsukudo-cho, Shinjuku-ku, Tokyo
03-3269-8111 (Pub. Ins., Eng.)

Jikei Medical University Hospital Sports Clinic
(Minato-ku, Tokyo; see page 343)

Keio University Hospital Sports Clinic
(Shinjuku-ku, Tokyo; see page 343)

Yokohama Kowan Hospital Sports Clinic
Yokohama Kowan Byoin Supotsu Kurinikku
横浜港湾病院スポーツクリニック
3-2-3 Shin Yamashita, Naka-ku, Yokohama-shi
045-621-3388 (Pub. Ins., Eng.)
Sports Clinic Offering Alternative Therapies

(Also see the alternative clinics listed on pages 278–85)

Global Sports Massage
Konno Bldg. 3 4 Fl., 3-2-2 Shinjuku, Shinjuku-ku, Tokyo
03-3358-6005 (Eng.)
At this official sports clinic for Olympic and other top athletes, nationally licensed practitioners offer sports conditioning, massage, acupuncture, and moxibustion. Call for the locations of many other branches.

Incidence and Treatment of Other Medical Conditions

If you should be diagnosed during your stay with one of the following conditions, you may be interested to know more about how common it is and how it is treated in Japan.

■ Recent research indicates that stomach (peptic) ulcers *i kaiyō* 胃潰瘍 and duodenal ulcers *jūnishichō kaiyō* 十二指腸潰瘍 are caused, in many cases, by the bacteria Helicobacter pyroli, shortened in Japanese to *pirori kin* ピロリ菌. It is estimated that over sixty percent of Japanese have this bacteria in their stomachs, and this is thought to contribute to the development of stomach cancer. So the good news is that an ulcer may be cured with a simple antibiotic. The bad news is that the Ministry of Health and Welfare has not yet approved the use of antibiotics for stomach ulcers, and so Japanese public insurance does not cover this treatment. If you have an ulcer, however, discuss antibiotic treatment with your doctor.

■ In Japan about eighty percent of patients who are afflicted with liver disease develop it from viral hepatitis; some also go on to develop liver cirrhosis and liver cancer. So it's important that people who are hepatitis carriers seek treatment. Although results do vary with the type and severity of the illness, hepatitis C generally seems to be responding well to interferon therapy here; testing involves a needle liver biopsy and blood studies, and treatment is with daily intravenous therapy which is given for two to four weeks and then gradually tapers off until the therapy is complete. Although there may be unpleasant side effects from the interferon during the course of the sessions, most of these disappear when the medication is stopped. Health insurance covers up to six months of interferon therapy.

Hepatitis B is not responding as well to interferon therapy, but health insurance covers up to one month of treatment. Other treatments for this form of hepatitis include the use of steroids and *kanpō* medicine.

■ Irregular heatbeat (dysrythmia) *fusei myaku* 不整脈 occurs when the heartrate goes above 140 or below 50 beats per minute, or there are palpitations or other irregularities. This condition can occur with normal hearts as a result of stress, but is also seen with cardiac disorders. In Japan, testing includes electrophysiologic studies *denkiseiri kensa* 電気生理検査, which are specific for dysrhythmias. After the evaluation, life-style changes alone—like quitting smoking or relieving physical and emotional stress—may be suggested, or more intensive treatment may be necessary. This condition is treated at cardiovascular medicine clinics *junkanki naika gairai* 循環器内科外来.

■ Cataracts, or opacity of the lens of the eye, is one of the most common complications of aging. In recent years there's been a revolution in the treatment of cataracts with the development of advanced surgical equipment and lenses. Japanese doctors also use the phacoemulsification surgical technique called *chōonpa suishōtai nyūkakyū injutsu* 超音波水晶体乳化吸引術, in which an ultrasonic device disintegrates the old lens. After the lens is removed, a permanent lens of plexiglas or acrylic is inserted through a small incision, with just one or two sutures being required. Japanese doctors are willing to let a patient decide when poor vision is affecting his life-style enough to have the surgery done.

■ Excimer laser surgery is performed as a treatment for nearsightedness at a few large hospitals and some private clinics but it is still in the clinical trial period, and is not covered by insurance. The laser itself is very expensive, which means that the treatment is too.

Understanding Your Diagnosis

If you are having trouble understanding your diagnosis or need further information on treatments available, the following organization may be able to help.

National Health Information Center
P.O. Box 1133, Washington, DC 20013 U.S.
1-800-336-4797/1-301-565-4167

http://nhic-nt.health.org/
Can direct you to further sources for virtually any disease or health issue.

You can also use a search engine on the Internet to further research your condition. Try typing in the name of the disease or disorder, or the URL of an appropriate resource in this chapter. See "How to Use This Book" for cautions on using medical information found on the Internet.

Support Groups for Other Conditions

Japan has support groups for many disabilities and disorders, including muscular dystrophy, ALS, neuralgia, rheumatism, gout, neurosis, whiplash, heart disease, kidney disease, spinal disorders, SMON, Parkinson's disease, Bechet's syndrome, and hemophilia. For the names, addresses, and telephone numbers of these and other groups, ask your doctor, or call one of the AMDA centers. Will probably require Japanese.

Ailments That Have No Direct English Translation

"When my eleven-year-old daughter woke up one morning with a swollen knee, we were very concerned and took her to various hospitals, trying to get someone to diagnose the problem. Finally at a famous hospital's sports clinic, we were told that it was 'tana shogai.' I looked though dozens of

medical texts and finally found it in a Japanese orthopedic book, but I could never find the English translation. I don't know if the problem was so rare that it wasn't included in medical dictionaries, or if it was a type of injury originally classified in Japan, and just had no English definition yet."

There are quite a few common ailments diagnosed in Japan that do not have a clear English translation. For instance, *katakori-shō* 肩こり症. Translating this loosely as "stiff shoulders" doesn't seem to do justice to the complexity of what it means in Japan. One family medical guide says that *katakori* sufferers are usually young women with a slight build that have muscle stiffness in the upper back around the shoulder blades. Stress may be one predisposing facter, and others may be ineffective eyeglasses, an irregular bite of your teeth, or doing detailed work (like an office job). The condition is thought to be hereditary since it seems to pass from mother to daughter. Self-help measures include application of heat, massage, maintenance of good posture, regular exercise, and—for any painful episodes—acupuncture.

Another diagnosis is *gojūkata* 五十肩, which some books translate as "frozen shoulder," and others call "periarthritis of the shoulder joint." It affects men and women alike who are over fifty, who suddenly develop pain and swelling in one shoulder. It is said to take six months to a year to recover completely, as the condition progresses from the acute to the chronic stages. Self-help includes exercising, taking aspirin, and applying heat.

Communicable Diseases in Japan

Considering the temperate climate, hygienic water treatment, and efficient public health system, living in Japan clearly presents few hazards in the form of communicable diseases to plague visitors from overseas. Serious communicable diseases like cholera, typhus, typhoid fever, and malaria are virtually nonexistent in Japan, and the few cases that are reported every year usually involve travelers returning from abroad. There have been no reported cases of smallpox, epidemic typhus, pest, polio, lassa fever, rabies, filariasis, yellow fever, or relapsing fever for years. Lyme disease *raimu-byō* ライム病, a common tick-borne disease in the U.S., is rare in Japan.

However, severe congestion in the large cities does create an ideal breeding ground for a variety of viruses, creating outbreaks of diseases that are relatively obscure or unheard of in the West, such as Hand, Foot, and Mouth disease and insect-borne diseases like *tsutsugamushi* disease or Japanese encephalitis. The chart on pages 200–205 will give you an outline of some of the more common communicable diseases.

Notes on Communicable Diseases in Japan

Some communicable diseases in Japan may be unfamiliar to you. Or you may be surprised by the treatments given in Japan for familiar diseases.

■ **Tsutsugamushi Disease:** Also known as scrub typhus, this is carried by ticks and is usually contracted by people who like to walk in grassy areas in the countryside—like farmers, hikers, and golfers. A similar type of disease also carried by ticks is being found in Shikoku island. Called Japanese spotted fever, its symptoms include high fever, skin rash, tiredness, and a small scab over the site of the bite. Check for ticks when walking outside, and be on the lookout for the distinctive scab or eschar that is a hallmark of these diseases.

■ **Japanese Encephalitis:** This mosquito-borne disease is endemic in Asia. Very few cases are reported in Japan each year, but this may be due to the fact that everyone is vaccinated, rather than there not being much disease. Although not everyone who is bitten develops symptoms, for people who do, the disease can be fatal. If you plan to spend some time hiking, camping, or spending time out in the countryside (especially around pig farms), you should probably consider being vaccinated. See pages 159–63 and 326 for information about the vaccine.

■ **Hepatitis B and C:** Japan is listed as a moderately endemic country for these diseases. The rest of southeastern Asia is considered highly endemic. Both are transmitted through activities that involve the exchange of blood, such as medical or dental treatments, sharing needles, acupuncture, tatooing and probably the biggest area of concern—sexual relations with an infected partner. In Japan about 100,000 people are infected each year with Hepatitis B. A vaccine is available for hepatitis B, but not for hepatitis C.

■ **Tuberculosis:** This was the leading cause of death in Japan in 1950. The rate of incidence has decreased dramatically since then, but the disease has not been eradicated; about 40,000 new cases are now reported annually. See pages 159–162 for information about the BCG vaccine.

■ **Strep Throat:** Before the advent of antibiotics, infections caused by the streptococcal bacteria, such as strep throat, which could develop into scarlet fever, rheumatic fever and glomerulonephritis, could be life-threatening emergencies, and evoked fear in all. Nowadays in the U.S., with the development of effective antibiotics, strep throat is quite common and is treated very matter-of-factly, with doctors recommending that parents keep their children home from school for twenty-four hours after the antibiotic has been started. In Japan, some of the fear associated with a streptococcal infection is still present, since scarlet fever (scarlatina) is still listed as being a designated communicable disease. This means doctors must report it to the local public health authorities within twenty-four hours, and that the patient's house must be fumigated. Because of these exaggerated regulations, doctors in Japan rarely diagnose scarlet fever (even if a rash is present) but call both strep throat and scarlet fever by the neutral name *yōrenkin kansenshō* (streptococcal infection). Strep throat is considered serious, and because it is not common, doctors treat the patient very conservatively, mandating ten days of bed rest.

■ **Infectious mononucleosis:** *Densensei tankakushō* 伝染性単核症 (nicknamed "mono" and "the kissing disease" in the U.S.), is primarily but not exclusively a disease of

Common and Less Common Communicable Diseases in Japan

English Name	Japanese Name	Causative Agent	How Spread
Pharyngo-Conjunctival Fever (pool fever)	咽頭結膜熱 *intō ketsumaku netsu*	Adenovirus	Very contagious; by direct or indirect contact—e.g., infected swimming pool water.
Japanese Encephalitis	日本脳炎 *nihon nōen*	Arbovirus	By mosquito. Use mosquito repellent; wear long sleeves, etc.
Scrub Typhus	つつが虫病 *tsutsugamushi-byō*	Rickettsiae tsutsugamushi or rickettsiae orientalis	By tick bite; remove tick immediately with tweezers. Use insect repellent if walking in fields or by a river.
Strep Throat or Scarlet Fever (scarlatina)	溶連菌感染症 *yōrenkin kansen-shō* or 猩紅熱 *shōkō netsu*	Group A streptococcus. Reported cases low; one of 13 diseases which must be reported within 24 hours	By air, e.g. breath of infected person. Uncommon in children under 3 and adults; usually school-age children.
Hepatitis, Viral Hepatitis B Hepatitis C (Hepatitis A, E, D are uncommon in Japan)	*uirususei kan'en* ウィルス性肝炎 *B-gata kan'en* B型肝炎 *C-gata kan'en* C型肝炎	B: Hepadna virus C: Hepatitis C virus	B, C: contact with blood, during medical or dental treatments, or sexual relations. B only: maternal-child. B: vaccine for those at risk; use condom. C: no vaccine.
Impetigo	とびひ *tobihi* (lit., "bushfire") i.e., can spread quickly	Steptococcal or staphylococcal bacteria	Contagious; contact with infected person and those with strep throat; prevalent in hot, humid weather.

Incubation Pd., etc.	Symptoms	Treatment and Notes
2–14 days.	Fever, malaise, pinkeye, sore throat, and swollen lymph glands for 10–14 days. Vision may be temporarily affected.	Corticosteroid eye medication. Prevent by using separate wash-basins and towels; wash eyes after swimming.
7–15 days. Partic. W. Japan and areas around slaughter-houses, Asia, E. Russia.	Many never develop symptoms (headache, confusion, vomiting) but for those who do, can be fatal or lead to serious neurological problems.	Vaccine available in summer months. (Incidence decreasing, but 55 cases in 1990, but only 4 in 1995.)
10–18 days. Asia and Southwestern Pacific. Incidence increasing annually.	Moist areas: groin, underarm; bite turns into blister, forming black scab 4–8 mm; no pain or itch, but swollen lymph glands, chills, fever; rash on chest and abdomen in second week.	Antibiotics (chloramphenicol, tetracycline) cure symptoms in 24–36 hours; untreated, may lead to pneumonia, encephalitis, and blood and cardiac problems.
2–5 days.	Sudden onset: sore throat, high fever; fine body rash in 12–36 hours. Swollen tonsils; tongue white with red bumps (strawberry tongue). Throat culture taken to confirm diagnosis; not all clinics have the lab facilities to do this.	Antibiotics prevent complications such as rheumatic fever. Japanese pediatricians treat very conservatively, mandating many follow-up visits and ten days of bed rest.
B: 45–160 days. C: 2 weeks to 6 months, with average 6–7 weeks.	B: Ranges from carriers with no symptoms, to jaundice and nausea, and an acute phase. Recovery in 3–4 months after onset of jaundice, but can lead to chronic hepatitis. C: Mild infection with jaundice, etc., but can lead to cirrhosis of liver and cancer.	B and C: Bed rest; small, frequent nutritious meals to prevent weight loss. Chronic hepatitis: steroid therapy, interferon, glycyrrhizin, and kanpō therapy; also experimental treatment with other antiviral medication.
7–10 days.	Often around mouth or nose, or skin abrasion or insect bite; single or groups of blisters break open and dry into thin yellow crusts; may cause pain and itching.	Antibiotic ointment, and if acute, oral antibiotic; soak crusts off before using ointment; cut nails short. Prevent with careful hygiene.

English Name	Japanese Name	Causative Agent	How Spread
Weil's Disease (or Leptospirosis)	ワイル病 *wairu-byō* レプトスピラ病 *reputosupira-byō*	Leptospira (thin, spiral, hook-ended microorganism)	Contact with leptospira in animal's urine (rat, dog, etc.), or contaminated water, soil, etc. Annual vaccine or Doxycycline for those at risk.
Tuberculosis	結核 *kekkaku*	Mycobacterium tuberculosis bacteria	Air-borne and highly contagious. Rate of TB in Japan is high compared with Western countries: 34.2 per 100,000. In 1995 42,958 registered cases.
Herpangina	ヘルパンギーナ *herupangina*	Coxsackievirus Group A	Fecal-oral; prevalent in summer to early autumn in children under 10.
Herpes Gingivostomatis (swollen gums) Herpes Labialis (cold sores or fever blisters)	ヘルペス性歯肉口内炎 *herupesu-sei shiniku kōnaien* 口唇ヘルペス *kōshin herupesu*	Herpes simplex type 1 virus (non-sexual type). Majority of Japanese have had exposure by age 20	By direct contact. After first infection, reactivation of latent virus may occur. First or recurrent infection may be brought on by strong sunlight or fever.
Epidemic Kerato-Conjunctivitis (EKC)	流行性角結膜炎 *ryūkō-sei kaku ketsumakuen* or はやり目 *hayarime*	Adenovirus	Very contagious; contaminated eye drops, shared towels, etc. Prevalent in summer.

Incubation Pd., etc.	Symptoms	Treatment and Notes
2–26 days, but usual range is 7–13 days. In Japan only about 50 cases reported in the last 20 years, but common in other parts of Asia.	Abrupt onset: 4–9 days headache, muscle ache, chills, fever, pinkeye. Second phase: no symptoms for 3 days, then reappears with neurological problems. Weil's Syndrome is severe form, with jaundice, hemorrhages, confusion, etc.	Antibiotics, e.g. Doxycycline. Diagnosis difficult because similar to meningitis, hepatitis, etc. Vaccine for children at risk, but not effective with all types of leptospira, esp. in Okinawa. 2 shots before 18 years; booster every 5 years.
2–10 weeks after primary infection, TB skin test will be positive.	Primary infection: few or no symptoms. In most cases infection is contained and healing occurs, but age is a factor—higher risks of infants developing extra-pulmonary TB, young adults developing pulmonary TB (chronic cough, bloody sputum); elderly may be susceptible to reactivated TB (weight loss, night sweats).	At least two medications over 9–12 months, usually INH and rifampin. Prevent with BCG vaccine, periodic TB skin testing, and medication for people who have had contact with TB patients. (See page 119 for information on BCG.)
3-6 days.	Fever and tiny blister-like spots with red ring on throat and tongue. In 24 hours blisters form small ulcers, which clear in 4–5 days.	Fever medication and diet of soft foods, with extra liquids.
2–12 days contagious; use lip balm with sunscreen to prevent recurrence.	Herpes gingivostomatis: usually in children aged 2–4 years; fever, swollen lymph glands and gums, and white sores in mouth and lips. Herpes labialis: cold sores around lips.	For mouth sores: fever medication, and soft foods. For cold sores: if no blisters, apply ice cube for 90 minutes to stop sores developing. For blisters: apply rubbing alcohol or antiviral cream until they dry up.
2–14 days.	Very red eye and pain; scar tissue may form on conjunctiva; low grade fever, headache, and malaise. May spread to cornea, temporarily affecting sight; can last 3–4 weeks.	Corticosteroid eye drops. In general, to prevent, wash hands carefully and regularly; dispose of any opened eye drops after 1 month.

Managing Specific Conditions

English Name	Japanese Name	Causative Agent	How Spread
Infantile Gastro-enteritis	乳児嘔吐下痢症 *nyūji ōto gerishō*	Rotavirus	Fecal-oral route; prevalent in late autumn and winter.
Erythema Infectiosum (or Fifth disease)	伝染性紅斑病 *densen-sei kōhan-byō* or りんご病 *ringo-byō*	Parvovirus B19—very common virus	Respiratory secretions and blood. Common in Japan, with large outbreak every six years.
Roseola (Exanthem Subitum, or Sixth disease)	突発性発疹 *toppatsu-sei hosshin*	Human herpes-virus 6	Unknown. Prevalent year-round in children under two.
Hand, Foot, and Mouth Syndrome (no relation to Hoof and Mouth disease in cattle)	手足口病 *te ashi kuchi-byō*	Coxsackievirus A16 (enterovirus)	Fecal-oral, and possibly oral route. Prevalent in summer to early autumn in children under 10.
Acute Hemorrhagic Conjunctivitis	急性出血性結膜炎 *kyūsei shukketsu-sei ketsumakuen*	Coxsackievirus A24 and enterovirus 70	Fecal-oral; flies, contaminated equipment at eye clinics.
Kawasaki Syndrome (Mucocutaneous Lymphnode Syndrome MCLS)	川崎病 *kawasaki-byō*	Possibly unknown strains of staphylococcus or streptococcus bacteria. Japan rate of 3,000 cases a year for the last 30 years is higher than other countries'	Unknown.

Incubation Pd., etc.	Symptoms	Treatment and Notes
2–3 days.	Children 6–24 months: vomiting, diarrhea, fever, abdominal pain; symptoms may last a week. Normal gastroenteritis lasts 24–48 hours.	No medication, but adequate fluids to prevent dehydration; intravenous fluids only in severe cases. Prevent by good hygiene.
Usually between 4 and 14 days; most infectious before onset; unlikely to be infectious after rash appears.	In children: bright red rash on face with a "slapped cheek" appearance, pale around the mouth, and a fine lace-like rash on arms moving down to thighs.	Supportive care; pregnant women should consult with doctor. Prevent by careful disposing of used tissues.
Estimated at 5–15 days.	As fever lasting 3–5 days subsides, fine rash appears that quickly fades, and is gone in 2–3 days.	Control fever with medication, etc.; encourage fluids. Convulsions may occur with high fever.
Usually 3–6 days.	Mild fever with blister-like sores in the mouth, and a fine rash, that may progress to a blister type on the hands and feet.	Fever medication and soft, easily-digested foods. Prevent with careful hand washing.
Usually 3–6 days.	Conjunctivitis, swelling, redness, congestion, pain in the eye; recovery usually complete in one week.	Corticosteroid eye drops may be prescribed. Prevent with careful hygiene.
Unknown.	Acute inflammatory disease, from birth to 8 years, with peak at 18 months. Starts with fever; may last 1–2 weeks, also pinkeye; body rash; swelling of hands and feet and lymph glands; red throat, cracked lips, and strawberry tongue; may last 60 days.	For heart: injections of gamma globulin; antibiotic therapy seems ineffective; aspirin is used to thin the blood.

adolescents in the U.S.; unclean or poor living conditions can also cause it to spread. In Japan, it's listed as a disease of 15- to 25-year-olds, which reflects the way that both dating patterns and poverty statistics differ in the two countries.

HIV and AIDS

Most communicable disease have been described in the chart on the preceding pages. But because of the special circumstances surrounding HIV/AIDS, we have devoted a separate section to it.

In Japan, through negligence on the part of the government, many hemophiliacs were infected with the AIDS virus by contaminated blood products in the mid-1980s. Details of the scandal which have come to light in recent years have created a deep sympathy for this group that was wronged by the bureaucracy. But at the same time, talking about the sexual transmission of AIDS is still considered shameful and taboo among the general public, and there is a great deal of prejudice towards HIV carriers and many unfounded fears about AIDS transmission.

Health and Welfare officials estimate that the actual number of HIV and AIDS patients infected by sexual transmission is probably seven times the official number of 3,000. Particularly worrisome is that since 1991 the rate among young heterosexuals is said to have increased dramatically. Because the numbers seem low, government efforts are concentrated on prevention and education. In Japan, since 1986 all donated blood is screened for the HIV antibody, so there is almost no risk involved in receiving a blood transfusion.

HIV Antibody Testing

Confidential testing for the HIV antibody is done free of charge at all public health centers. A number system is used, and you must pick up the results (positive *yōsei hannō* 陽性反応 or negative *insei hannō* 陰性反応) personally; centers will not send them by mail. Since most centers only provide weekly or bimonthly testing, call ahead in Japanese to ask the dates and times; in some cases you may need to make an appointment. If you are planning to take the test, bear in mind that the antibody may not be produced until up to three months after infection has occured; test results are only reliable if three months have passed since your possible exposure.

Confidential testing can also be done in English at most of the international clinics with varying fees. Most doctors offer pre-test counseling, and if the results are positive, you will be referred to a counseling center for post-test counseling as well, and to a hospital for treatment. Testing can be done at many hospitals for a fee, but not always with the same degree of confidentiality.

Treatment and Insurance

If you test positive for the virus, although it may take years to actually develop the disease, new research indicates that aggressive treatment right from the beginning may allow the virus to be contained or possibly eradicated. Optimal care can be received with a HIV experienced physician or hospital that can acurately monitor your immune system and administer the medications. Medicine will probably be a combination of at least two drugs and an additional protease inhibitor. In Japan, Retrovir (AZT), Videx (ddl), zalcitabine (ddC), (3TC), (IDV), and the protease inhibitors have been approved, and are covered by national health insurance. The cocktail treatment is also used. Full medical coverage using approved drugs is available for AIDS treatment. Starting in April 1998, HIV carriers were designated as physically handicapped and are eligible for public welfare services, depending on the progression of AIDS symptoms.

Problems may arise in finding a hospital or doctor to treat you, especially in an emergency. Maintaining privacy and preventing discrimination in the workplace are serious concerns in Japan, particularly since diagnosis and medications could possibly be reported to your company if you are covered by Employees' Health Insurance. The Ministry of Health and Welfare has asked each prefectural government to designate at least two hospitals where people with HIV or AIDS can receive care. However, hospitals are reluctant to be designated as care facilities. Even hospitals that have agreed to cooperate refuse to have this information made public, for fear of scaring away other patients. To find an appropriate doctor and hospital, it's probably best to consult with the telephone hotlines listed below or the public health department. See also the hospices listed on page 330.

HIV and AIDS Support Groups, Hotlines, and Resources

See also pages 239–40 for more counseling services.

Tokyo English Life Line (TELL) HIV/AIDS Hotline

03-3968-4073; Mon., Wed., Thurs. 7:00 P.M.–10:00 P.M.

Free, confidential information about HIV transmission and testing from trained counselors, referrals, and telephone counseling for HIV-affected persons. TELL recommends that anyone considering testing receive both pre- and posttest counseling.

HIV Seropositive Persons Support Group

Call TELL for the current number.
Biweekly support group meetings.

Japan HIV Center English Hotlines

03-5259-0256 (Tokyo)

0720-43-2044 (Osaka)
Sat. 1:00 P.M.–6:00 P.M.

One of the largest volunteer support groups nationwide, with offices in Tokyo, Osaka, Nagoya, Kyushu, and Shikoku. They support anyone who is suffering from HIV/AIDS regardless of means of infection. In addition to providing information and counseling by phone, they also offer various support groups. New members, volunteers, and donations to support activities are welcomed.

Tokyo Metropolitan Government's 24-Hour Telephone Information Service on AIDS

0120-08-5812 (Eng.)/0120-49-4812 (Thai)
Prerecorded information on various resources, including where to go for testing in Tokyo.

Tokyo Metropolitan Testing and Counseling Office
Minami-Shinjuku Kensa Sodan-shitsu
南新宿検査相談室
Tokyo Minami-Shinjuku Bldg. 3 F1.
2-7-8 Yoyogi, Shibuya-ku, Tokyo
03-3377-0811 (J. only); Mon.–Fri. 4:00 P.M.–6:00 P.M.
Bring a translator. Tests are anonymous and free of charge. By appointment.

Kyoto YWCA Women's HIV and AIDS Hotline
Josei no Tame no HIV/AIDS Denwa Sodan
075-414-3747; Mon. 1:00 P.M.–9:00 P.M. except hols.
Information and counseling on HIV and AIDS; also available in English.

AMDA Centers (see back endpapers) and the **HELP Asian Women's Help Shelter** (see front endpapers) may be able to give advice in lan-guages other than English and help you find an appropriate caregiver.

International Medical Center of Japan
Kokuritsu Kokusai Iryo Senta
国立国際医療センター
1-21-1 Toyama, Shinjuku-ku, Tokyo
03-3202-7181
03-5273-5418 (AIDS Clinical Center direct line)
http://www.imcj.go.jp/
Testing and treatment. Every weekday, by appointment. English, Portuguese, Thai translators.

Project Information for People with HIV/ AIDS, Family, Friends, and Caregivers
1-800-822-7422/1-415-558-9051 (U.S.) Mon.–Sat. 10:00 A.M.–4:00 P.M.
http://www.projinf.org/

American Foundation for AIDS Research
1-800-392-6327/1-212-806-1600 (U.S.) Mon.–Fri. 9:00 A.M.–5:00 P.M.
Information on treatments.

Organ Transplants/Brain Death *zōki-ishoku* 臓器移植 / *nōshi* 脳死

In Japan the legal definition of "brain death" has been hotly debated for some years, and it wasn't until the fall of 1997 that legislation was passed authorizing organ transplants from brain dead donors. Even so, the strict conditions attached to the procedures seem to have stalled the process from moving forward rapidly. Donors must be 15 years old or older—automatically barring children from becoming donors, and in most cases, receivers. The donor must have given written permission in advance, and there most be no objection from any of the donor's close relatives. Further, the patient must be confirmed brain dead by two doctors who are not involved in the organ transplant.

Other obstacles to organ donation and transplant include slow distribution of donor cards, donor cards that are too complicated to complete properly and easily, and few facilities that are permitted to or prepared to perform the transplants. The largest barrier seems to be that there is not widespread acceptance among the Japanese public of the idea of organ transplantation from brain-dead patients.

Registering to Be an Organ Transplant Donor

The Japan Organ Transplant Network *nihon zoki ishoku network* 日本臓器移植ネットワーク is the only group in Japan licensed to act as an intermediary for organ transplants. Donor cards (written in Japanese only) are supposed to be available at post offices nationwide, but distribution is slow.

Organ Donor Card (Translation of Back of Card)

Please circle as many of the number(s) 1, 2, and 3, as express(es) your wishes concerning organ donation. If appropriate, circle the name of the organ(s) you wish to donate.

■ 1. I hereby agree to be diagnosed as brain dead and wish to donate the circled organs for transplant. Organs that I do not wish to donate are crossed out with an X.

Heart, Lungs, Kidneys, Pancreas, Intestines, Others

■ 2. I hereby agree to donate the circled organs for transplant at death only after my heart has stopped beating. Organs that I do not wish to donate are crossed out with an X.

Kidneys, Eyes, Pancreas, Others

■ 3. I do not wish to donate any organ.

Date:
Signature of holder of card:
Signature of family member:

Japan Eye Bank Association
Nihon Gankyu Ginko Kyokai
日本眼球銀行協会
Shinsei Bldg. #405, 2-8 Ogawa-machi, Kanda
Chiyoda-ku, Tokyo
03-3293-6616

Since corneal transplants can be done after the patients heart has seized, a separate registration system is used. There is a bank in each prefecture. Call in Japanese for the local contact number.

Donations That You Can Make While You Are Still Living

Blood Donation   kenketsu 献血

Donating blood in Japan is much the same as in any other country of the world. Walk into one of the hundreds of Red Cross donation centers nationwide (or one of their mobile buses) and although it depends a bit on your age and weight since there is some variation, generally 400 ml of blood is given at one sitting. As you relax on a comfortable bed or chair, you will quickly be set up to the tubing and have your blood taken, and after receiving your well deserved glass of orange juice, probably feel that you have contributed to the benefit of your fellow man. Afterwards you will be sent detailed results of tests on such things as your blood count or cholesterol level. These results, however, will not include any information about whether you are HIV-positive or not (the Red Cross tests for it, but will not include the information since they don't want to encourage people to use this as an HIV testing center.)

Before donating, however, you must fill out a questionnaire (which may be in Japanese). Because of the need to guarantee the recipient a safe blood supply, there is a trend now worldwide for requiring a detailed questionnaire to be completed prior to donating. In Japan you will not be allowed to donate if you indicate that you:

■ are donating with the purpose of testing for AIDS.
■ have had sexual relations with someone of the same sex during the past year
■ have injected narcotics intravenously during the past year

■ are a carrier of hepatitis B or C, or are infected with HIV
■ have received a blood transfusion or an organ transplant
■ have had a sexually transmitted disease, or malaria

Other questions include items about tatoos, infectious mononucleosis, etc. so unless your Japanese reading ability is very good, it might be better to bring someone along to translate for you. Some donation centers, but not all, have the form translated into English. The number of people who are donating in recent years has decreased, so blood is always needed. Don't let the questionnaire deter you from making a donation.

If you are going to have planned surgery, it's possible that you can donate blood for your own sake, to have on hand in case you should need a transfusion. Known as *jikoketsu yuketsu* 自己血輸血 this would be the safest procedure, since it guarantees that you will have no adverse reactions. Speak with your doctor ahead of time to see if hospital policy allows it.

Bone Marrow Donation

A bone marrow transplant, or the infusion of bone marrow cells into a patient, is used to treat some types of leukemia, aplastic anemia, and severe immunodeficiency. This is almost always a life-saving procedure. Donors are usually found among the patient's family members, and if he is lucky enough to have a twin, he's guaranteed a perfect match. Unfortunately, though, some patients are not so lucky, and need to depend on a donor bank to find compatible marrow.

If you decide to register to become a donor, the first step is simple: just fill out the registration card and have a blood test. If by chance your marrow matches that of a needy patient, keep in mind that you can be directly responsible for saving a life. Granted, the process is not nearly as simple as giving blood. You must first undergo counseling and a physical exam, and then sign a legal document of intent; a member of your family must sigh too. You can not retract your offer after this point. The actual extraction of the bone marrow (called "harvesting," in transplant lingo) requires a four- to five-day stay in the hospital. You will probably be given a local anesthetic, since this is said to be most common; then your bone marrow will be removed with a needle, usually from your hip (iliac) bone. Later your marrow will be transplanted into the recipient. An English brochure is available.

Contact: Japan Marrow Donor Foundation
0120-37-7465 (J.only); fax 03-3355-5090 (Eng.)

For details on vaccines and on diseases contracted only by children, see pages 155–56 and 158–63.

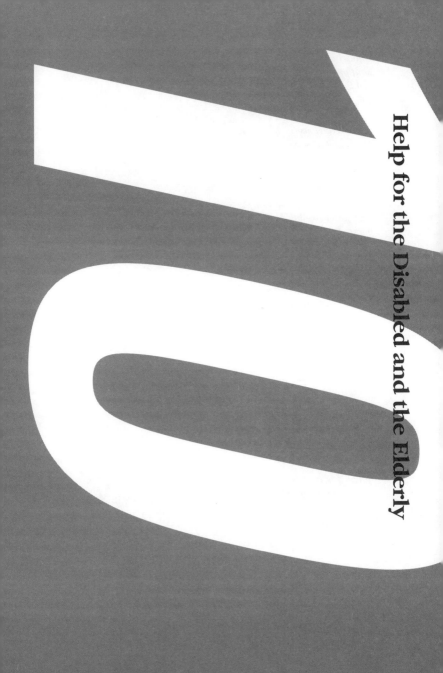

10

Help for the Disabled and the Elderly

"I have three children, and when the doctor said my sixty-eight-year-old Japanese mother-in-law would need constant supervision, I panicked. However, after a bit of research I found that, since a physician had recommended it, her Japanese public health insurance would pay most of the cost of hiring a helper. I found one through a home-helper agency introduced by the welfare department at my local city office. My mother-in-law also now stays at a nearby public day-care center four days a week from 10:00 in the morning to 3:00 in the afternoon, when a bus picks her up and brings her home. The center staff serves lunch and helps her take a bath. She gets great care and keeps busy with daily activities there. It only costs me ¥900 per day."

Help for the Disabled & the Elderly

The day may come when either you or someone you love requires special care, and it may even come while you are in Japan. Whether you have given birth to a child with a disability, need a place for your bedridden father-in-law, or have a visitor from home who is wheelchair-bound, an idea of what kinds of help are available may ease your burden somewhat.

The system is designed primarily to help the Japanese, but registered foreign residents who have permanent physical or mental disabilities and are covered by Japanese public insurance can also take advantage of special welfare services, medical benefits, and other forms of financial assistance. But certain national programs apply to all residents, regardless of area, insurance coverage, or visa status (see page 84). Further assistance can come from support groups or other groups in the community. Whether you have insurance or not, you can use public consultation centers, which can put you in touch with public and private resources in your area.

Programs can vary greatly in different areas. Many are run by local governments, some of which simply have more financial and human resources than others. Also, since public services are free or low-cost, long waiting lists for them are common, and as a result many people are forced to turn to private services. Hopefully the situation will improve with the present focus on this part of the system.

The Disabled

Japan is not noted for its attention to the needs of the disabled, and most people who use wheelchairs will find the road somewhat rough. Historically, having a family member with a disability was considered shameful, and attempts to hide evidence of imperfections in the family from society were all too common. Even today, many disabled people hesitate to venture out, for fear of being shunned or of inconveniencing others. Existing laws do not sufficiently protect the rights of or prohibit discrimination against the disabled.

But attitudes are changing. Exposure to programs abroad has opened the eyes of many Japanese to the benefits and the means of integrating those who are differently-abled into society. Parents are challenging schools that initially refuse to enroll their wheelchair-confined children. Often it is the handicapped themselves who are the most vocal—calling for, among other things, elevators in stations, ramps on buses, wheelchair-accessible lavatories, and wider employment opportunities. The increasing size of the aged population—a large percentage of whom are in some way disabled—is also contributing to the pressure to create a society that can address the needs of all its citizens.

Registration of Disabilities

If you have Japanese public insurance, first register your disability at your local government welfare office *fukushi jimusho* 福祉事務所. To do this, you will need a designated doctor's written assessment *tokutei no shindan-sho* 特定の診断書. In the case of registration of a physical disability, the welfare office will issue a Handbook for the Physically Disabled *shintai shōgai-sha techō* 身体障害者手帳, and for a mental disability, a Handbook of Love *ai no techō* 愛の手帳. The handbook notes the degree of your disability (with first-degree being the most serious), and will be your passport to receiving public financial assistance and services. The handbook often takes as much as a month from the time of your application to arrive, but in cases of acute need you may be able to start receiving some services even before it arrives.

Tokyo Metropolitan Rehabilitation Center for the Physically and Mentally Handicapped
Tokyo-to Shinshin Shogai-sha Fukushi Senta
東京都心身障害者福祉センター
3-17-2 Toyama, Shinjuku-ku, Tokyo

03-3203-6141, 03-3208-1121 (for children's needs)
Rehabilitation and treatment center. A designated center for the medical assessment required for the registration of disabilities.

Consultation for the Disabled

Once you've registered your disability, the welfare office may direct you to the public health center, or to a health and welfare center *hoken fukushi sentā* 保険福祉センター specializing in the care of the disabled and elderly, so that you can begin to look into your resources. You'll probably need to speak Japanese or to bring along someone who does (some local governments can call in volunteer interpreters). These centers offer information and counseling on medical care, home nursing, special equipment, education, jobs, and even marriage. Instruction, training, and legal advice may also be available.

The information services listed on the back endpapers and the counseling centers on pages 175 (for children) and 239–40 may also be of help.

Financial Assistance for the Disabled

A lot of paperwork is involved, but national, prefectural, and local governments all provide allowances. Your local welfare office can give you details on all of these financial assistance programs as well as others and tell you where to apply (recipients are usually required to have been resident in the district for at least one year). In addition, some disabilities qualify for reductions of or exemptions from income, resident, automobile, or other taxes. Other discounts include reduced public transportation fares and highway tolls.

Assistance for Medical and Nursing Expenses

Forms and amounts of assistance available vary with income level, degree of disability, and area in which you live, but part or all of the difference between the actual cost of medical care/equipment and the amount covered by insurance will be paid (this applies only to those enrolled in Japanese public insurance and only to forms of care which are covered by it). You'll be issued a certificate for payment of disability-related medical fees *shinshin shōgai-sha iryō-hi jukyū-shashō* 心身障害者医療費受給者証. If you present this with your health insurance certificate when you receive medical care at designated medical institutions, the government will pay the facility directly. If you receive services at other facilities, or purchase equipment which is covered, you can apply for reimbursement at the local welfare office.

Some areas also provide extra assistance for psychiatric inpatient care, disposable diapers, and even home haircuts.

See page 62 for more programs for those under age eighteen; for work-related disabilities and accident compensation, see page 59.

Special Allowances

Depending on the degree of disability, several allowances from the national government are available to those not living in institutions, whose household income is below a certain level. These include the *tokubetsu shōgai-sha teate* 特別障害者手当 (for disabled adults), the *shōgai-ji fukushi teate* 障害児福祉手当 (for disabled children) and the *jidō fuyō teate* 児童扶養手当 (for children of a disabled father). For those over age twenty, there is also a special national pension *shōgai kiso nenkin* 障害基礎年金.

It may be possible to receive other allowances from your prefectural or local government. For example, the Tokyo Metropolitan Government now offers a monthly allowance known as the *jūdo shinshin shōgai-sha teate* 重度心身障害者手当 for various kinds of disabilities.

Depending on a family's income, financial assistance may be available to assist in remodeling the home for a disabled member, and obtaining all kinds of equipment for home care.

Getting Around

Getting around in Japan is becoming easier for the disabled than it was even a few years ago. Both the national and local governments are increasing the number of buses able to accommodate wheelchairs, and are installing escalators and elevators in train stations (including all the stations on the *shinkansen* bullet train lines). A device that carries wheelchairs up and down stairs is available at some train stations. For the blind, traffic lights play tunes at major crossings, and the floors of train stations have raised-bump pathways leading to wickets as well as ticket machines that are inscribed in Braille.

Many local governments cooperate with taxi companies to provide transportation for the disabled. If your disability qualifies you for this service, you'll receive a supply of tickets monthly or annually to use with specified taxi companies. If you need a wheelchair or are completely bedridden, the tickets will be for a special taxi equipped with a lift (*rifuto-tsuki fukushi haiyā* リフト付き福祉ハイヤー). To learn whether you qualify, contact your local welfare office.

If you are looking for a wheelchair, you may want to visit a showroom or a public consultation center to try out various sizes and features.

Resources

Tokyo Metropolitan Technical Aid Center

Tokyo-to Fukushi Kiki Sogo Senta
東京都福祉機器総合センター
Central Plaza 13–14 Fl., 1-1 Kagurabashi
Shinjuku-ku, Tokyo
03-3235-8571

Currently the newest and largest exhibition of wheelchairs and other equipment (beds, baths, etc.) for caring for the bedridden and disabled, especially the elderly. Also, classes on home care using barrier-free model apartments, and model walkways for practicing the use of wheelchairs. Numerous catalogs of sale and rental companies in Japan.

Access International

アクセス・インターナショナル
03-5248-1151, fax 03-5248-1161
(Tokyo showroom)
06-536-5515, fax 06-536-5595
(Osaka showroom)
http://www2.channel.or.jp/access

U.S.-made wheelchairs, communications equipment, and software. Stock is geared toward Japanese market, but the company can order non-adapted U.S. models and large sizes. No rentals. Call in Japanese or fax in English for catalog and information.

Nihon Abilities

日本アビリティーズ
03-3460-2341, fax 03-3460-3275 (Tokyo)
06-934-6241, fax 06-934-6240 (Osaka)
Imports all kinds of equipment from around the world. Stocks various sizes and models. Rental

possible of certain items. Showrooms in several major cities around Japan. Call in Japanese or fax in English for catalog and information.

Travel

If you're traveling in Tokyo, one very useful guide for wheelchair users is *Accessible Tokyo*, compiled by the Japanese Red Cross Language Service Volunteers. For a free copy, write to the Red Cross at 1-1-3 Shiba-Daimon, Minato-ku, Tokyo, or fax 03-3432-5507, with a note about your reasons for wanting the book. You can also check it out on the Internet:
(http://www.jwindow.net/OLD/LWT/TOKYO/REDCROSS/redcross_index.html).
The booklet explains how to rent a wheelchair, grades major tourist areas, hotels, and stations in terms of their accessibility, and gives information on parking and other necessities.

When you are sightseeing, note that entry and parking fees are waived at some public parks, gymnasiums, and museums for those who show a handbook for the disabled.

Tokyo Station Traveler's Emergency Rest Center

Kyukyu Engo Senta 救急援護センター
Marunouchi South Exit
03-3287-1400 (J. only)
8:00 A.M.–8:00 P.M. all year round
Rest area with nurse but also a center for planning trips for the disabled. Information on wheelchair-friendly roads, inns, hotels, and public transport, as well as on helpful volunteer groups in most parts of Japan.

Trained Dogs mōdōken 盲導犬, pātonā doggu パートナードッグ

Japan still lags behind other industrialized nations in the use of guide dogs for the blind and partner dogs for those who are without the use of their arms or legs, but the situation is gradually improving. Note that Japanese dogs are trained in English—well, Japanese English, with the accompanying accent.

Guide dogs are in great demand, and the wait for one can be as long as a year or two. If you need a guide dog, first contact your local welfare office. The Nihon Modoken Kyokai (03-3375-6201) loans out dogs through local governments around the country. You can also try Eye Mate Kyokai (03-3920-6162). If you want a partner dog, contact the Patona Doggu o Sodateru-kai (0426-66-2825).

You can also bring your trained dog from overseas—guide dogs do not need to be kept in quarantine. Just be sure that your dog has a rabies shot at least thirty days before arriving (bring the certificate) and a stamped certificate of good health from your government's department of agriculture. If you are a tourist, you will need a letter of guarantee from a Japanese living in Japan. Before the dog can enter the country, you must also submit an itinerary to the airport quarantine office indicating your contact address and telephone in Japan.

Finding Specialized Medical Care

Your family doctor can recommend a specialist, usually at a university or specialty hospital. Support groups (on page at left) may also be a useful resource. You can also try asking at your local public health center, or at a consultation center for the health and welfare of the physically disabled *shintai shōgai-sha kōsei sōdan-sho* 身体障害者厚生相談所 or the mentally disabled *seishin renjaku-sha kōsei sōdan-jo* 精神連弱者相談所. Note that every prefecture in Japan has several public hospitals specializing in different areas of medical care for the disabled. Public health centers can direct you to these, as well as to dental clinics for the disabled.

Home Care for the Disabled

If you are taking care of a physically disabled person at home, you may want to visit the Tokyo Metropolitan Technical Aid Center (page 216) or a similar center in your area for ideas. Consult your local welfare office too. Attend classes at your public health center or your prefectural consultation office for the elderly *kōrei-sha sōgō sōdan sentā* 高齢者総合相談センター. Every prefecture also has a center for teaching home nursing skills *kaigo jisshū/fukyū sentā* 介護実習・普及センター; here you can learn a lot just by watching (or take along an interpreter).

If you don't speak Japanese, try contacting the Foreign Nurses Association (see the endpapers). They may have a member in this specialty who can at least give you some tips over the phone.

Partial government subsidies of accommodation and transportation costs are available to qualifying families taking care of disabled relatives at home, in order to provide caregivers with a short break, but these must be applied for months in advance. Provision is made for the disabled person to stay in a public facility during this time.

Families who have a seriously disabled child living at home may be eligible for free home-help services. The period and frequency of use depends on the family's income and needs. Ask about these benefits at your local welfare office.

Public Services for the Disabled

Services vary in each area, so check at your local welfare center for the disabled. However, note that scarcity of space, equipment, and caretakers may put you on a waiting list. The following are typical services:

Emergency Signaling System

Regardless of income, those with a first- or second-degree physical disability living alone at home may be entitled to an apparatus which makes direct contact with the Fire Department in case of emergencies, twenty-four hours a day. Also provides a telephone and/or help with paying phone bills for qualified low-income adults.

Equipment

Canes for the blind, artificial eyes, artificial larynxes, Braille pens, glasses, hearing aids, artificial limbs, wheelchairs, etc. may be provided, as may such household items as special beds.

Hygiene

Mobile baths (*junkai nyūyoku-sha* 巡回入浴車) and professional beauticians (*riyō gyōsha* 理容業者) may be available, as may a diaper service and a laundry service for bedridden (*netakiri* 寝たきり) patients.

Escorts and Companions

Escorts and helpers for the physically disabled are sometimes available, as are companions for the blind.

Rest and Relaxation for the Disabled

Registered disabled residents and their escorts can stay at holiday hostels for the disabled (*shinshin shōgai-sha kyūyō hōmu* 心身障害者休養ホーム) free of charge a couple of times a year. Transportation is often provided.

Alternative Therapies

Free coupons are often provided for such alternative therapies as acupuncture or shiatsu.

Resources

■ At least one news program broadcast each day on the regular television channels offers sign language interpreters.

■ Some public libraries have Braille books and audio books.

■ Television schedules in Japanese-language newspapers indicate which TV programs are adapted for people with disabilities. Look for the following symbols:

㊉　sign-language interpretation

㊢　closed-captioned for the hearing impaired

㊙　closed-captioned for the visually impaired, with additional narration explaining the action.

The Tokyo Metropolitan Welfare Hall for the Handicapped

Tokyo-to Shogai-sha Fukushi Kaikan
東京都障害者福祉会館
5-18-2 Shiba, Minato-ku, Tokyo
03-3455-6321
Holds public events to increase community awareness, such as bus hikes, bazaars, and handicraft exhibits.

The Braille Library of Japan

03-3209-0241

The Helen Keller Society Braille Library of Tokyo

03-3200-0987

The Braille Library of the Japanese Federation of the Blind

03-3200-0011 (Tokyo), 06-772-0024 (Osaka)

The Hearing Disabled Information and Cultural Center

fax 03-3356-2389
Captioned videos for the hearing impaired.

Recreational Facilities for the Disabled

Japan is just beginning to recognize the value of participation by the disabled in sports. The following are just a few of the sports facilities around the country that make provisions for use by the disabled.

Factory Smile Ski School
Echigo Yuzawa, Niigata
080-68-26425 (Ask for Jay Kato)
Ski school open to all disabled skiers. Excellent reputation for helping disabled skiers build self-reliance and self-esteem. Head instructor with experience in Canada.

Comprehensive Sports Center for the Disabled
Tokyo-to Shogai-sha Sogo Supotsu Senta
東京都障害者総合スポーツセンター
03-3907-5631 (Kita-ku, Tokyo)

Yokohama Rapport
Shogai-sha Supotsu Bunka Senta Yokohama Raporu
障害者スポーツ文化センター　横浜ラポール
045-475-2001 (Kohoku-ku, Yokohama)
Largest sports facility of its type in the country. Of-fers instruction and state-of-the-art equipment. Also welcomes those who are not disabled.

Kyoto City Sports Center for People with Disabilities
Kyoto-shi Shogai-sha Supotsu Senta
京都市障害者スポーツセンター
075-702-3370 (Sakyo-ku, Kyoto)

Additional Resource

Japan Association of Sports for the Physically Disabled
Nihon Shintai Shogai-sha Supotsu Kyokai
日本身体障害者スポーツ協会
03-3204-3993
Information on sports facilities and special sport-ing events for the disabled around Japan.

Support Groups for the Disabled
Check with TELL or look in the announcement section of your English-language newspaper for current contact numbers. If you can speak Japanese and participate in a Japanese group, your search may be made easier. Also ask your doctor or local welfare office, or one of the AMDA centers (see the endpapers) about support groups.

For educational opportunities for disabled children, see pages 174–75 and 177–78.

The Elderly
One of the greatest problems facing Japan is its rapidly aging population. The average life expectancy of the Japanese is presently the highest in the world, while the birthrate is the lowest. In 1996, the percentage of the population over the age of sixty-five stood at 15.1. The government estimates that senior citizens will comprise more than a quarter of the country's total population by the year 2020. If current trends in elderly health continue, the numbers of bedridden elderly and of senior citizens suffering from dementia will nearly triple by that same year. The government is taking great strides to meet the needs of the aging population, but it is a difficult proposition.

Plan Ahead
Whether you will be taking care of elderly relatives here or spending your own golden years in Japan, it's best to plan ahead.

Where you live can make a big difference. Consider living in an easy-care house or apartment near public transportation, shopping, and medical facilities in a city that offers ample services for the elderly. The local government may provide loans or compensate you for remodeling your home to make it safer or more accessible. Maintain good relations with your neighbors, since you never know when you might need one another, and familiarize yourself with the services for the elderly in your community. Since home care appears to be the wave of the future, consider how you will provide it. This is a challenge for everyone, but often even more so for international families, whose members tend to be scattered around the world. Private nursing homes are usually comfortable but costly, especially if you want a private room. Public homes, while less expensive, rarely provide either privacy or adequate maintenance of the facility and often have long waiting lists, sometimes of as much as three years.

Even with all the benefits available, old-age savings can easily be depleted by those costs that are not covered by public insurance. Look into health insurance benefits and consider taking out extra policies for cancer, private hospital rooms, extra nursing care, advanced medical care, and other conveniences that are not covered. Watch for changes in the insurance system. The planned compulsory nursing care insurance will not cover everything. To protect assets, listen to the experiences of friends and relatives, consult a lawyer specializing in the legal problems of the elderly, a financial adviser, and a social worker at your local welfare office.

One last thought. To help keep senior citizens actively participating in society, government offices have created departments that help the elderly find employment. These are the *kōrei-sha shokugyō sōdan-shitsu* 高齢者職業相談室 for those seeking regular employment and the "silver human resource centers" *shirubā jinzai sentā* シルバー人材センター for those wanting part-time occupations. Many have suggested that this kind of work can be a good way to stay mentally and physically fit.

Insurance for the Elderly

Health Insurance System for the Elderly (HISE)

For detailed information on HISE, see pages 77–78. Note that the government is considering reforming this system. In the future, co-payments made by the elderly may rise, to between ten and twenty percent of the cost of medical care. The government may also launch a system (not limited to the elderly) based on set fees for a complete course of treatment, rather than the present set fees for individual procedures. This will limit the number of procedures, tests, and the like which are covered in the course of treatment of any one condition.

Nursing Care Insurance

For Japanese public insurance, see pages 78–79; for private insurance plans, see pages 80–83.

Consultation for the Elderly

For medical problems, the best sources of information most directly related to your specific needs are likely to be your physician and the medical social worker at the hospital where you are being treated.

There are also numerous other consultation resources. Japanese language ability (or an interpreter) is usually necessary to use the following types of consultation services.

General Consultation Centers for the Elderly

Each prefecture has one of these centers *kōrei-sha sōgō sōdan sentā* 高齢者総合相談センター, which also serves as a hotline (in Japanese), reachable from push-button phones by pushing the pound sign, followed by the number 8080 (#8080). This telephone code is used in every prefecture. Those without push-button phones can ask their public health center for the regular telephone number of their local hotline. Hotline centers vary in capacity, but are usually staffed by a team of lawyers, doctors, nurses, social workers, clinical psychologists, physiotherapists, and occupational therapists ready to answer questions and discuss problems related to pensions, legal matters, welfare programs, and medical care—especially rehabilitation, home remodeling, and care for those with senile dementia. Not all specialists are available at all times.

Tokyo Center for the Promotion of Active Life
Tokyo-to Iki-Iki Raifu Suishin Senta
東京いきいきらいふ推進センター
Central Plaza 7 Fl., 1-1 Kagurabashi, Shinjuku-ku Tokyo

03-3269-4177
The #8080 hotline in Tokyo is based here. Training, counseling, information, and advice on caring for the bedridden, and on nursing services and facilities for the elderly.

Welfare Offices for the Elderly and/or Welfare Consultation Centers

These offices go by various names, but if you ask for the *rōjin fukushi jimusho* 老人福祉事務所 or *fukushi sōdan sentā* 福祉相談センター, you should be directed to the right place. Ask for these at your city or ward office. Centers of this type introduce local services, welfare programs, and welfare and private facilities, and also help you to make plans for care. They will also supply or rent equipment, some of which they may have on display. To make use of public welfare, bring your health insurance certificate, elderly person's medical care certificate, and nursing care insurance card, if applicable. These centers stock various pamphlets on equipment, services and facilities, and are useful even if you plan to use only private services.

Welfare Centers for the Elderly *rōjin fukushi sentā* 老人福祉センター

Found in most neighborhoods, these offer professional consultation on general matters, and provide various recreational, educational, and bathing services free of charge to the elderly in the community. Your local municipal office can provide more information. Free bus service is often available.

Private Industries

Companies selling or renting equipment for home care often provide consultation. Consultation offices can also be found in some large department stores that carry home care goods.

Home-Care Support Centers   *zaitaku kaigo shien sentā*   在宅介護支援センター

Home-care support centers provide a professional twenty-four–hour consultation service on caring for the bedridden elderly at home and on related services and facilities. These centers also display equipment. Consultation is free of charge.

Centers for Senile Dementia Patients   *rōjin-sei chihō shikkan sentā*   老人性痴呆疾患センター

These centers offer twenty-four–hour emergency consultation on the care of patients with senile dementia, in addition to inpatient care. Found in some hospitals with psychiatric departments and sometimes in independent clinics that offer this as one of several specialties. These often allow more space per person than do other facilities.

Support Groups

Japan has support groups (in Japanese) for those taking care of the elderly at home. Ask at your local public health center, or call an AMDA center.

Financial Assistance for Care of the Elderly

In some areas, including Tokyo, people between age sixty-five and sixty-nine who are not covered by employees' health insurance are eligible for the same health insurance benefits as those aged seventy and over (see HISE, pages 77–78), provided that their income is below a specified amount. Ask at the senior welfare section of your local government office for details on how to apply, before you turn sixty-five. You will be issued a medical welfare recipient certificate (*fukushi iryō-shō* 福祉医療証), which you must present, together with your health certificate, whenever you receive medical care. The certificate is valid for one year, renewable in July at the time of the review of your income for the previous year.

In some areas, those who have been residents for a year or more, and bedridden for more than six months can receive (regardless of their income level) a one-time gift (*neta-kiri rōjin mimai-kin* ねたきり老人見舞金) of about ¥12,000. Other allowances *kōrei-sha fukushi teate* 高齢者福祉手当 ranging from ¥30,000 to ¥55,000 may also be available, with the amount depending on the length of time bedridden, income level, age, and other factors.

Some local governments provide an annual allowance to families caring for a bedridden or senile person aged sixty-five or older. Income and residence tax deductions may also apply. Some also provide monetary compensation *jūtaku seibi shikin yūshi* 住宅整備

資金融資 to people remodeling their homes to accommodate bedridden or senile elderly family members.

Assistance for low-income, long-term–bedridden elderly can also include services such as futon drying *shingu kansō sābisu* 寝具乾燥サービス, diaper delivery *kami o-mutsu no takuhai sābisu* 紙おむつの宅配サービス, and provision of such special equipment *nichijō seikatsu yōgu no kyūfu* 日常生活用具の給付 as motorized beds.

Medical Care for the Elderly

The Japanese public insurance system provides very low-cost medical care to the elderly. The patient pays only the regular premium and a nominal co-payment at the time care is received. The care of welfare patients is completely free. Because medical care is so inexpensive, clinic waiting rooms often serve as social gathering spots for the local elderly.

Because they see so many elderly patients on a regular, even casual, basis, doctors are sometimes accused of failing to give serious enough consideration to the problems of the elderly. The government is now trying to remedy this flaw in the system, while still providing the elderly with readily available, low-cost care.

One advantage to growing old in Japan is the availability of oriental medicine and therapies. Since older people tend to suffer from multiple ailments, coordinating medications can be a problem. The great advantages of using oriental medicine are the low incidence of side effects and the holistic approach (see "Alternative Healing").

The elderly in Japan can receive treatment not only at ordinary hospitals, rehabilitation centers, and specialty centers or advanced treatment departments, but also at various kinds of facilities specially designed for them.

Hospitals for the Elderly

In the past, hospitals for the elderly *rōjin byōin* 老人病院 did not necessarily specialize in geriatrics, but rather were hospitals in which more than 60 percent of the patients were elderly. They were not particularly designed or staffed for caring for the elderly, and treatment tended to rely on medication and bed rest, rather than the nursing care and rehabilitation which is generally most needed by geriatric patients. This situation is now being addressed. As an incentive for hospitals to discharge patients in a more timely fashion, the government has now set the fees which hospitals are allowed to charge so that they are progressively lower the longer the patient stays. Japan now also has geriatric specialty hospitals *kōreisha senmon byōin* 高齢者専門病院 as well as units in general hospitals that specialize in geriatric care and are staffed by specialists in conditions common among elderly patients (stroke, heart disease, cancer, senile dementia, etc.).

Elderly patients with chronic conditions who have passed the acute stage of their disease and who no longer need active medical treatment so much as simple daily nursing can be treated in Special-Permit Hospitals for the Elderly *tokurei kyoka rōjin byōin* 特例許可病院. Within this category, the facilities that are especially suited for long-term care, with larger staffs in nursing and rehabilitation, and fewer physicians than other hospitals, are called *nyūin iryō kanri shōnin byōin* 入院医療承認病院, or nursing care–intensive hospitals *kaigo kyōryoku-ka byōin* 介護強力化病院.

Patients suffering from senile dementia can receive medical treatment or nursing care at hospital units specializing in this condition *rōjinsei chihō shikkan senmon chiryō byōtō* 老人性痴呆疾患専門治療病棟. Elderly patients who have stable chronic conditions such as rheumatoid arthritis or high blood pressure but require long-term inpatient care are sometimes treated in care-oriented hospital units *ryōyō-gata byōtō* 療養型病棟 specially designed for this purpose.

Intermediate Care Facilities for the Elderly *rōjin hoken shisetsu* 老人保健施設

An intermediate stage between inpatient hospital treatment and home care, these facilities provide short-term stays or day-care physical therapy, medical care, and basic nursing for the bedridden elderly and those needing various forms of rehabilitation, nursing, and assistance. Patients must be enrolled in the HISE. Those suffering from senile dementia must be able to participate in group living situations to be admitted. Stay is limited to three months.

Nursing Homes

When nursing homes were first introduced in the late nineteenth century by Christian and Buddhist organizations, they were criticized as undermining the tradition of children caring for elderly parents. However, the number of nursing homes and assisted-living houses has been increasing in recent years as fewer young women wish to take care of aging parents or parents-in-law, and the number of elderly living with adult children is decreasing. Changes in hospital care have also influenced this trend.

Public nursing homes usually require one year's residence in the district for admission. Apply through the local welfare office; a welfare officer will usually be sent to determine what type of home is suitable. Although they are very reasonable, public homes often have long waiting lists and may restrict the resident's freedom and independence.

Special Nursing Homes for the Elderly
tokubetsu yōgo rōjin hōmu 特別養護老人ホーム
Welfare homes for the elderly who are bedridden or suffering from dementia and the severity of whose condition makes it difficult to provide proper care at home. A clinic and a rehabilitation room with at least one part-time doctor are standard. No income limit; fees are set on a sliding scale based on income.

Nursing Homes for the Elderly
yōgo rōjin hōmu 養護老人ホーム
These facilities are basically the same as special nursing homes, but for those with a low income. Meals and other daily necessities are provided. Typically, four people share a twelve-mat room. Most are publicly run, and residents pay no fees.

Care Houses (moderate-fee nursing-care homes) *kea hausu* ケアハウス
Public residential nursing homes for those aged sixty and over who are unable to live alone but do not suffer from dementia or need full-time assistance. Private rooms with space for wheelchairs. Consultation, meals, and other services are provided. There are no income limits, but

people who are on public welfare or who do not pay city taxes are not admitted.

Private Homes for the Elderly
yūryō rōjin hōmu 有料老人ホーム
Admission to private homes is usually limited to those aged sixty or over, but each facility sets its own rules. Some homes are only for the healthy, while others can accommodate people who are bedridden or suffering from senile dementia. Meals and daily necessities are provided. These are usually more luxurious than public nursing homes. Although systems vary, fees include a one-time entrance fee in addition to a monthly charge. A refund policy sometimes repays part of the entrance fee on a sliding scale when a resident dies or moves away.

Group Care Homes for Senile Dementia
chihō-sei rōjin no gurūpu hōmu 痴呆性老人グループホーム
Geared to the elderly who have serious disabilities or severe senile dementia. Small staff-resident ratio, as the number of residents generally remains between six and nineteen, as opposed to the usual fifty. Residents can maintain a high degree of independence, and those who have had trouble in hospital or larger homes often do much better in these facilities. These homes are now receiving government subsidies and are increasing in number.

Home Care for the Elderly

"I've been taking care of my husband, who has Parkinson's disease. Our doctor visits him twice a week, and my local government provides all the materials I need to take care of him, as well as monthly financial aid. In addition, through his national health insurance, two people come every week to help with care and a public nurse comes twice a month. Thanks to their visits, I'm able to go out with my friends sometimes to relax."

Contact facilities or services directly, or through a home-care support center.

Home-Care Equipment *rōjin nichijō seikatsu yōgu* 老人日常生活用具
In response to the rapid aging of society, companies selling and/or renting home-care equipment are springing up everywhere. Supply or loan of equipment from local governments is also possible; fees are set on a sliding scale according to income.

Resources

Tokyo Metropolitan Technical Aid Center
(Shinjuku-ku, Tokyo; see page 216)

Elderly Service Providers Association
Shiruba Sabisu Shinko-kai
シルバーサービス振興会
Petro House 3 Fl., 4-5-21 Kojimachi, Chiyoda-ku Tokyo
03-5276-1600, fax 03-5276-1601
Researches elderly services and administers the government-affiliated "Silver Mark" system—a mark of excellence awarded to providers of services for the elderly such as mobile bath operators, home-care equipment rental companies, nursing homes, and other home care services. Provides information on Silver Mark companies and on companies offering home-help services.

Nihon Silver Care
048-432-7733 or 048-834-0055 (J. only)
Sells and rents equipment including special beds, walkers, wheelchairs, sensor lights, bedside commodes, and intercoms. Free catalog.

Access International and **Nihon Abilities**
(see page 216)

Physician House Calls   *hōmon shinryō* 訪問診療

Doctors—particularly those from neighborhood clinics—will sometimes make house calls to bedridden elderly patients. Patients pay the amount not covered by insurance, plus the cost of travel.

Home-Visit Nursing Care Stations

Under the instructions of the patient's doctor, these stations *rōjin hōmon kango sutēshon* 老人訪問看護ステーション send out nurses to care for the bedridden and elderly who require medical assistance at home. The nurses check on bedridden, or potentially bedridden, elderly who are enrolled in the HISE. Emphasis is on observation of the person's condition, and guidance in rehabilitative nursing care. Presently limited to three days a week, unless the person is in the last stages of cancer or certain other designated diseases such as multiple sclerosis. Patients must pay travel costs and must also compensate for extra hours or for visits made on holidays. Some areas can now provide twenty-four-hour nursing services if necessary.

Home Helpers   *hōmu herupā* ホームヘルパー

Provided under public insurance and welfare for the bedridden elderly or those suffering from dementia. Fees charged depend on the family's income; if the family income is so low that the family is not required to pay taxes, services may be provided free. The housekeeper-type helper (*kaji enjo-gata* 家事援助型) advises on daily matters and helps with meals, laundry, house cleaning, shopping, and simple daily chores. Rules vary, but public assistance, if any, allows for visits once or twice a week, for no more than three hours at a time. The other type is more a personal care nurse (*shintai kaigo-gata* 身体介護型), helping with physical care and personal hygiene. This type of helper works about three hours or less a day, and no more than six days a week.

Home-care support centers or welfare consultation centers introduce individual helpers or home-helper agencies (*kasei-fu shōka-ijo* 家政婦紹介所 or *hōmu herupu sā-bisu* ホームヘルプサービス) in the community. Those hired directly from private companies tend to offer wider-ranging services, but also to charge more. Japanese is likely to be the only language used. Some communities have volunteer interpreters who help, at least in the beginning.

Instruction at Home   *hōmon shidō* 訪問指導

Public health centers and other community organizations offer lectures on the prevention of adult diseases as well as demonstrations of how to care for the elderly at home.

Some districts also send public health nurses to teach the bedridden elderly or their family at home. Instruction is by a team of visiting public health nurses, clinic or hospital nurses, nutritionists, and dental hygienists, under the guidance of a doctor, and focuses on community services available, what to do in an emergency, how to care for the patient's daily needs, and how to prevent senility. These visits may also include advice on making the home safer by installing railings, enlarging bathrooms, and adding other conveniences. There is no fee for this service.

In some areas, the caregiver relative and the elderly patient bedridden for at least three weeks can check into a local nursing home or medical facility for a week of training *hōmu kea sokushin jigyō* ホームケア促進事業. Each pays a small fee to cover the cost of meals.

Short-Term Stay Centers *shōto sutei* ショートステイ

Private and public facilities provide temporary, limited care of the elderly when the family caregiver is sick or needs to attend a wedding, funeral, or other event. The maximum stay is usually seven days, but in certain circumstances this can be extended to three months. Fees at public facilities depend on the type of center, and whether the stay is necessary or optional.

Some centers allow overnight stays *naito kea* ナイトケア for patients whose families are temporarily unable to care for them at night.

Short-term stays are also possible at some hospitals, intermediate care facilities, private nursing home, and group care homes.

Day-Care Centers *dei sābisu* デイサービス

For those who are in fragile health and need help with daily activities, public and private day-care centers provide lunches, baths, physical training, counseling, physical exams, sleeping areas, and other services. Bus service is available. Day-care also possible at some Intermediate Care Facilities for the Elderly and hospitals.

Bath Services

Public baths *sentō* 銭湯 often offer the elderly use of rooms on the premises for social gatherings at no cost during the daytime on certain days of the week. Those who want to stay and bathe may do so, often at a discount, depending on the generosity of the bath manager.

A specially designed mobile bath is available in some areas for home visits to help bathe bedridden or disabled residents. Usage under the public welfare system is generally limited to three times a month, with a small fee being charged according to income. Privately-owned mobile bath services charge much more per visit, but may be used more frequently.

Emergency Care for the Elderly

Emergency care for the elderly is not very different from any other emergency care, but some facilities provide special forms of care. A hotline consultation center (#8080 from a push-button phone; see page 221) or twenty-four–hour home-visit nursing-care station (see page 226) can provide the necessary information. For further information on what to do in an emergency, see pages 45–51 and the front endpapers.

For information on hospice care, see pages 329–31.

"In our home country we were each other's best friend. In addition, we both had other friends we could rely on and who we shared different interests with. In Japan, however, we found ourselves isolated, dependent on each other, insecure, and jealous. We found we needed more space from each other."

"If one more person looks at me like I'm from the moon or asks me how old I am, I think I'll punch them … On my day off, all I want to do is stay in my apartment and watch videos."

"When I first arrived in Japan, it seemed the only time I left the house was to go shopping. Then we got a puppy who had to be walked three times a day. People naturally stopped and made conversation during the walks. It was a great way to meet people, and there was no more coming home to an empty house."

Mental Health

Any health problem is an extra challenge when you're surrounded by unfamiliar circumstances, but psychological concerns can be especially troublesome. Living in Japan, you'll probably experience some degree of culture shock, and you'll also certainly find yourself under greater stress in general. These conditions sometimes lead to emotional problems or uncover past trauma. Whatever the problem is, recognizing the symptoms and working on a solution is important. Sometimes counseling or other professional help is necessary.

Culture Shock

Many of the insights in the following are based on Joy Norton and Tazuko Shibusawa's book, *Coping and Beyond: The Japan Experience*, which we highly recommend and which will soon be republished by Charles E. Tuttle under a different title.

A foreign language, new foods, different customs, smaller spaces, schedule changes—emotional responses to these shifts in life-style bombard the newcomer to Japan. Your old sixth sense of "what to do, when, and how" no longer works. If you do not have a basic familiarity with the language, even daily activities like commuting, banking, and shopping can become major hurdles. "Culture shock" is the anxiety and stress you feel at having to function "normally" in a place where all the basic ground rules have shifted. Uncomfortable as this may be, it's also a normal part of adapting to a new culture.

People react to the stress of coping with a different culture in different ways. You may notice a general uneasiness without a clear cause—a kind of free-floating anxiety—or you may have panic attacks. You also may feel less confident, worry more about your health, and become more easily angered, afraid, or suspicious.

Adjusting to Japan and a new life-style is not the only issue. You also might be missing the home, family, friends, routine, and occupation or profession you left behind. Finding substitutes in Japan can take a great deal of courage and perseverance. How you cope usually depends on your experience and what resources you have. Your usual abilities to solve problems are challenged, and if you're having trouble communicating, finding help can be doubly hard. All of this together may leave you with a sense of helplessness.

If your immediate family is with you, you may find that they can't provide the support they used to. They may be struggling too much with their own adjustment to be able to help.

Couples and Culture Shock

Couples experience culture shock in different ways and for various reasons. If you're both working, you may find you have less energy to spend on home life and child care. If you don't have a career, you may become isolated and feel insecure, fatigued, and ineffective, especially if no one acknowledges your accomplishments in adjusting to Japan. If your spouse is working, he or she probably works long hours to meet new job demands, but gets support, feedback, and satisfaction from it. If you're accustomed to socializing together, the Japanese custom of stag entertainment can intensify your loneliness. Many couples find the usual roles in their relationship change—some grow closer, while others find that the strain creates destructive patterns between them.

Children and Adolescents and Culture Shock

Children and adolescents express culture shock in many ways. Some children become resentful, withdrawn, passive, and depressed. Others express their feelings by becoming aggressive or rebellious. Your children may be angry at you for making the move. Not only do they have the added stress of making new friends, but they will also have to adjust to a lack of play space and perhaps less attention from their working parent(s). They may have a different amount of independence—whether more or less—which can also be a source of stress. For adolescents, leaving friends behind may be especially difficult. And finally, if your adolescents are already self-conscious, standing out as a non-Japanese may be particularly uncomfortable.

Women and Culture Shock

Women who are competent in their own country often feel that their skills are not valued here, and consequently feel significantly less important, less of an individual, and less effective.

"At home I used to work an eight-hour nursing shift, then take care of my two young children, prepare dinner for my husband, do the housework, and study for a master's degree. Here, I'm lucky if in a day I accomplish the food shopping and maybe find some simple item that I lost in the move and that I've been searching for all month."

"Not only am I the only foreigner in my company, but I'm also the only woman manager. The weirdest thing is going out to dinner with a group of colleagues (all men) and sitting through the really stupid jokes that they start to make as they get a few beers down. They definitely are not comfortable with talking about anything serious, but just like to ask a lot of questions about my personal life and comment on the way I look. Then they giggle and say, 'Uh-oh! Seku-hara (sexual harrassment). I better watch out or the American will sue me!" I often wonder if I wouldn't be better off back at my desk working into the night, but then again, if I want any sort of future with this company ..."

While you're adjusting, these feelings can intensify until you form new patterns.

Culture Shock and Single Life

Single people and recent university graduates face the issue of competency in new roles and new living and working environments. As a single person, you might be completely isolated from other non-Japanese and be disoriented—"sinking" rather than "immersed" —in Japanese culture. In this situation it's easy to feel you have lost control, and are helpless and incapable. In addition, there is the attention you attract simply by being a non-Japanese. To escape the pressures of having to adapt, you may withdraw into your home and read, watch videos, or sleep more than usual.

Bicultural Families and Culture Shock

Foreign spouses of Japanese may be deeply immersed in Japanese culture and still experience much of the same dilemma. This is particularly true if you are a foreign wife of a Japanese, since your stay in Japan may be more permanent, and the consequences of maladjustment greater. Seemingly trivial matters can become major issues when trying to adjust to life in Japan, where tradition and rituals of daily life are so important.

"I was a capable housewife until I came to Japan and had to live with my Japanese mother-in-law. Suddenly, I couldn't do anything right. I cut vegetables with the wrong knife. I didn't hang out my wash properly or air the house at the correct time. My ways took less time and energy, but they weren't the tried and true ways of the traditional Japanese wife. I felt trapped!"

Phases of Culture Shock

You might not notice that you're experiencing culture shock. It can come as a mild depression, six months after you thought you had adjusted. Depression and relationship problems are the most frequently identified problems of people seeking counseling and may be a reflection of culture shock. Different phases of culture shock can be identified, but they don't always occur in the same sequence for everyone:

The Honeymoon

This period is often filled with excitement, curiosity, and a heightened awareness of the similarities between home and Japan. "People are people wherever you go."

Initial Culture Shock

The initial shock includes confusion, disorientation, and frustration as you are bombarded with the unfamiliar. You may feel as though you're "going crazy," but it's more likely the result of being overwhelmed with so many new experiences at once.

Superficial Adjustment

A stage of superficial adjustment often follows, as you begin to feel successful and able to function in the Japanese culture.

Depression and Isolation

As you notice the deeper cultural differences, you begin to question your personal set of values and sense of self. This can make you feel hopeless and alienated.

Reintegration and Compensation

Eventually, you gain control by reintegrating and compensating. You may rebel against the now familiar basic attitudes and values of the Japanese and become more assertive.

Autonomy and Independence

The final stage, when you begin to combine aspects that you like in your culture and the Japanese culture in a way that increases your happiness and benefits others.

Coping with Culture Shock

Once you identify and accept culture shock, you can begin a healthy adaptation to the Japanese culture. Welcome it as an opportunity to grow as an individual and/or family.

The first step to coping with culture shock is to accept that developing new skills is a normal and necessary part of adaptation. Also, recognize that experiencing stress is a positive sign that you are becoming involved in this new culture. Your goal is not to eliminate stress, but to manage it so you can better adapt. To find new coping skills, make yourself open to new ideas and behaviors and be willing to experiment. Although you may not feel flexible and adventurous, it's necessary to take risks to discover what works in Japan.

Tips on Handling Culture Shock

■ Become aware of and accept your feelings and reactions

Be willing to laugh at the situation and often at yourself. Be willing to forgive. Learn to tolerate ambiguity and enjoy not knowing what to expect. Be secure in yourself and things will usually work out, even if everything else is unpredictable.

■ Develop social supports beyond your immediate family

Knock on the doors of churches, clubs, schools, special interest groups, and organizations catering to the foreign community. You'll often find welcome support from others in the same situation or veterans with tips to share. Sharing your views can also help them.

■ Study Japanese

Efforts to study and use Japanese will increase your independence and self-confidence. Take some language classes: an increasing number of cities offer Japanese classes, and there are also numerous private schools. Many Japanese people are not interested in speaking their own language with foreigners. Try to be friend not only more "internationalized" people, but also someone who doesn't speak a word of English. On the other hand, remember that friendships among Japanese are usually formed over long years together in the same classroom, neighborhood, or company, and don't be surprised if it seems to take forever to "break in."

■ Keep in touch with your support systems at home

Write to family and friends; send tapes and videos.

■ Get to know your city and its people

Buy a map of the city. Learn to use the public transportation system. Get off the train at a place you've never been, and wander around, see what's there.

■ Guard against depression

Resist withdrawing by reading too many books or watching too many videos. Think about how you really want to spend your free time, and try to do things that you enjoy that are also positive for you.

■ Avoid submersing yourself in work as a substitute for human support

Combat isolation with a balance of relationships differing in degrees (casual, close, and intimate) and in nature (business and social).

■ Get to know your neighbors, shopkeepers, hairdressers, etc.

Even if it's simply seeing a familiar face, having some friendly contact with people every day helps you to feel more a part of the community. Invite deeper friendships by reaching out to people who have been just casual acquaintances.

■ Set up realistic, limited, attainable goals for your adjustment

Pace yourself, accepting your limitations. Be happy with small successes. Don't overextend yourself and then burn out. Expose yourself to a few challenges at a time. As you adjust, your increased interaction with the new culture can offer many enriching rewards.

■ Make a schedule to get out of the house

Shop on Monday, go to the park on Tuesday, etc.

Health Maintenance

How you take care of yourself on a daily basis influences your management of stress and your ability to adapt and live in another culture. Good health is the most important tool you have for helping you to function in a different culture. In a new environment, however, keeping healthy can be a challenge. The following guidelines may help:

■ Exercise

Exercise is essential to release many of the tensions accompanying your new life. Regular exercise, even for short periods, is crucial. Jogging, yoga, tennis, martial arts, aerobics, swimming, and other sports are all available in Japan (see pages 315–18). You may need to modify your usual program to fit in with what's available here. Home video exercise programs are efficient, if you have the space. Simplest of all is walking, which you can do anytime, and which also helps you explore new places.

■ Maintain a regular diet

This can be a challenge when you're dealing with new foods, cooking styles, facilities, and perhaps very different time schedules. Japan has many nutritious fast foods, but keep a balanced diet in mind (see "Nutrition"). Also remember that trying to manage stress may make you more vulnerable to substance abuse. Don't cause further problems for yourself by overindulging in alcohol, tobacco, caffeine, or other substances.

■ Be aware of your health

In times of stress, your immune system is less effective, so see a doctor if you have any health concerns. Living in a new environment also means unfamiliar pathogens, increasing the likelihood of illnesses and allergies. A high percentage of newcomers have to consult a doctor during their first three months because of this vulnerability. Reduce stress by recognizing this possibility and seeing a doctor early for even minor medical problems.

■ Have fun

Finding humor and making room for fun in a foreign culture is an excellent way of coping with stress. There are usually many reasons to laugh and smile.

■ Get rest and relaxation

To function at your peak, you need adequate rest and relaxation. Make time for relaxing activities like traveling, brief vacations or retreats, social activities, home entertainment, or family holidays. For extra relaxation you might also like to try meditation or a hot spring bath, or treat yourself to some of the therapies mentioned in "Alternative Healing."

■ Find a good friend

Confiding in a trusted friend has proven to be one of the best stress relievers—speak out about your experiences and your feelings, even if there are no easy answers to the things you're worried about.

■ Keep a journal

This can be a useful way of chronicling your experiences in Japan. It can monitor your progress and help you gain insight and perspective. It also can be an outlet for emotional expression and a great creative activity. Write about the books you read, sketch the people you see on the train, or paste in pictures or articles from the newspaper.

■ Boost your ego

Boost your morale by keeping up your skills, perhaps in new roles, like teaching or consulting, or in new contexts, such as groups or organizations. You can also learn new skills that could help you develop untapped talents. Increasing your sense of self-worth is important; one way to do it is to make a contribution to society—for example, by volunteering to do something that you excel at anyway.

■ Accept yourself

Accept yourself and the adventure of adaptation and enjoyment will soon follow.

Support Resources

Coming to a new culture may raise unresolved issues from your past. Being far from your country, family, and relationships may start you thinking and wanting to explore more in yourself. You may expect that you'll behave differently because you're in another culture, and then be disappointed to find that you're still repeating old behavior patterns that don't work in Japan. Those who want to change or explore more deeply often find that community or professional support is a great help in managing cultural adjustment.

Hotlines

Several telephone hotlines provide crisis counseling and/or information to the foreign community (see the endpapers).

Community and Group Support

Support is offered at various community groups and associations, and at your office or place of worship. English-language newspapers, journals, magazines, and newsletters carry announcements of activities. These organizations may also help you get adjusted:

Welcome Furoshiki (Oak Associates)
Tokyo and Yokohama areas 03-5472-7074
Osaka, Kobe, Kyoto areas 06-441-2584
Nagoya area 052-836-9261
Free community service providing a warm welcome to foreign residents of any nationality. A representative knowledgeable about living in Japan visits your home with a packet of gifts and information all wrapped up in a *furoshiki.*

Tokyo Family Network
03-3710-1331
http://www.cyber.ad.jp/tfn
Helps newcomers and residents meet others with common interests by providing neighborhood contacts and local information.

Call one of the information services listed on the endpapers or in "Regional Resources" for the current phone numbers of the following community and support groups.

Self-Help Support Groups
Including Alcoholics Anonymous (page 242); Adult Children of Alcoholics; Al-Anon; Co-dependency Anonymous; Overeaters Anonymous; and the Pre-natal and Infant Death Support Group (page 275).

Special Concerns Support Groups
Including the Adoptive Parents Support Group; HAPA (Half-Asian); and Hostess Net.

Religious Groups
Including the Tokyo Union Church; Tokyo Baptist Church; the Franciscan Chapel Center; the Jewish Community Center; and Islamic centers.

Service-oriented Groups
Including the College Women's Association of Japan (CWAJ); the International Ladies' Benevolent Society; International Social Service of Japan; the Japan Red Cross Society; and Refugees International Japan.

Professional Interest Groups
Including the Society of Writers, Editors and Translators (SWET); the Japan Association of Language Teachers (JALT); the Foreign Nurses Association in Japan (FNAJ); your country's Chamber of Commerce; Foreign Executive Women (FEW); and Foreign Women Lawyers Association.

Women's Support Groups and Resources

Association of Foreign Wives of Japanese
045-753-7485, also fax; Chris Ishikawa, Asst. Membership Secretary
president@afwj.org (or)
membership-sec@afwj.org
http://www.bekkoame.ne.jp/~ycishikawa/
Active support network for foreign women married to Japanese men. Groups nationwide. Has a very active e-mail discussion group.

Filipina Wives of Japanese Association
7-302 Pilot Homes, 1-14 Mihama Takasu
Mihama-ku, Chiba-shi, Chiba-ken
043-278-9551 (Contact: Fanny Kyo)

Yokohama Women's Association for Communication and Networking
Landmark Tower 13 Fl., 2-2-1-1 Minato Mirai
Nishi-ku, Yokohama-shi
045-224-2002 (J. only)
Small library, inexpensive meeting spaces.

HELP Asian Women's Shelter
03-3368-8855 (Eng., Tag., Thai—but not all languages everyday)
Crisis counseling and emergency housing for women of all nationalities. Helps to resolve crises with medical and social service support.

Tokyo Rape Crisis Center
03-3207-3692
Can introduce lawyers, help with police, etc. Leave message in Japanese on machine.

Mizura
2-1-613 Aoki-cho, Kanagawa-ku, Yokohama-shi
045-451-3776 (office) Mon.–Fri. 9:00 A.M.–6:00 P.M.
045-451-0740 (free counseling) Mon.–Fri. 2:00–5:00 P.M., 7:00–9:00 P.M.; Sat. 2:00–5:00 P.M.
Phone office in Japanese to make an appointment, and translators can be arranged. Women's telephone counseling on any subject. Short-term shelter for all women needing help. Not a hostel.

Saalaa Women's Shelter
Aoba P.O.Box # 13, Yokohama-shi
045-901-3527 Mon.–Fri. 10:00 A.M.–6:00 P.M. (Eng., Tag., Thai., Sp.)
Emergency shelter where foreign women (including illegal aliens) escaping from bad situations can stay for up to a month; counseling also available.

Women's Center Osaka
1-3-23 Gamo, Joto-ku, Osaka-shi
06-933-7001 (information) Mon.–Sat. 10:00 A.M.–5:00 P.M. (J. only)
06-930-7666 (health counseling) 1st, 2nd, 3rd Thurs. 1:00–8:00 P.M. (J. only)
Women's health counseling and health services center, with an emphasis on self-help. Also diaphragm fitting and acupuncture training.

Resources for Intercultural Couples

Association for Multicultural Families
fax 0422-79-4498 (Yoshiko Delehouzee)

Network of multicultural families around Japan. Published 国際結婚ハンドブック *Kokusai Kekkon Handbook* (see "References and Further Reading").

Asian People Together
075-451-6522 (J., Eng., Kor., Thai)
Mon. 3:00–6:00 P.M., Thurs. 3:00–8:00 P.M.
Volunteer group at Kyoto YWCA provides telephone counseling on the concerns of daily life (face-to-face on request).

Kokusai Kekkon o Kangaeru Kai
All-Japan: 3-8-2-612 Abiko-Higashi
Sumiyoshi-ku, Osaka-shi
anakama@gol.com
Kansai: 1-6-26-103 Miyamadai, Tarumi-ku
Kobe-shi: 078-753-2430
Association of Japanese women married to foreign men offers encouragement and friendship.

Mishuk-no-Kai
Buna no Mori Nai, 2-20-5 Naka Aoki
Kawaguchi-shi, Saitama-ken
048-258-0039, fax 048-258-9505
http://www.sainet.or.jp/~
Network for couples in which one partner is Japanese and the other is from an Asian or developing country. Quarterly information magazine; send ¥80 with your name and address to receive a sample copy.

Marriage and Self Encounter Programs
Fr. Donnon Murray, O.F.M. of the Franciscan Chapel Center

03-3401-2141, fax 03-3401-2142
Non-religious program, two overnights, in English or in Japanese for self-discovery and to deepen family life. Marriage Encounter is for married couples. Self Encounter is for anyone, married or single.

Volunteering
To volunteer in your neighborhood, contact your local welfare council volunteer center *shakai fukushi kyōgikai borantia sentā* 社会福祉協議会ボランティアセンター. Every town has a welfare council. Your local international information services (see "Regional Resources") or the following may also be of help:

Japan Hospital Volunteer Association
03-3581-7851 (in Japanese)
Push around moving libraries, talk to bedridden patients, take patients for walks, etc. Non-Japanese volunteers have been active at several hospitals including the National Cancer Center in Tsukiji, Tokyo. Most groups offer volunteer insurance policies to cover liability. Contact for further information on groups.

Volunteering in the Tokyo Area, Foreign Executive Women (FEW)
Lists volunteer groups in the Tokyo, Yokohama, Chiba and Saitama areas. To order, call TELL for the current FEW number or check out the FEW web site: http://www.few.gol.com

Counseling

The importance of choosing a therapist who can meet your counseling needs and with whom you feel comfortable cannot be overestimated. Read again the section in this book on choosing a caregiver. Since therapists and clients are all individuals, finding the right match may require some exploration.

Large university hospitals sometimes have an English-speaking professional who can counsel you. Japanese public insurance allows only for brief assessments of short-term outpatient psychotherapy. If you know your diagnosis and what medications work for you, it is wise to talk about these things at the beginning of the session. If you need longer therapy, you'll usually be hospitalized or referred to a private counselor. Special centers for the treatment of various conditions such as alcoholism (see page 241–44) are available, though not all are in English.

Often, it is most helpful to talk with a counselor who shares your cultural background. And if the problem is cross-cultural issues, you'll want someone who is familiar with the other culture as well. In some areas you can find Western independent counselors or counseling centers staffed, at least partially, by Western therapists. Most non-Japanese counselors are not licensed or certified in Japan, but should be licensed/certified elsewhere, or at least eligible for such licensing/certification. The recently-established International Mental Health Providers Japan, which requires its clinical members to have these qualifications, serves as a network for these counselors, as well as for Japanese mental health professionals targeting the foreign communities around Japan.

Suggested Counseling Services

For information on counseling specifically for children, see page 175.

The following are counseling centers and independent counselors, long-term and active in the international community. This is not a comprehensive list. Most of the counseling centers, the information services (see the endpapers and "Regional Resources"), and sometimes your public health center can give you further references. All offer counseling in English, and are experienced in dealing with cross-cultural issues. Several of the centers also offer educational services and workshops for personal development and specific mental health issues. Costs vary, and not all services are covered by public or even private insurance. Some therapists will counsel over the phone or the Internet, especially for clients in outlying areas. All require appointments.

Pastoral counselors are available through churches, or call TELL.

TELL Community Counseling Service

2-20-2 Tokiwadai, Itabashi-ku, Tokyo
03-3968-4084 (Individual, group, and family therapy)
Affiliated with the Samaritans, this center offers face-to-face counseling by professionals on a flexible fee basis. Consulting psychiatrists are available for clinical supervision and consultation to the staff. Individual, couples, marital, family, and group counseling services are offered. Also community education, workshops, and lectures. Referrals to appropriate counselors, including those outside the practice.

Tokyo Psychotherapy Center

2-1-15-705 Takanawa, Minato-ku, Tokyo
03-3280-5776, also fax
Masafumi Nakakuki, M.D., F.A.P.A., C.G.P.
Bilingual and bicultural psychiatrist certified in both the U.S. and Japan. Nearly 30 years practice in the U.S. Treats anxiety, depression, panic psychosomatic disorders, marital problems, etc. Japanese insurance not accepted.

Counseling International

3-2-13-411 Nishi-Azabu, Minato-ku, Tokyo
03-3408-0496, fax 03-3456-5970
U.S.-trained and -licensed psychotherapists, authors of *The Japan Experience: Coping and Beyond*, offer cross-cultural counseling, and confidential consultation in psychotherapy, crisis intervention, careers, etc. By appointment only; 24-hour answering machine. Telephone counseling for out-of-town residents; fees set on a sliding scale according to income. May–October counseling in the Nagano area, 0262-55-5755.

St. Luke's International Hospital

03-3541-5151 (see page 344)
Psychiatrist on staff.

Tokyo Medical and Surgical Clinic

(Minato-ku, Tokyo; see page 33)
Psychiatrist available on certain days.

AMI Counseling

3-17-5, 5 Fl. Shiroganedai, Minato-ku, Tokyo
03-3448-1272, also fax (Eng., Fr.)
U.S.-licensed clinical psychologist. Full range of long- or short-term psychological services for individuals and couples. Lectures and workshops also offered. Fees on a flexible scale.

Aurora Counseling Center

Medical Friend Bldg. 1F, 3-2-4 Kudan-Kita
Chiyoda-ku, Tokyo
03-5275-3638, also fax 010-705-9120
Also Japanese, German, French, Dutch, Tagalog. Clinical psychologists offer counseling for depression, neurosis, marriage problems, etc. Psychiatrist adviser.

Institute of Psychoanalytic-Systems Psychotherapy

Highland Bldg. 3 Fl., 2-5-19 Higashiyama
Meguro-ku, Tokyo
03-3760-3631
Individual, group, family, and couples psychotherapy. Adult and children.

Ikebukuro Counseling Center

RS Bldg. 2 Fl., 1-25-4 Minami-Ikebukuro
Toshima-ku, Tokyo
03-3980-8718, fax 03-5431-1035
http://www.gol.com/hozumiclinic/counselinge.html
Individual, family, and group counseling, individual and group dance movement therapy and psychotherapy services. Japanese and foreign therapists. Fees on a sliding scale.

Jim McRae, Ph.D.

Offices in Takadanobaba and Roppongi, Tokyo
03-3983-0582, fax 03-3983-2533
California-licensed psychotherapist. Psychotherapy and counseling with adults and couples in Tokyo since 1983. Fees on a sliding scale based on income.

Shoko Sasaki, M.S.

Yoyogi Terrace 211, 1-32-27 Tomigaya
Shibuya-ku, Tokyo
03-3466-1481 (J., Eng.)
U.S.-trained psychologist and family therapist. Individual/family therapy for relationship problems, improvement of communication skills, etc.

Ron Shumsky, Psy.D.

3-2-13-412 Nishi-Azabu, Minato-ku, Tokyo
Also at the Bluff Clinic, Yokohama-shi (see page 34)
0423-82-1263, also fax
Psychotherapy with children, adults, and families.

The Psychotherapy and Healing Practice

1-2-22-903 Shimomeguro, Meguro-ku, Tokyo
03-3491-8144
http://www2.gol.com/language/dana/
Prem Dana Takada is an Australian clinical psychologist with a specialty in depression and eating disorders. Individual and family therapy.

Betsey Olsen, Ed.D.

Musashino area (on Chuo and Inokashira lines)
0422-47-1824, also fax
U.S.-licensed psychologist. Individual and family psychotherapy.

International Counseling Center

Kobe Kaisei Hospital
(Nada-ku, Kobe-shi; see page 348)
078-856-2201 (direct line)
http://www.venus.dti.ne.jp/~marten/#web
Non-profit, non-sectarian organization offering long- and short-term counseling by Western-trained psychotherapists for depression, stress, anxiety, alcoholism, relationship problems, etc. 24-hour answering machine. Also Japanese, European languages.

Aoibashi Family Clinic

Shimodachiuri Agaru, Karasuma-dori,
Kamigyo-ku, Kyoto-shi
075-431-9150 (J., Eng.)
International marriage and crisis counseling.

Resolutions Counseling Service

19-16 Uyama-cho, Hirakata-shi, Osaka-shi
0720-67-4437
http://www.resolutions.org
U.S.-trained social worker (Kelly Lemmon-Kishi) offers counseling and psychotherapy for individuals, couples, and families for depression, anxiety, etc. Specializing in trauma, especially sexual violence and disaster response.

Treating Addictions

Since individuals with these disorders tend to deny or hide that they have a problem, it is often the role of the parent or a friend to insist that they seek help early.

Nicotine *nikochin* ニコチン

Japan lags behind many other countries in discouraging the use of tobacco, and an inordinately large percentage of the population smokes. Since many doctors themselves smoke, they seem hesitant to instruct patients to give it up. But with the increased rate of lung and other cancers nationwide, and the increased risk that smokers have for angina, heart attack, and respiratory diseases like emphysema, Japan is waking up to the dangers of tobacco smoke. Also, with recent strains on the insurance system, the government and insurance companies are looking for ways to reduce illnesses. Employers are being encouraged to introduce incentives for employees to stop smoking, more offices are going smoke-free, doctors are offering outpatient smoking cessation clinics, and the Japanese Ministry of Finance now allows life insurance companies to a give a deduction for non-smokers.

Several times a year the Tokyo Adventist Hospital (see page 344) offers in Japanese a smoking cessation program *nyū-in kin'en shidō* 入院禁煙指導, an inpatient group therapy; outpatient programs in English are offered on a regular basis by Edward Fujimoto. Dr. Mayumi Abe at the smoking cessation outpatient clinic *kin'en gairai* 禁煙外来 at both Mitsui Memorial Hospital (see page 343) and the department of respiratory diseases at Tokyo Women's Medical College Hospital (see page 344) offers smoking cessation programs combining counseling with the use of prescription nicotine gum *nikoretto* ニコレット. Most quit smoking within three months. Dr. Abe speaks English, but the nurses who work under her and record your medical history do not. Dr. Gabriel Symonds (see Tokyo British Clinic, page 33) considers the use of nicotine gum to be counterproductive, and uses nothing but face-to-face consultations in his smoking cessation treatment (as many consultations as it takes until you quit, for a single set fee). Other hospitals have programs similar to these.

Nicotine patches aren't available in Japan yet. Cigarette holders that reduce the amount of smoke inhaled are available at most drug stores.

Unless utilized to treat a disease, smoking cessation treatments are considered preventive medicine, and are therefore not covered by Japanese public insurance.

Alcoholism *arukōru chūdoku* アルコール中毒, or *arukōru izonshō* アルコール依存症

In Japan, with its high social tolerance for alcohol-induced behavior and business practices which include pouring each other drinks until everyone is ready to slide under the table, it's sometimes difficult to evaluate what is normal. But if you or your family detect signs like blackouts, secretive drinking practices, aggressive behavior, etc., and you can't cut down on your own, you'll want to seek help before a crisis develops.

Depending on the severity of your illness and whether you will require tranquilizing drugs to lessen the symptoms of withdrawal, your choice of a therapist or a medical doctor may vary. Find someone you feel comfortable with and who has experience treating this condition. Those who don't know how to treat alcoholism can actually perpetuate the problem by incorrect advice and insufficient counseling. In Japan, help can be found in psychiatric departments or special outpatient clinics for alcohol dependency syndrome at large hospitals. Most programs are in Japanese, but hospitals may also have English-speaking doctors who can offer some help on an individual basis. Included in the therapy are physical checkups, group therapy, and useful techniques for reducing embarrassment at having to refuse drinks altogether. Dr. Satoshi Tanaka and Dr. Tomofumi Sone, in their book *Getting Sick in Japan*, give these tips for politely refusing alcohol in Japan.

1) "*Ishi ni tomerarete imasu.*" (A doctor ordered me not to drink.)
(The doctors suggest that you say this while touching your upper abdomen as though in pain. Japanese businessmen often suffer from stomach pains due to stress or excessive drinking, and this will be acceptable.)

2)"*Kuruma de kimashita no de...*" (I drove here, so ...)

3) "*Shūkyō-jo no riyū desu.*" (For religious reasons.)

4) "*Shuran-desu.*" (I'm a physically abusive drinker.)

(If you look muscular, the doctors say that this last will work well.)

Another simple, tested way to avoid drinking is to order *oolong-cha* (Chinese tea) or a soft drink early in the evening, and stick with refills of that. When people offer you beer, just point to your glass and say "*Kore de ii desu*" (I'm fine).

Group support in English can come from Alcoholics Anonymous meetings in the foreign communities. Al-Anon groups are available to help family members. Call TELL (see the endpapers) or one of the following.

Alcoholics Anonymous Japan General Service Office (JSO)
03-3971-1471 (Eng.)
http://www.geocities.com/Tokyo/Ginza/6783/a aindex.html
03-3590-5377 (J. only)
http://www4.justnet.ne.jp/~serenity/
Introduces AA groups around Japan, in English or Japanese.

ASK Human Care
アスク・ヒューマン・ケア
Sogno 21 Bldg. 2 Fl., 3-19-3 Hama-cho
Nihonbashi, Chuo-ku, Tokyo
03-3249-2551, fax 3249-2553
Information on support groups and treatment centers for all kinds of addictions (alcohol, drugs, gambling, sex, etc.) around Japan. Also, counseling and annual bilingual lectures by noted foreign specialists in addiction treatment, open to caregivers and the general public. Published and accepts orders for *Adikushon*『アディクション』(Addiction), edited by Arukoru Mondai Zenkoku Shimin Kyokai, 1995, a book listing 260 facilities nationwide treating addiction and self-help groups for addicts.

Kokuritsu Kurihama Byoin
国立久里浜病院
National Kurihama Hospital
5-3-1 Nobi, Yokosuka-shi, Kanagawa-ken
0468-48-1550
Japan's main institution for dealing with alcoholism. English-speaking physicians for outpatient treatment.

Drug Addiction, see Children's Health, page 172–73.

Gambling (pachinko, mah jong)

Gambling becomes an addiction when you no longer play to win, but rather crave the exciting tension of the game itself, without giving any thought or consideration to the financial risks you are taking. Most gambling is restricted in Japan, except for horse racing *keiba* 競馬 and bicycle racing *keirin* 競輪. Since pachinko, or Japanese-style pinball, requires cash to play, it provides a safety net for an addictive gambler. Yakuza-controlled mah jong games present the biggest danger for losing large sums of money in Japan. There are stories of Japanese salarymen taking out large loans at exorbitant interest rates to pay their gambling debts, eventually losing their homes and possessions. If you need help, seek counseling. There may also be an English-speaking support group nearby; check with TELL.

Eating Disorders *sesshoku shōgai* 摂食障害

The scientific term in Japanese for anorexia nervosa is *shinkeisei shokuyoku suishō* 神経性食欲推症, but in conversation the words *anorekishia* アノレキシア, or more often *kyoshokushō* 拒食症, (literally, "food refusal syndrome") are usually used. Bulimia (binge eating followed by purging) is termed *burimia* ブリミア but is generally called *kashokushō* 過食症 (literally, "overeating syndrome"). These are most often the problem of teenage girls, but can carry over into or even begin in adulthood. They are increasingly common in Japan, and the Japanese medical system is struggling to offer appropriate help.

For both these disorders, the main treatment is talking with a doctor or counselor; medication is only supplementary. If not dealt with early, treatment becomes increasingly difficult and can often take several years, which is an especially heavy burden here, since Japanese health insurance does not provide for much counseling.

Counseling is available at the psychiatric department or an outpatient clinic for eating disorders (*sesshoku geka* 摂食外来) or for adolescents (*shishunki gairai* 思春期外来) at university hospitals. Some have English-speaking pychiatrists. See also the resources below and on pages 239–40. TELL can direct you to English-speaking support groups.

Nippon Anorexia Bulimia Association
(NABA)
日本アノレキシア（拒食症）ブリミア
（過食症）協会
4-9-12-212 Kami-Kitazawa, Setagaya-ku, Tokyo
03-3302-0710 (J. only)

Support group, telephone counseling, workshops, and publications for those suffering or recovering from anorexia, overeating, bulimia, and other eating disorders, and also for family members. In Japanese. Network around Japan. Annual membership fee.

Other Addiction Resources

See also Counseling Centers and therapists on pages 239–40.

Homecoming Educational Program
2-2-10-605 Hiranuma, Nishi-ku, Yokohama-shi
045-313-3281
U.S.-trained counselors. Non-medical, out-patient, individual, and group counseling for all kinds of addictions including eating disorders. Referrals to inpatient programs in North America if necessary.

Can Do Harajuku (Director Kyoichi Miyazaki)
1-11-1 Jingumae, Shibuya-ku, Tokyo
03-3423-2501 (Eng.)
U.S.-trained therapists offer total healthcare and counseling in English and Japanese for drug, tobacco, and alcohol abuse or addiction, and eating disorders. New Start Program (including a high-fiber, low-cholesterol diet) for a healthier

approach to food. Facility in Hakone for one-week or overnight healthy life-style training. Also recommended for heart disease treatment and degenerative disease prevention. Free introductory consultation. (Weimar Institute, Dr. Onishi; based on the Seventh-Day Adventist healthy living style.)

MAC and DARC Alcoholism and Drug Rehabilitation Centers
(Maryknoll Fathers)
Ueno P.O. Box 56, Taito-ku, Tokyo
03-5685-6128 (Fr. Roy Assenheimer)
Support and counseling by former addicts. Many branches around Japan. All programs in Japanese.

Japanese Psychotherapy

Historically, the Japanese have left the care of the emotionally disturbed to the family. Professional counseling, rehabilitation programs, and pharmaceutical treatment of psychological disorders are all relatively new. Many Japanese are still reluctant to seek professional help, especially for minor problems. One reason is the stigma which has been attached to mental instabilities.

If you visit one of the counseling services mentioned above, you will find the therapies used are identical or very similar to those in the West. If you choose to go elsewhere, you will find many of the same therapies, but also a greater emphasis on medication. This is probably due at least partially to the Japanese insurance system, which does not reward physicians for their time. Whether a physician sees a patient for ten minutes or for an hour makes no difference in terms of the amount of money he or she receives, which makes lengthy psychotherapy economically difficult for the caregiver. As a result, first-time sessions tend to be at least an hour, while subsequent visits are much shorter and are mainly devoted to reviewing the effectiveness of the medication, with a minimum of supportive therapy. Medications may be different from those now popular in the West, and at present Prozac, Zoloft, Paxil, and Zoast are unavailable here. As for other therapies, much attention has recently been paid to Small Garden Therapy *hako niwa ryōhō*, and occupational, recreational, dance, art, music, and karaoke therapies are especially popular. Although Freudian psychoanalysis is generally known in Japan, and psychologists and psychiatrists who practice this and other Western techniques are in the majority, other therapies native to Japan such as Morita therapy and Naikan psychotherapy may also be used, usually in combination with Western therapy techniques.

Morita Therapy Morita ryōhō 森田療法
Morita therapy has been used for over sixty years to treat a group of neuroses called

shinkeishitsu 神経質. The term *shinkeishitsu* is used in Japanese to describe anyone who is highly sensitive, and does not necessarily refer to a pathological condition.

According to the Morita theory, people suffering from *shinkeishitsu* become overly introspective and perfectionistic. Morita therapy tries to get the patient to accept the environment and the self as is (*aru ga mama*), and to convince the patient that no one is perfect. In contrast to Freudian psychology, which seeks to alter the patient's feelings, Morita therapy urges the patient to get on with living and to let the emotions fix themselves. Treatment usually consists of complete bedrest for the first four to seven days, followed by immersion in constructive activities involving manual labor.

Resource

Seikatsu no Hakken Kai
4-41-12 Otsuka, Bunkyo-ku, Tokyo

03-3947-1011, fax 03-3947-1018
Morita therapy study group.

Naikan Psychotherapy *naikan ryōhō* 内観療法

Naikan psychotherapy was first developed in 1954 as corrective therapy for prison inmates and delinquents. It tells the patient to abandon selfish, destructive behavior, and to ask society (parents) for forgiveness. The patient is encouraged to recognize his/her debt to society (parents), and work to repay it. This is the opposite of Freudian psychology, which asks the patient to forgive society (again, parents) for wrongs committed against the patient. The patient sits in isolation for one to two weeks, meditating on past experiences and considering what debts he has incurred and which have been repaid. A therapist visits every hour or so to listen to the patient's confessions. The aim is to transform the patient from an arrogant, self-centered person to a humbler, more industrious citizen.

Resource

Yonago Research Center
Yonago Naikan Kenshujo
米子内観研習所
1-2-24 Sanbonmatsu, Yonago-shi, Tottori-ken

0859-22-3503 (J. only), fax 0859-22-1446
By appointment; referrals from Tottori University
as well as from other patients.

Constructive Living

Constructive Living is a Westernized Japanese system of personal growth developed by American David Reynolds, who has been heavily influenced by Morita Therapy, Naikan Psychotherapy, and other oriental therapies.

David Reynolds
047-333-5830
Instruction and further information.

Meditation

The Zen Buddhist practice of *zazen*, quiet sitting combined with meditation and breath control, has been used for centuries to cure neuroses and is still sometimes used today.

Dogen Sanga
Tokyo University Buddhist Youth Association
Tokyo Daigaku Bukkyo Seinenkai
東京大学仏教青年会
3-33-5 Hongo, Bunkyo-ku, Tokyo
03-3813-5903 (J. only)
Zazen and classes in Buddhism.

Shoun-ji
松雲寺
306 Nakagawara-cho, Ikeda-shi, Osaka-fu
0727-53-3587 (Mr. Yasunaga Sodo)
Zazen meetings at 6:30 P.M. on Sundays;
beginners at 6:00.

See also *Tokyo Whole Life Pages* ("References and Further Reading").

Inpatient Psychiatric Treatment

Most people find that serious mental disturbances are best treated in their own country, where language and cultural barriers are not a problem. Japan has very limited resources for the appropriate treatment of non-Japanese patients requiring psychiatric hospitalization. Communication difficulties, differences in customs, and a lack of experience with non-Japanese, not to mention legal concerns, may sometimes influence Japanese hospital staff to refuse admission outright to foreign patients.

People who do seek treatment here will find Japan does have English-speaking psychiatrists who can offer consultation and treatment and facilitate a hospital admission. These doctors can be found, through the centers on page 239–40, in university hospitals and often in large public mental hospitals, including those listed on the following page.

As mentioned above, attitudes and methods can differ somewhat from those now common in the West. Differences are most pronounced when it comes to inpatient treatment. Japan does have some good facilities for treating the mentally ill, but poor conditions have prevailed in many psychiatric units. Especially in private institutions seeking financial gain, there has been a tendency to keep patients unnecessarily sedated and isolated in locked hospital wards without proper rehabilitative care. Electric shock treatment has been used excessively or underused, and there have been consistent reports of physical abuse, maltreatment, and overcrowded conditions.

In the past few years, however, recognition of the importance of treating mental illnesses in a nurturing environment has brought some changes. In 1988 the government passed the Mental Health Law, which aims to protect the human rights of the mentally ill and to promote their rehabilitation and reintegration into the community. It has given local governments and social welfare organizations the right to establish rehabilitation facilities for the mentally ill with the aim of helping patients return to the community. Private institutions are also looking in new directions. Although Japanese society still struggles with long-standing prejudices against the mentally ill, these and other efforts are gradually changing attitudes as well as forms of treatment.

Emergency Admission

The most important thing is to seek help early, before your condition turns into an emergency. Psychiatric hospitals in Japan claim that too many foreign people arrive at the hospital seriously ill and suicidal. Many mental problems can be solved in a few sessions with a counselor on an outpatient basis. However, if left untreated, these emotional disturbances can sometimes result in severe mental illnesses.

If you are already in treatment and experience an emergency (suicidal thoughts or mental breakdown), call your therapist first for help in arranging emergency treatment or a referral to the appropriate resource. If you have not been receiving care, contact your primary physician for a referral.

Otherwise, in a psychiatric emergency, call the police on 110 (not the fire department or ambulance: 119). The police will help you get to a hospital, usually a police-affiliated hospital or a municipal mental health hospital.

People arriving at an emergency hospital on their own will also be evaluated for admission, and this might be the best course to take if you can't reach a familiar counselor and wish to avoid police involvement. Be aware, however, that not all hospitals with psychiatric units will handle emergencies. The hotlines and information services listed on the endpapers can help you find a facility that will accept you. Don't go without confirming that there is a psychiatrist on duty who can treat you. Psychiatric hospitals accepting emergency cases in the Tokyo area are listed below. Most cities have no one facility, but work on a rotation system.

Emergency Psychiatric Hospitals

For further reference, call one of the hotlines (see the front endpapers), your municipal foreign relations office (see "Regional Resources"), your public health center, or the police.

Tokyo Metropolitan Matsuzawa Hospital
Toritsu Matsuzawa Byoin
都立松沢病院
2-1-1, Kami-Karasuyama, Setagaya-ku, Tokyo
03-3303-7211
The oldest and largest public psychiatric hospital in Japan, Matsuzawa has an emergency ward, though it often takes time for the hospital to agree to take an emergency case; stay of up to 3 months possible.

Tokyo Metropolitan Umegaoka Hospital
Toritsu Umegaoka Byoin
都立梅ヶ丘病院
6-37-10 Matsubara, Setagaya-ku, Tokyo
03-3323-1621
For children.

Tokyo Metropolitan Bokuto Hospital
Toritsu Bokuto Byoin
都立墨東病院
4-23-15 Kotobashi, Sumida-ku, Tokyo
03-3633-6151
Public hospital; one-night stay only—patients are referred to a private hospital the following day.

Tokyo Metropolitan Fuchu Hospital
Toritsu Fuchu Byoin
都立府中病院
2-9-2 Musashidai, Fuchu-shi, Tokyo
0423-23-5111
Public hospital; one-night stay only.

For services and assistance for those with mental disorders and disabilities, see "Help for the Disabled and the Elderly."

For help with child abuse, see page 178.

2

All About Drugs and Drugstores

"The first time I took my daughter to a Japanese doctor for treatment of a bad cold and cough, I came home with six different medicines. One was for bringing up phlegm from her lungs, another to calm the cough and let her sleep, another for fever, another in case the other medicines upset her stomach, and the other a packet of vitamins. I've forgotten what the last one was. Since then I've had no reason to change my initial impression that the Japanese are a grossly overmedicated people."

"My overall impression after twenty years in Japan is that the major problem in treatment is the drug dosage. My husband, a generously-proportioned American, dislocated his shoulder and was taken to a local hospital. While waiting for the doctor, he was given the usual dose of pain medication, but it was too small to ease the pain. The nurses refused to give him any more until the doctor arrived."

Distinctive Features of the Pharmaceutical System

The most infamous feature of the pharmaceutical system is that doctors and dentists, like pharmacists, can sell medications and make a profit on them. This is probably a carryover from an old tradition in oriental medicine in which practitioners made and also sold their own medications. A doctor practicing Western medicine may also prescribe Chinese medications (see pages 277–80), which may be covered under public insurance plans.

In general, doctors take little time to explain the drugs that they are prescribing, although polite foreigners may get a lengthier explanation than usual.

"I will always remember one private doctor who treated my son for a bad cold. When I asked him what he was prescribing, he became very angry and said that he saw a hundred patients every day and did not have time to explain the medications to each one."

The patient is simply supposed to trust that the doctor is prescribing the correct drug for his or her condition.

By law, the maximum supply of medications that can be prescribed per medical examination is fourteen days for any newly prescribed medications (these need to be checked for efficacy), certain heart disease drugs (the patient needs to be closely followed), anti-cancer drugs, and Chinese medications *kanpō yaku* 漢方薬. For other drugs (with some exceptions), the prescription can cover thirty days. However, in reality prescriptions are often written for just three- or four-day periods and then you must return for another doctor's visit and another prescription. This is especially true with antibiotics. Although the doctor's explanation that he wants to check on the efficacy of the drug is probably true, it is also true that the doctor or hospital will make money on each visit and each prescription. If you know that you will not be able to return when the prescription runs out, tell the doctor, and he or she will probably increase the days covered. In any case, you are expected to keep returning when your medication runs out until the doctor says you are cured. Refills *saichōzai* 再調剤 are not supplied at pharmacies in Japan. Occasionally you will not need to see the doctor to get a new prescription. Depending on the doctor, the medication, and/or the disease, the nurse may be able to get the doctor's signature on a new prescription for drugs you are taking regularly, without making you wait to see the doctor. As soon as you arrive at the department reception window, ask whether this is possible.

But you should be aware that racial and ethnic differences can affect the way that drugs are metabolized in the body. The rate of metabolism and excretion of medications from the body also varies from one person to another. Differences have also been identified in the effects of heart medications, diuretics, tranquilizers, and antidepressants. For this reason, the Japanese custom of writing prescriptions for just three or four days may work for your good, since the return visit gives the doctor the opportunity to make sure that the medication he has prescribed for you is working as it should.

Types of Medication

analgesic *chintsū zai* 鎮痛剤

antacid *seisan zai* 制酸剤

antiarrhythmic *kōfuseimyaku zai* 抗不整脈剤

antibiotic *kōseibusshitsu* 抗生物質

antidepressive *kōyoku utsu zai* 抗抑うつ剤

antidiarrheal *geridome* 下痢止め

anti-emetic *seito zai* 制吐剤

antifungal *kō-shinkin zai* 抗真菌剤

antihistamine *kō-hisutamin zai* 抗ヒスタミン剤

anti-inflammatory *kōenshō-zai* 抗炎症剤 or *shōen zai* 消炎剤

antiparasitic *kaichū kujo zai* 回虫駆除剤

antipyretic *genetsu zai* 下熱剤

antiseizure *kōtenkan zai* 抗テンカン剤

antiseptic *shōdoku zai* 消毒剤

antitussive *sekidome* せき止め

beta blocker *beta shadan zai* ベタ遮断薬

blood pressure reducer *ketsuatsu kōka zai* 血圧降下剤

bronchodilator *kikanshi kakuchō zai* 気管支拡張剤

cancer chemotherapy agent *kōgan zai* 抗がん剤

cold medicine *sōgō kanbō yaku* 総合感冒薬

cortisone *coruchizon* コルチゾン

cough expectorant *kyotan zai* 去たん剤

cough suppressant *sekidome zai* 咳止め剤

digitalis *jigitarisu* ジギタリス

diuretic *rinyō zai* 利尿剤

hormones *horumon* ホルモン

insulin *insurin* インスリン

iodine (Betadine) *kiyōdochinki* 希ヨードチンキ

laxative *ge zai* 下剤

multivitamins *sōgō bitamin* 総合ビタミン

nasal decongestant *hanazumari no kusuri* 鼻づまりの薬

nitroglycerine *nitoroguriserin* ニトログリセリン

oral hypoglycemic *keikō tōnyōbyō-zai* 軽口糖尿病剤

sedative *chinsei zai* 鎮静剤

sleeping medication *suiminchinsei zai* 睡眠鎮静剤

steroid *suteroido zai* ステロイド剤

sulfa drug *surufa zai* スルファ剤

tranquilizers *torankiraizā* トランキライザー or *seishin antei zai* 精神安定剤

vitamins *bitamin* ビタミン

Forms of Medication

Drugs are prescribed in many forms—tablets, powders, suppositories, intravenous infusions, injections, etc.—but not necessarily in familiar ways. For instance, suppositories are often prescribed for children in Japan to reduce fever.

Powdered medication, which is meant to be swallowed in one gulp, is popular in Japan. If you cannot manage the gulp, buy *oburāto* papers オブラート made of edible gelatin (also available in drugstores) and carefully wrap the powder into a small, capsule-like form to be swallowed.

Avoid taking tablets with strong green tea, because the tea may slow absorption of the medication, especially iron supplements.

capsule *kapuseru* カプセル

ear drops *tenjiyaku* 点耳薬

eye drops *tenganyaku* 点眼薬

eye ointment *gannankō* 眼軟膏

gargle medicine *ugaigusuri* うがい薬

inhalant *kyūnyūzai* 吸入剤

injection *chūsha* 注射

nose drop *tenbiyaku* 点鼻薬

ointment or cream *nankō* 軟膏,
  kurīmu クリーム

pill *ganyaku* 丸薬

powder *konagusuri* 粉薬

rectal suppository *zayaku* 坐薬

sublingual tablet *zekkajō* 舌下錠

syrup *shiroppu* シロップ

tablet *jōzai* 錠剤

troche, lozenge *torōchi* トローチ

vaginal suppository *chitsu zayaku* 膣座薬

Generic Drugs

In Japan there is no system of generic prescription drugs (non–brand-name drugs that have the same chemical content as brand-name drugs but are cheaper). Patients have no choice as to the brand of medicine they will take, as the law requires that the prescription be filled exactly as the doctor has written it.

Antibiotics

Antibiotics are usually prescribed for very short periods of just two or three days. This is a great surprise if you have been taught that most bacterial infections take seven to ten days of antibiotic treatment to clear up completely. The reason given for the two- or three-day prescription is that the doctor wants to see if the antibiotic is working as it should. You are to keep returning for more medication until the doctor determines that you are completely cured. Even if the pain goes away and it looks as though the infection has healed, you are supposed to keep returning to the outpatient clinic until the doctor tells you that the infection is completely cured.

Another reason for a short-term prescription of antibiotics may be patient pressure. The doctor may feel he has to do something even when antibiotics are not really called for. Some doctors, for instance, prescribe antibiotics for a cold, even though a viral cold is not cured by antibiotics. Patients and parents often insist on a medication even in cases in which the body would probably heal naturally.

Pain Medications

Pain medications are prescribed modestly, or not at all. Foreigners of a generous build will need to remind their doctor of their increased dosage needs.

Reading Your Medicine Packet

The pharmacist will give you your prescription medications in a paper bag with instructions for taking the medicines written on it. The following vocabulary should help you understand these instructions as well as the labels on nonprescription drugs.

用療 *yōryō* dosage

用法 *yōhō* directions

成人, 大人 *seijin, otona* adult

溶液 *yō eki* solution

水 *mizu* water

〜ごと *-goto* every ~

1日2回 *ichinichi nikai* 2 times a day

1日3回 *ichinichi sankai* 3 times a day

1日4回 *ichinichi yonkai* 4 times a day

1日3回8時間毎 *ichinichi sankai hachijikan-goto* 3 times a day every 8 hours

1時間毎 *ichijikan-goto* every hour

隔日 *kakujitsu* every other day

必要に応じて *hitsuyō ni ōjite* as necessary

食前 *shoku zen* before meals

食後 *shoku go* (about 30 minutes) after meals

食間 *shokkan* between meals (about 2 hours after last meal)

眠時 *minji* at bedtime

半分 *hanbun* half

経口的 *keikō-teki* by mouth

医師の指示通り *ishi no shiji dōri* as instructed by your doctor

Side Effects *fukusayō* 副作用

It is extremely important that you ask the doctor and/or the pharmacist if any of the drugs you take has any potential side effects. You can also call the pharmaceutical section (*yakumu-ka*) of your prefectural government in Japanese for this information.

Obtaining Medications

Hospital or Clinic Pharmacy *byōin no yakkyoku* 病院の薬局

It is common to receive two or three types of medicine together in one packet. By law only the name of the patient, the dosage, and the form of the medication need be noted on it. Some doctors as a matter of course still direct that all identifying labels be removed from the medication itself, so it's doubly important to ask what each medication is and to write a description of it on the pharmacy envelope (for instance, "red for cough" or "oval white tablet for headache"). Happily, more and more pharmacists are prepared to cheerfully give detailed information on the drugs they dispense. See pages 70 and 75 for information about Japanese health insurance coverage of prescription medications.

Outside Dispensing Pharmacy *chōzai yakkyoku* 調剤薬局

A new type of pharmacy which fills prescriptions, these stores constitute a first attempt by the Ministry of Health and Welfare to separate the act of prescription from the sale of drugs. However, these pharmacies are still not popular with physicians or patients, because it takes the doctor longer to write out the prescription and the patient longer to receive the medications, and it costs slightly more. This pharmacy is designated by a sign saying 処方せん受付 (*shohōsen uketsuke* "prescriptions filled") and a yellow sign with the words 保険薬局 (*hoken yakkyoku* "health insurance–designated pharmacy") written in black letters. This kind of pharmacy is usually located within a short distance of the medical facility that issued the prescription. You may be asked whether you want your prescription filled at the medical facility's pharmacy or at the outside dispensing pharmacy. Sometimes you may have no choice but to go to the outside pharmacy. In any case you will be given a copy of your prescription and a map showing the location of the outside pharmacy, which will stock all the drugs prescribed by neighboring hospitals or clinics.

Stick to the pharmacy recommended by the clinic or hospital. Pharmacies stock a limited supply of medications, and other stores may not be able to fill the prescription. Make sure that you write down the descriptions of the drugs before leaving the pharmacy. This pharmacy may also sell over-the-counter drugs.

Nonprescription Pharmacy kusuriya 薬屋

This type of pharmacy sells nonprescription drugs (see pages 257–61), vitamins, sanitary items, personal toiletry items, beauty products, cleaning supplies, baby supplies, etc. Unless it is an outside pharmacy, it does not fill prescriptions. Although the manager must be a pharmacist *yakuzaishi* 薬剤師, the staff selling the various products and over-the-counter drugs do not have to be. For less serious illnesses you may elect to go to a nonprescription drugstore and ask for some appropriate medication, but the salesperson may not have any professional medical knowledge. If you do not find the non-prescription medication that you want, but the medication is available in Japan, you may be able to order it through this type of drugstore.

Another kind of drugstore is the *yakuten* 薬店. The manager is not a pharmacist, but has a special license to sell a limited variety of over-the-counter drugs. It may be difficult to distinguish the *yakuten* from a nonprescription pharmacy.

Handy Tips

■ To avoid a wait: Leave your prescription at the hospital pharmacy. Return later in the day to pick up your medications. If the prescribed medication is an over-the-counter drug, buy it at a local drugstore, but remember that if you do buy it there, it won't be covered by public insurance.

■ To avoid being prescribed unnecessary drugs: Tell the doctor that you have a stock of simple medications at home.

■ To save money: If you use an over-the-counter drug regularly, go to a doctor and get a prescription which will be covered by insurance and will cost much less than when purchased at the nonprescription drugstore.

Pharmacies

The following pharmacies stock a wide variety of foreign products or cater specifically to the foreign community, and may have greater access to imported drugs than do other facilities.

National Azabu Drug Store
4-5-2 Minami-Azabu, Minato-ku, Tokyo
03-3442-3495 Daily 9:30 A.M.–7:00 P.M.
Has pregnancy and ovulation tests with instructions in English. English telephone counseling available; mailing service.

Mimi Pharmacy
2-29-21 Dogenzaka, Shibuya-ku, Tokyo
03-3463-6419 Daily 9:00 A.M.–midnight

English-speaking pharmacist with particular interest in oriental medicine. Appointment necessary.

American Pharmacy
Hibiya Park Bldg. 1 Fl., 1-8-1 Yurakucho
Chiyoda-ku, Tokyo
03-3271-4034
Mon.–Sat. 9:30 A.M.–7:30 P.M.; first Sun. and hols. 11:00 A.M.–5:00 P.M.

Has pregnancy test with instructions in English. English-speaking pharmacists available; mailing service throughout Japan.

Medical Dispensary
(with Tokyo Medical and Surgical Clinic)
32 Mori Bldg., 3-4-30 Shiba-Koen
Minato-ku, Tokyo
03-3434-5817 Mon.–Fri. 9:00 A.M.–5:30 P.M.;
Sat. 9:00 A.M.–1:00 P.M.; closed Sun. and hols.

Hill Pharmacy
4-1-6 Roppongi, Minato-ku, Tokyo
03-3583-5044; 9:00 A.M.–7:00 P.M.; closed Sun. and hols.
045-641-0886 (Branch in Motomachi, Yokohama); 9:00 A.M.–7:00 P.M.; 3rd Mon. sometimes closed.

Pharmacy Madonna
3-7-11 Ooka, Minami-ku, Yokohama-shi
045-743-5251
Consultations in English.

Seishindo Pharmacy
1-8-7 Okano, Nishi-ku, Yokohama-shi
045-314-9009; 9:00 A.M.–7:00 P.M.; closed Sun. and hols.

Osaka Hankyu Department Store
8-7 Kakuda-cho, 3 Fl., Kita-ku, Osaka-shi
06-361-1381; Mon.–Sun. 10:00 A.M.–7:30 P.M.
Skin-care room with pharmacist on hand to answer questions. Call to make appointment for free counseling. Regular drugstore on first floor.

Using Home Country Prescriptions in Japan

Prescriptions from your home country cannot be filled in Japan. Show your old prescription to your Japanese doctor, who will then write you a new prescription.

Medications from Outside Japan

Medicines can be brought into Japan in a one month's supply (or the smallest amount sold retail—for example, a bottle of pills containing a three-month supply) of prescription medications and a two-month supply (or the smallest amount sold retail) of nonprescription medications. Do not take the medications out of the boxes or original packaging. Have your doctor include a letter with the drugs stating that they are for your personal use. *Narcotics or stimulants cannot be brought into Japan.*

The same is true for medications ordered through the mail. A word of caution: you will want to be sure the company that you are ordering from is reputable. This can be a problem particularly when you use the Internet since there are now no controls placed on online commercial activity. You'll also want a physician in Japan who is familiar with the medication to give you periodic checkups and to be there in case of an emergency.

If you have problems or questions about bringing medications into Japan, you can contact the following agency at the Ministry of Health and Welfare:

Pharmaceutical Safety Bureau,
Surveillance and Guidance Section
Iyaku Anzen Kyoku Kanshi Shido-ka
医薬安全局看視指導課
03-3503-1711, ext. 2768 (J. only)

Mail-Order Medicines

John Bell and Croydon
50–54 Wigmore Street, London W1H OAU U.K.
44-171-935-5555, fax 44-171-935-9605
British nonprescription drugs; medical supplies.

Puritan's Pride
1233 Montauk Hwy., P.O. Box 9001, Oakdale, NY
11769-9001 U.S.
1-800-645-1030, fax 1-516-471-5693
http://www.puritan.com

Amway Products
Nihon Seimei Minami-Azabu Bldg.
2-8-12 Minami-Azabu, Minato-ku, Tokyo
(toll-free) 0120-123777 (J. only)
03-3928-9357, fax 03-3928-4226
(Contact: LoAnne Olson in Eng.)
Natural food supplements, water and air treatment systems, non-polluting laundry products,
cosmetics for sensitive skin, toothpaste, etc. Call
for catalog.

See also **Foreign Buyer's Club (FBC)** on the
endpapers.

Door-to-Door Salesmen

One day you may open the door to greet a smiling sales representative who wants you to
subscribe to a home medicine box service. The deal is that you keep a medicine box filled
with a variety of nonprescription drugs (like hot and cold packs, cold medicines, pain medications, throat lozenges, band-aids, Chinese medicines for digestive troubles and other
ills) in your home, with no obligation to use any at all. Every three to six months a representative will return to check the contents of the box, receive payment for any packets you
have opened, and replenish the box. Called Toyama Kusuriya or Toyama Kusuribako because the business originated in Toyama Prefecture, this traditional style of drug selling is
still being used and appreciated by Japanese families today.

Nonprescription Drugs *shihan-yaku* 市販薬

The following over-the-counter drugs are for short-term minor ailments. Not all will be
available at every drug store. For persistent or severe symptoms, consult a doctor.

The manufacturer's name is indicated in parentheses after the brand name. Please
note that nonprescription medications list the composition *seibun* 成分 of the drug on the
label in different ways. Some list the total amount of the ingredients in each dose, others
in the total recommended dosage per day.

Abbreviations: **tab.** = tablet; **x** = times; **hr.** = hour; **cap.** = capsule; **yrs.** = years

MEDICATIONS FOR COLDS AND HAY FEVER
None of the following cold medications contain
aspirin. Nonprescription antihistamines may
cause drowsiness; prolonged use may raise
blood pressure. Consult a physician before giving
cold medications to a child under two.

Antihistamine and Decongestant Types
Restamin Kowa
レスタミンコーワ (Kowa 興和)

Contains: Antihistamine only (Benadryl)
Dosage: Adults 3 tabs.; 11–15 yrs. 2 tabs.; 5–11
yrs. 1 tab. Up to 3x a day.

Arerugiru-jo
アレルギール錠 (Sankyo 三共)
Contains: Antihistamine (Chlor-Trimeton),
Vitamin B-6, calcium, licorice, anti-inflammatory
Dosage: Adults 3 tabs. 2–3x a day; 7–14 yrs. 2
tabs. 2x a day; 4–6 yrs.1 tab. 2x a day.

Contac 600 SR

コンタック600SR (Smith Klein)

Contains: Antihistamine (Chlor-Trimeton), decongestants, expectorant.

Dosage: Adults 1 cap. Every 12 hrs.; contraindicated in those with glaucoma or high blood pressure.

Benza Bi-en Yo

ベンザ鼻炎用 (Takeda 武田)

Contains: Antihistamine (Chlor-Trimeton), decongestants, caffeine, serrapeptase

Dosage: Adults 1 cap. Every 12 hrs.; contraindicated in those with glaucoma or high blood pressure.

Antitussive Types

SS Bron Eki Ace

エスエスブロン液エース (SS エスエス製薬)

Contains: Expectorant (as in Robitussin), antitussive (Codeine), antihistamine (Chlor-Trimeton), caffeine

Dosage: Adults 5 ml; 11–14 yrs. 3.3 ml; 8–12 yrs. 2.5 ml. 3x daily; if necessary, every 4 hrs. up to 6x a day.

Contac Sekidome SR

コンタックせき止めSR (Smith Klein)

Contains: Antitussive, antihistamine, decongestant, expectorant.

Dosage: Adults 1 cap. Every 12 hrs.

Shin Sekidome Aneton Shiroppu

新せき止めアネトンシロップ
(Pfizer ファイザー)

Contains: Antitussive (Codeine), antihistamine, decongestant, plus stabilizers and red dye.

Dosage: Adults 10 ml; 11–15 yrs. 6.5 ml; 8–11 yrs. 5 ml; 5–8 yrs. 3.4 ml; 3–5 yrs. 2.5 ml; 1–3 yrs. 2 ml; 3 mos.–1 yr. 1 ml. Every 4 hrs., but no more than 5x a day; contraindicated in those with glaucoma and high blood pressure.

Antipyretic Types (to lower temperature)

Pabron S Jo

パブロンS錠 (Taisho 大正)

Contains: Antipyretic, expectorant, antitussive (Codeine), antihistamine, decongestant, caffeine, vitamins B-1 and B-2, Lysozyme

Dosage: Adults 3 tabs.; 11–14 yrs. 2 tabs., 5–10 yrs. 1 tab. 3x a day after meals; contraindicated in those with glaucoma and high blood pressure.

Contac Sogo Kanbo Yaku

コンタック総合感冒薬 (Smith Klein)

Contains: Antipyretics, antitussive, antihistamine, decongestant, Vitamin C, caffeine

Dosage: Adults 2 tabs.; 7–15 yrs. 1 tab. 3x a day after meals; contraindicated in those with glaucoma and high blood pressure.

Nose Drops

For stuffy nose; all contain antihistamine. Avoid frequent use for more than 4–5 days.

Paburon Tenbi

パブロン点鼻 (Taisho 大正)

Dosage: From 7 yrs. to adult 1–2 drops each nostril. Up to 6x a day.

Shin Nabel Tenbi Eki (for children)

新ナベル点鼻液(幼児用) (Chugai 中外)

Dosage: Over 2 yrs. 1–2 drops, 4–6 hrs. apart.

Nazar Supre

ナザルスプレー (Sato 佐藤)

Dosage: From 7 yrs. to adults, spray into nose every 3 hrs. as needed, up to 6x a day.

Gargle Medications

Isojin Ugai Gusuri

イソジンうがい薬 (Meiji 明治)

Contains: Iodine

Dosage: Mix 2–4 ml (up to the 1st or 2nd lines on cup) with 60 ml water; gargle. Repeat several times a day for sore throat.

Pain Relief Medications

For headache, muscle, joint, menstrual pain; not for stomach or intestinal distress. Also for reducing inflammation and fever.

Type 1: Aspirin has been associated with Reye's syndrome, a very serious brain disease, when given to children with chickenpox or influenza; can cause upset stomach.

Bayer Aspirin

バイエルアスピリン (Eizai エーザイ)

Contains: Aspirin 0.5 g (each U.S tab is 0.3 g)

Dosage: Adults 1 tab.; children 1/8 tab. per year of age. Every 4 hrs.

Bufferin A

バファリンA (Lion ライオン)

Contains: Aspirin 330 mg and buffering agent

Dosage: Adults 2 tabs. Twice a day at least 6 hrs. apart.

Type 2 Ibuprofen (as in Advil); can cause upset stomach; should be avoided by pregnant women or people allergic to aspirin.

Nurofen
ニューロフェン (Taisho 大正)
Contains: Ibuprofen 75 mg
Dosage: Adults 2 tabs. 3x a day
Also Eve イブ (SS エスエス), Suparomin スパロミン (Sampo 三宝) with the same strength.

Type 3 Acetaminophen (as in Tylenol); less likely than aspirin to cause stomach irritation.

Children's Bufferin CII
小児用バファリンCII (Lion ライオン)
Contains: Acetaminophen 33 mg
Dosage: 3–7 yrs. 3 tabs.; 7–11 yrs. 4 tabs.; 11–15 yrs. 6 tabs. 3x a day.

Also **New Children's Isomidon** 新小児用イソミドン (SSエスエス) with same strength.

Alpiny A Zayaku
アルピニ A 坐剤 (SS エスエス)
Contains: Acetaminophen 100 mg
Dosage: Up to 2 yrs.1/2 supp.; 3–5 yrs. 1 supp; 6–12 yrs. 1–2 supp. 1x daily; rectal suppository.

Teirin
テーリン (Wakodo 和光堂)
Contains: Acetaminophen 125 mg and caffeine
Dosage: Adults 2 tabs., 8–15 yrs. 1 tab. 1–3x a day.

VOMITING AND DIARRHEA MEDICATIONS
Drink alternating sips of a sweetened carbonated beverage (Sprite, etc., but not Coca-Cola or diet drinks) and clear salty soup or drink sports drinks; add fruit juices for diarrhea.

Buscopan A
ブスコパン A (Nihon Boehringer Ingelheim 日本ベーリンガーインゲルハイム)
Contains: Antiemetic (to prevent nausea)
Dosage: Adults 1 tab. 3x a day, at least 4 hrs. apart.

Shin Biofermin
新ビオフェルミン (Takeda 武田)
Contains: Lactobaccilus; helps to regulate stomach, intestines after diarrhea, etc.
Dosage: Adults 3 tabs.; 5–14 yrs. 2 tabs. 3x a day after meals.

Sato Geri Dome Nai Fuku Eki
サトウ下痢どめ内服液 (Sato 佐藤)
Contains: Kaolin, a simple adsorbent, and others
Dosage: Adults 30 ml. 3x a day after meals.

Constipation Medications
Also Increase fluids, fruits, vegetables, bran; exercise.

Colac
コーラック (Taisho 大正)
Contains: Bisacodyl, a stimulant
Dosage: Adults 2 tabs. before sleeping. (Swallow whole, do not chew.)

Ichijiku Kancho
イチジク浣腸 (Ichijiku Seiyaku イチジク製薬)
Small glycerine enema. May be used by all ages for constipation. Available in three different sizes.

STOMACH, INTESTINAL CRAMP MEDICATIONS
Consider appendicitis if pain and/or nausea persist for more than 24 hours. The following contain antispasmodics to calm cramps, and antacids to neutralize stomach acids.

Sankyo Chintsu Chinkei Ichoyaku
三共鎮痛鎮ケイ胃腸薬 (Sankyo 三共)
Dosage: Adults 3 tabs.; 11–15 yrs. 2 tabs.; 5–11 yrs. 1 tab. 3x daily, at least 4 hrs apart.

Takeda Chintsu Chinkei Ichoyaku
タケダ鎮痛鎮ケイ胃腸薬 (Takeda 武田)
Dosage: Adults 3 tabs.; 11–15 yrs. 2 tabs.; 5–11 yrs. 1 tab. 3x a day after meals.

Kolantyl A
コランチルA (Shionogi 塩野義)
Dosage: Adult 1 packet. 3x a day with meals.

See also **Buscopan A** (this page).

ACID INDIGESTION MEDICATIONS
See doctor if symptoms persist over long period.

Takeda Ichoyaku 21
タケダ胃腸薬21 (Takeda 武田)
Dosage: Adults 3 tabs.; 11–14 yrs. 2 tabs.; 5–10 yrs. 1 tab. 3x daily after or with meals.

Maalox Plus
マーロクス　プラス　(Yamanouchi 山之内)
Dosage: 10–30 ml per dose

Also **Kolantyl A** (see previous page)

NAUSEA OR MOTION SICKNESS MEDICATIONS
May cause drowsiness.

Travelmin Senior/Junior
トラベルミンシニア / ジュニア
(Eizai エーザイ)
Dosage: Senior—1 tab. 30 mins. before travel;
repeat as necessary every 4 hrs. up to 3x a day.
Junior—5–10 yrs. 1 tab.; 11–14 yrs. 2 tabs.
Repeat if necessary every 4 hrs., up to 3x a day.

Senpa (chewable)
センパー (Taisho 大正)
Dosage: Adults 1 tab.; 7–14 yrs. 1/2 tab. 1x a day.
Take 30 mins. before travel.

SKIN ALLERGY MEDICATIONS
For allergies (cortisone cream/ointment). Apply
sparingly 2x–4x a day. Don't use over a long
period.

Rari-A Kurimu/Nanko cream/ointment
ラリーエイクリーム / 軟膏 (Zenyaku 全薬)
Contains: Dexamethasone 0.5 percent

Flucort F (cream)
フルコートF (Tanabe 田辺)
Contains: Antibacterial plus steroid

Berica Kurimu
ベリカクリーム (Shionogi 塩野義)
Contains: Prednisolone 1 percent plus Vitamin E

ANTIBIOTIC CREAMS
For minor skin infections, burns, cuts, abscesses.
Apply sparingly to affected area.

Dorumaikochi Nanko (ointment)
ドルマイコーチ軟膏 (Zeria ゼリア)
Contains: Antibiotic plus hydrocortisone

Kuromai-P (Ointment)
クロマイーP軟膏 (Sankyo 三共)
Contains: Antibiotic plus prednisone

FUNGUS MEDICATIONS
For athlete's foot, ringworm, etc.

Scorpio Kurimu/Eki (cream or liquid)
スコーピオクリーム / 液 (Eizai エーザイ)
Apply 2x–3x a day.

Takkuru W Eki/Nanko (liquid or ointment)
タックルW液 / 軟膏 (Sankyo 三共)
Apply 2x a day.

Tamuchinki Powder Spray B
タムチンキパウダースプレーB
(Kobayashi 小林)
Shake well and apply 2x–3x a day.

LICE MEDICATIONS (for head and pubic hair)

Sumisurin Powder
スミスリン (Sumitomo 住友)
Spread about 7 g of the powder through the hair
to the scalp; cover head with towel and leave
for about 1 hr. Wash hair thoroughly and repeat
every other day, a total of 3x–4x. Note that anti-
lice shampoo has not yet been approved for
sale. See FBC, in the back endpapers.

ANTISEPTIC SOLUTIONS
For cleaning and disinfecting of cuts and abra-
sions.

Makiron マキロン (Yamanouchi 山之内)
Contains: Anesthetic, antihistamine, antiseptic,
and anti-inflammatory

Isojin S イソジンS (Meiji 明治)
Contains: Iodine (Betadine). Apply to affected
part; note that this stains the skin brown.

INSECT BITE MEDICATIONS

Muhi S ムヒS (Ikeda Mohando 池田模範堂)
Contains: Antihistamine, plus others

Una Kowa A ウナコーワA (Kowa 興和)
Contains: Antihistamine, plus others

Kinkan キンカン (Kinkando 金冠堂)
Contains: Ammonia water, plus others

EYE DROPS
For tired, blood-shot eyes. Do not use when hard
contact lenses are in place. Infections need
antibiotic drops—prescription is required.

Shin Smile 新スマイル (Lion ライオン)
2 drops, 3–6x a day.

Airisu アイリス (Taisho 大正)
2–3 drops, 3–5x a day.

Shinsumarin Deluxe (Allergy)
新スマリン・デラックス（アレルギー）
(SS エスエス)
Contains: Antihistamine, plus others. 1–3 drops,
3x–6x a day for allergies.

Muscle/Joint Ache Medications
Directions: Rub into affected area 3x–4x a day.

Salomethyl Nanko (ointment)
サロメチール軟膏 (Tanabe 田辺)

Indomethacin Eki (lotion)
インドメタチン液 (Banyu 萬有)

Mobilat Nanko (ointment)
モビラート軟膏 (Maruho マルホ)

Multivitamins
Multivitamin products are expensive; order
through a company in your country or one of the
companies on page 257. *Nikochinsanamido* (ニ
コチン酸アミド) is niacinamide (a B vitamin)
and not nicotine.

Nyujiyo Popon S (liquid for children)
乳児用 ポポンS (Shionogi 塩野義)
Dosage: From birth to 3 mos. 0.5 ml 1x a day; 4
mos. to 1 yr. 0.5 ml. 2x a day; 1–5 yrs. 0.5 ml. 3x
a day. Contains 9 vitamins.

Shin Popon S
新ポポンS (Shionogi 塩野義)
Dosage: Adults 2 tabs. a day; 6–15 yrs. 1 tab. a
day after breakfast or supper. Contains 10 vitamins plus calcium.

Panvitan Hai
パンビタンハイ (Takeda 武田)
Dosage: Adults 3 tabs. /day; 11–14 yrs. 2 tabs./
day; 5–10 yrs. tab./day. Take whole with water
after meal; don't chew. Contains more than 10
vitamins and minerals.

Contraceptive Products (see pages 101–102)

Other Drugstore Products

Ammonia water *anmonia sui* アンモニア水
Bicarbonate of soda *jūsō* 重曹
Brewer's yeast *bi-ru kōbōseizai* ビール酵母製
   剤 by Ebios and Wakamoto
Disinfectant *shōdoku yaku* 消毒薬
Glycerin *guriserin* グリセリン
Hydrogen peroxide *okishidōru* オキシドール
Lanolin *ranorin* ランノリン
Mentholated products *mentoru ganyū seihin*
   メントル含有製品
White petroleum jelly *hakushoku waserin* 白色
   ワセリン

For Hair
shampoo *shanpū* シャンプー
   for itchy scalps *kayumi-yō* かゆみ用 and
   dandruff *fuke-yō* フケ用
   for damaged hair *itanda kami-yō* 傷んだ髪
   用 or *damēji hea-yō* ダメージヘア用
conditioner *rinsu* リンス
styling gel *hea sutairingu jeru* ヘアスタイリ
   ング ジェル
dye, color *kezome, hea karā* 毛染め, ヘアー
   カラー

For Ears
ear plugs *mimisen* 耳栓
earpick, Japanese-style *mimikaki* 耳かき
ear swabs *menbō* 綿棒

For Nose
face masks *masuku* マスク
inhaler *kyūnyū ki* 吸入器

For Skin
sun block products *san sukurīn* , UV *yōhin*
   サンスクリーン, UV用品
sun block lip cream *san sukurīn rippu*
   サンスクリーンリップ
sensitive skin care products *binkan hada no*
   tame no yōhin 敏感肌のための用品
underarm deodorant *asedome* 汗止め
soap *sekken* 石けん
   medicated *yakuyō* 薬用
   body soap *bodī sōpu* ボディーソープ
   baby soap *akachan yō* 赤ちゃん用
   facial soap *kaoyō* 顔用
razor *kamisori* カミソリ
shaving cream *higesoriyō kurīmu* ひげ剃り用
   クリーム

aftershave *higesori ato no rōshon* ひげ剃り後のローション

depilatories *datsumō kurīmu* 脱毛クリーム

medicated *yakuyō* 薬用

insect repellant *mushi yoke* 虫よけ

Sanitary Products *seiri yōhin* 生理用品

sanitary napkins *seiriyō napukin* 生理用ナプキン

(Note that the overnight kind are the most absorbent オーバーナイト or 夜用 or 長時間用)

tampon *tanpon* タンポン

Super スーパー

Super Plus スーパープラス

Regular レギュラー

Beginner ビギナー

Ache and Pain Relievers

ice bag *hyō nō* 氷嚢

chemical compress *shippuyaku* 湿布薬

Note that hot compresses *onkan* 温感 are packaged in red, orange or yellow; cold compresses *reikan* 冷感 are packaged in blue or green.

pocket hand warmers *hokaron* ホカロン

magnetic (bead) patches to increase circulation to sore muscles *tokuhon pippu erekiban* トクホンピップエレキバン

hot water bottle *yutanpo* 湯たんぽ

Urine Tests

Home Tester ホームテスター
by Taisho for sugar and protein

Tes Tape A テステープA
by Shionogi for sugar

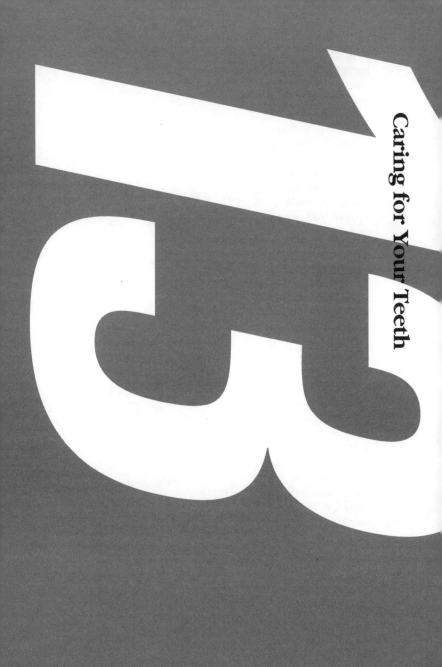

13

Caring for Your Teeth

"We leave teeth under the pillow for the tooth fairy, but in Japan I learned another custom. If the tooth is an upper tooth, a child throws it beneath the narrow wooden veranda running along the side of the house, in the hope that the new tooth will grow down straight and strong. If the tooth is a lower one, then it is flung high onto the roof in the hopes that the new tooth will grow up straight and strong."

"Our local dentist is not what you would call forthcoming in explaining what's going on. And like all dentists here, you can't go in just one time to get your teeth cleaned —it's a two- or three-visit process. But professionally he is very good, and he has the best "touch" of any dentist I've ever had. My daughter had to have root canal surgery at the age of four. Her experience was such that she enjoys going to the dentist. I am always comforted to find exactly the same advice being offered when I check with our dentist back home."

Finding a Dentist *haisha* 歯医者

After six years of dental school, the dentist receives his or her diploma. Depending on the university, some dentistry students don't need to take a final practical dental technique test. Even the national qualifying examination does not include a practical test. It is compulsory, though, to do one year of postgraduate study before starting a practice. But most dentists go on for a further two or three years of education and clinical training at a hospital affiliated with their dental university. Although the government encourages dentists to continue to participate in educational programs, the quality and type of treatment you receive will vary according to the talents and enthusiasm of the individual dentist. Professional dental societies also have their own, five-year programs of further study, resulting in a certificate of recognition. You may see these certificates at dental clinics, although dentists are not allowed to advertise this information outside as it is felt dentists with this qualification would have an unfair advantage.

Dental hygienists *shika eisei-shi* 歯科衛生士 must complete a two- or three-year specialized course after high school and then pass a national exam in order to be licensed. They must work with a dentist and cannot work independently.

Finding a good dentist is a challenge shared by both Japanese and foreigners living in Japan. You may have to visit several before most of your criteria are met. Get a recommendation from a friend before you go, and make sure that you both agree on the meaning of a "good" dentist.

Dental clinics for business people may be a good place to find dental care. Although there are no signs which label them as such, you will find them in the business areas of cities. Appointments are more or less kept to schedule, the atmosphere is professional, and national and employees' health insurance plans can be used.

Dental clinics for foreigners in the larger cities offer good care, appointment systems, foreign language skills, and the more thorough cleaning methods you may be accustomed to. However, they often do not take national and employees' health insurance, although private insurance forms will be completed for a small fee.

Another option is to use the dental hospitals affiliated with dental universities, which provide practical experience for new dentists. Although treatment is usually good, the time spent in the waiting room and the time it takes to complete the treatment session may be long. These hospitals also offer emergency services on holidays and weekends.

Types of Dentists

When a dentist is ready to start a practice, he chooses one of three types of dentistry: general dentistry *shika* 歯科; pediatric dentistry *shōnishika* 小児歯科; or orthodontics *kyōseishika* 矯正歯科. The general dentist undertakes all types of dental care for both adults and children, with the exception of orthodontics.

Pediatric Dentistry

Pediatric dentistry concentrates on prevention and early care of dental caries in baby teeth and on teaching good dental hygiene practices to children. Pediatric dentists encourage regular checkups when the teeth are examined for early cavities, obvious tartar is removed, and resin sealants or fluoride paint is applied, if requested.

Orthodontics *kyōsei* 矯正

Dentists specializing in orthodontics provide straightening of the teeth for both children and adults. In Japan there is a popular belief that the alignment of one's teeth is a gift from one's parents and so crooked teeth do not necessarily have to be straightened. Although some children with crooked teeth do wear braces *kyōsei-kigu* these days, they are not common. Young adults, however, are now opting to get their teeth straightened.

There are two types of therapy used in orthodontics. The first is known as mechano-therapy, and has to do with the kind of appliances used on the teeth. The Edgewise appliance is used in Japan, as in many other countries. The Begg appliance, which is still being used at Nihon Dental University Hospital in Tokyo, is gradually being replaced by the Edgewise appliance.

The second type of therapy is functional therapy, concerning the movement and placement of muscles and tendons. Both the Activator and Fraenkel appliances are used.

In almost all cases (with the exception of treatment to correct a cleft palate or cleft lip) orthodontic treatment is not covered under insurance plans, and is very expensive. A recent quote was around ¥700,000 to ¥800,000 for treatment to straighten teeth. Japanese parents are warned as a matter of course that they should start saving a million yen when their child is born, in case she needs braces someday. Repair of jaw deformities would include a combination of orthopedic care (covered by insurance) and orthodontic care (not covered unless performed at designated hospitals). Other uses of orthodontics (following injury in an accident, for example) would probably be covered by accident insurance, although resulting malocclusion problems may pose difficulties for getting insurance reimbursement (see page 82).

Although orthodontic treatment has just a fifty-year history in Japan, Japanese orthodontists are proud that they have contributed to orthodontics worldwide with two discoveries. Bonding materials now used worldwide were first perfected in Japan. Another discovery, titanium-nickel alloy with both shape memory and superelasticity, is a great contribution to the forming of brace wires.

Finding an orthodontist may be a problem if you live far from a large city. Your regular dentist may be able to introduce you to an orthodontist. Alternatively, ask at a dental university or a public health center. Since orthodontic treatment can take many years to complete, it is a good idea to make sure, before you start treatment, that treatment can be continued abroad if you are thinking of moving within two years or so.

Oral and Maxillofacial Surgery *shika kōkugeka* 歯科口腔外科

This is a new specialty which treats oral cavity diseases and conditions such as oral cancer, soft tissue changes, dento-facial injuries, jaw deformities, dental implants, wisdom teeth extraction, and temporomandibular joint (TMJ) disorders.

Oral and maxillofacial surgeons must pass the Japan Association of Oral Maxillofacial Surgery exam after completing eight years of postgraduate clinical practice at their dental university hospital. These surgeons practice at large general dental university hospitals.

Preparing for the Dental Clinic Visit

Dental clinics do work on an appointment system, but this does not mean that there will be no waiting time. Also, when you call to make an appointment, check if the dentist will be able to care for your problem. Refer to the section on Outpatient care pages 28–32.

Visiting a Dental Clinic

You may be asked to fill out a questionnaire, which will include questions on your present health and your health history, in particular with reference to heart disease, diabetes, jaundice, allergies, pregnancy, and any medications you may be taking. If there is no questionnaire, talk to the dentist about these points yourself, rather than waiting for him to ask.

In the treatment room there may be a whole row of chairs occupied by patients at various stages of treatment. Most of the patients will be staring stoically straight ahead. Take it like the Japanese do—consider it as a Zen meditation session, and try to imagine the area around the chair as your own private space. You may be expected to take off your slippers before sitting down (tall patients may find that their legs hang out over the foot of the chair). Women will usually be given some kind of protective drape for the legs.

"Dentists take too many X-rays," and "Dentists take too few X-rays," are common complaints in Japan. In fact, there seems to be a wide range of views among Japanese dentists about the necessity and timing of X-rays—always ask the reason for an X-ray if your dentist decides to take one. Some dentists are lax about providing a lead apron *purotekutā* プロテクター to protect your body when X-rays are taken. Don't hesitate to request one if it is not provided.

Local anesthesia tends to be used sparingly for minor dental work. A little pain is thought to be normal, and even to build character. However, if you don't agree with this philosophy, tell the dentist before he starts any treatment, "*Kyokubu masui o kakete kudasai,*" "Please use a local anesthetic."

Bring a pocket mirror with you to view the dental repairs in case you are not offered a mirror at the end of each treatment. Dental hygienists may give a demonstration of the correct way to brush your teeth after your treatment.

Treatment

Treatments available include a long list of familiar-sounding dental repairs and therapies—simple fillings *tsumemono* 詰め物, *jūtenzai* 充填材; larger biting surface crowns *shikan* 歯冠, or *kinzokukan* 金足冠; inlays *inrē* インレー; bridges *buridji* ブリッジ; tooth extraction *basshi* 抜歯; false teeth *ireba* 入れ歯 or *gishi* 義歯; etc. Some clinics may also do dental implants *inpuranto* インプラント or *jinkōshine* 人工歯根.

All but the simplest cavities will be filled with an inlay. The dentist will drill and take a mold of the hole at one visit and fit the inlay the next visit. Each visit will be short, since only one tooth will be repaired per visit. This is the usual routine (probably related to the health insurance payment schedule), and there doesn't seem to be anything one can do to speed it up.

Not all treatments are available under the national and employees' health insurance plans (*hoken* 保険); the ones that are not must be paid for privately (*jiyūshinryō* 自由診療). Fillings done with a silver and gold mixture (*kingin* parajiumu 金銀パラジウム), a silver and nickel mixture (*amarugamu* アマルガム), or a resin (*rejin* レジン) are covered by insurance. However, gold (*kingōkin* 金合金) fillings and white ceramic caps (*seramikku jaketto* セラミックジャケット) must be paid for privately. (Note that resin fillings tend to shrink away from the sides of the tooth, allowing dental decay to set in again.) Be sure to let the dentist know what kind of material you want, or you may end up with a metallic grin. Ceramic caps are generally about ¥80,000 each. Repair work can also be done partially using insurance and partially paid privately.

False teeth can be covered by health insurance, but some dentists only offer false teeth on a private payment basis. The base of false teeth paid for by insurance is made of plastic resin, which is more easily stained and broken. False teeth paid for privately have a more durable metal base; these false teeth are also made to match your natural tooth color as closely as possible, and innumerable fittings ensure a perfect fit.

Evaluation of the Dentist

Check that the dental office, especially the instruments and equipment, is clean. The Japan Dental Association has recommended the use of gloves *gurabu* グラブ to prevent the spread of AIDS and hepatitis C. However, the association has no enforcement power, and each dentist is free to do as he or she wishes. Note whether the dentist changes his gloves or washes his hands between patients.

A good dentist should listen to your explanation of the problem, carefully examine your teeth, and then tell you just what he plans to do, and why, before starting treatment. Various options and prices—including the difference in price between treatment that is covered by insurance, and treatment that is not—should be discussed openly.

Evaluating the treatment you receive is difficult, but a filling should fit perfectly, with no rough edges, and should not be felt when biting or chewing. Caps should cover the tooth down to the gum line, to prevent cavities from forming between the cap and the gum. A good dentist will talk to you about preventive dental care, and encourage you to come in again for follow-up care. Don't be surprised if it takes visits to several different dentists before you find one that meets your expectations.

Payment

Complete payment is usually expected at the end of each visit. However, if you are undergoing a very expensive treatment, like the fitting of a full set of false teeth, a special time-payment schedule may be arranged.

If you cause a car accident in which your or the other driver's teeth are damaged, your car insurance will cover the cost of the necessary dental repairs. However, if you have no car insurance, you will be personally liable for all expenses. If someone hits you in a fight and the incident is witnessed by others willing to testify, the other party is liable. If you collapse or fall down, without anyone else's being involved at all, your treatment will be covered.

Preventive Dentistry for Children

Like most health care in Japan, preventive dentistry begins at the public health centers. Regular dental examinations for infants and children are offered, the schedules varying according to ward and city. At well-baby examinations, teeth are examined and their condition noted in the Mother and Child Health Handbook (see page 118). At the same time, mothers are given advice on dental care for their children. Three points are stressed:

■ Healthy teeth are an integral part of a healthy body, starting with a well-rounded diet consisting of enough calcium and other minerals, crunchy vegetables and fruits (to supply vitamins and to massage the gums and exercise the jaw), low sugar intake, and restriction of snacks. You may have noticed a drawing of a smiling tooth under an umbrella on some chewing gum, snack, or dessert wrappers. This indicates that the gum or food is sugarless.
■ Proper brushing for three minutes, three times a day after meals.
■ Early treatment of tooth problems.

For schoolage children, preventive dentistry is offered through the school system. Dentists examine teeth at schools twice a year, through the end of senior high school. No dental care is offered at international schools.

Preventive Dentistry for Adults

Adult preventive dentistry is also provided through public health centers. Preventing periodontal (gum) disease *shishū-byō* 歯周病 is stressed since tooth loss in adults is more often caused by gum disease than by dental decay. (Periodontal specialists *shishū-byō senmon-i* 歯周病専門医 are found in dental university hospitals.) Proper brushing and a good diet are especially encouraged. The World Health Organization's 80/20 campaign (supporting the goal of retaining twenty natural teeth through the age of eighty) is publicized, but within a framework of total health. Although the campaign's goal is a worthy one, it will not be easy to achieve in Japan—recent surveys showed an average of 4.5 healthy teeth in people aged over eighty.

Tooth Cleaning, Scaling *sukēringu* スケーリング

Checkups (which include some consultation on preventive care) usually involve just a quick removal of obvious tartar from around the gums *haguki* 歯茎. A more thorough scaling is available at dental university hospitals. Regular dentists may also do this scaling, but during several appointments, a few teeth at a time—again, probably because of the health insurance payment schedule. The deep, thorough, American-type cleaning (scaling) of teeth done at one sitting by a dentist is available from some dentists familiar with American dental practice. A few Japanese dentists have started to offer a service called *dentaru dokku*(デンタルドック), which includes tooth cleaning (scaling) for about an hour and preventive care checkup for a fee of around ¥10,000. Ask your local dentist if he offers this treatment.

Resin Sealant *shīranto* シーラント

Resin sealant (which is covered by public health insurance) can be applied to the chewing surfaces of children's molars by pediatric dentists. Should be reapplied periodically.

Fluoride *fusso* フッ素

Fluoride paint can be applied to the teeth at public health centers (see the schedule printed in your local health news bulletin) and at pediatric dentists, both for a fee.

"I took my son to a dentist recommended by my neighbor. The dentist was very polite and answered all my questions. He checked my son's teeth carefully, but in the end could not do what I had really come for—to have my son's teeth painted with a fluoride solution. The dentist had very few young patients and so did not keep that medication in stock. I was shocked that something so basic was not to be found in every dentist's office. Later I was angry at myself for not checking when I called for an appointment."

Fluoridated Water

Fluoridated water is not part of preventive dental care in Japan. The Japanese have never accepted the addition of fluoride to the water to prevent cavities, because of concerns about unknown long-term side effects and a general philosophy of not forcing people to take any unwanted medication. All drinking water in Japan is treated so that it contains no more than 0.8 ppm (parts per million) fluoride. Depending on the area, the fluoride content of drinking water may be very low, or up to 0.8 ppm in areas near natural hot springs. In comparison, the United States has set a maximum limit of 4 ppm, recommending between 0.7 and 1.2 ppm. In Britain, opinion is still divided about whether the addition is beneficial; the Netherlands and Germany have banned the practice. Oral fluoride tablets are also unavailable.

Fluoride *fusso* フッ素 toothpaste (W and W by Lion; G.U.M by Sunstar, and Clinica

DFC by Lion) is widely available. Colgate is sometimes available. Foods such as soybeans, *miso*, fish, small shrimp, shellfish, seaweed, coffee, and tea contain small amounts of natural fluoride.

Tooth Care Aids

The following are available at most drugstores:

■ Toothpaste for sensitive teeth and gums: Sensodyne by Kobayashi; DM Denta Medics by Lion; Delicate by Sunstar.

■ Toothpaste for:
swollen gums (*haguki ga harete iru* 歯ぐ きが腫れている)
bleeding gums (haguki ga *shukketsu shite iru* 歯ぐきが出血している)

■ Interdental brushes (インターデンタルブ ラシ)

■ Dental floss *itoyōji* 糸ようじ is found at most drugstores, in regular spools, or in picks shaped like small cheese cutters.

■ Check Tablets (*ha chekku* 歯チェック) by Sunstar let you see if you are brushing your teeth correctly. First brush your teeth, then chew the tablet with the front teeth and spread over teeth with tongue. Rinse out your mouth and spit; do not swallow. Red areas show where food residue and plaque remain on the teeth. Finally, brush and floss again to completely clean the teeth.

■ Denture soak (*ireba senjōzai* 入れ歯洗浄剤): Polident by Kobayashi; Pika by Rohto; Liodent by Lion, and others

Dental Clinics

Many large hospitals also have dental departments *shika* 歯科. See the section of "Regional Resources" for your area for more suggested hospitals and for the number to call in an emergency to find the emergency facility nearest you. For all dental work (even emergencies), an appointment system is used.

Usui Dental Clinic
2-12-1-104 Kagurazaka, Shinjuku-ku, Tokyo
03-3260-7448 (Pub. Ins.)
Small friendly clinic; "great touch."

Nakashima Dental Office
4 Fl. Roppongi U Bldg.
4-5-2 Roppongi, Minato-ku, Tokyo
03-3479-2726 (Pub. Ins., Eng., some Sp.)
U.S.-trained general dentist; scaling; very friendly.

Yamazaki Family Dentistry
5-5-15 Kamiuma, Setagaya-ku, Tokyo
03-3418-6611, also fax (Pub. Ins., Eng.)
General dentistry.

Jason Wong Dental Clinic
1-22-3 Kamiosaki, Shinagawa-ku, Tokyo
03-3473-2901 (Eng.)
General dentistry.

Shinjuku Orthodontics and Pediatric Dentistry

1-28-3 3 Fl. Kabukicho, Shinjuku-ku, Tokyo
03-3200-8661 (Eng.)
U.S.-trained. Also at **Azabu Orthodontics**
03-5449-3308

Tanaka Dental Clinic
1-1-1 Minami-Aoyama, Minato-ku, Tokyo
03-3475-1188 (Pub. Ins., Eng.)
General dentistry; highly recommended.

Royal Dental Clinic
Komuro Bldg. 2 Fl., 4-10-11 Roppongi
Minato-ku, Tokyo
03-3404-0819 (Pub. Ins., Eng.)
General and pediatric dentistry.

Tokyo Clinic Dental Office
32 Mori Bldg., 3-4-30 Shiba-Koen
Minato-ku, Tokyo
03-3431-4225 (Eng.)
U.S.-trained. General and pediatric dentistry; orthodontic referrals.

Japan Orthodontic Center
Toho Seimei Bldg. 21 Fl., 2-15-1 Shibuya
Shibuya-ku, Tokyo
03-3499-2222 (Eng.)
Practice limited to orthodontics.

Aspen Orthodontic Clinic
Miyake Bldg. 6 Fl., 1-4-14 Kichijoji Hon-cho
Musashino-shi, Tokyo
0422-21-8888 (Eng.)
Orthodontics.

Yamamoto Dental Clinic
2-3-8 Nigawa-cho, Nishinomiya-shi, Hyogo-ken
0798-54-0863 (Pub. Ins., Eng.)
U.K.-trained orthodontist specializing in cleft lip, etc.

Nakamura Dental Clinic
Higashioji-Kitaojidori, Kyoto
075-711-0242
Trained in Western dental practices.

Suwa Dental Clinic
Long Hill 2 Fl., 3-3-10 Kaiden, Nagaokakyo-shi
Kyoto-fu
075-955-4118 (Pub. Ins., Eng.)

Yamamoto Dental Clinic
Yanase Bldg. 5 Fl., 2-6-6 Kita-Nagasadori
Chuo-ku, Kobe-shi
078-391-2025 (Pub. Ins., Eng.)
General dentistry.

Kitano Dental Office
1-1-1 Kita-Nagasadori, Chuo-ku, Kobe-shi
078-331-3522 (Pub. Ins., Eng.)
U.S.-trained general dentist.

Chang Dental Clinic
1-8-18 Takamiya, Minami-ku, Fukuoka-shi
092-526-6331 (Pub. Ins., Eng., Kor.)
General dentistry.

France Dental Clinic
Sasshin Bldg. 6 Fl., Minami 2-jo, Nishi 3-chome
Chuo-ku, Sapporo-shi, Hokkaido
011-251-6022 (Pub. Ins., Eng., Fr.)
General dentistry.

Dental University Hospitals

Dental university hospitals offer some or all of
the following: general dentistry, scaling, implants, dental and facial surgery, dentistry for
high-risk patients including pregnant women,
dentistry for the handicapped, and emergency
care. Call in advance for an appointment.

**Tokyo Dental University Ichikawa General
Hospital**
(Ichikawa-shi, Chiba-ken; see page 343)

Nihon Dental University Hospital
Nihon Shika Daigaku Shigaku-bu Fuzoku Byoin
日本歯科大学歯学部付属病院
2-3-16 Fujimi, Chiyoda-ku, Tokyo
03-3261-5511 (Pub. Ins., Eng.)

Tokyo Medical Dental University Hospital
Tokyo Ika Shika Daigaku Shigaku-bu Fuzoku Byoin
東京医科歯科大学歯学部付属病院
1-5-45 Yushima, Bunkyo-ku, Tokyo
03-3813-6111 (Pub. Ins., Eng.)

Osaka Dental University Hospital
Osaka Shika Daigaku Fuzoku Byoin
大阪歯科大学付属病院
1-5-17 Otemachi, Chuo-ku, Osaka-shi
06-943-6521 (Pub. Ins., Eng.)

Dentistry for the disabled (see page 217)

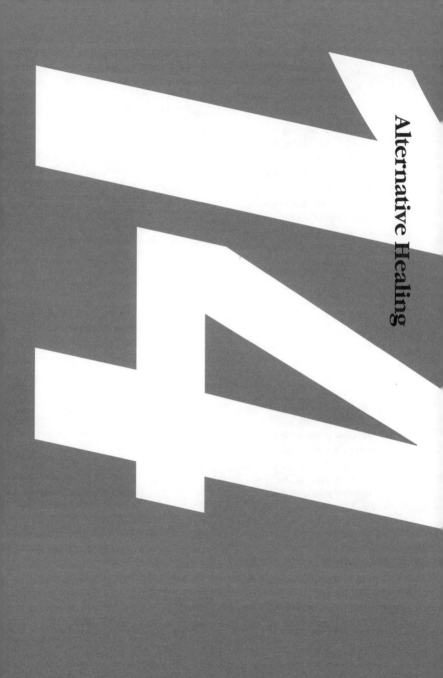

Alternative Healing

"I have found shiatsu particularly useful in curing old sports injuries."

"Every time I came back to Japan, a nagging problem with dry skin would reappear. I tried all kinds of skin creams and ointments and nothing seemed to help until I visited a Japanese herbal medicine store. The pharmacist asked a few questions and then mixed up a powder for me. Sure enough, the problem cleared up within a few weeks. The next time I went in, thinking to get the same medication, I saw a different pharmacist, who insisted on giving me something else. After a while the same old problem came back. I went back to the first pharmacist, who gave me some more of the original mix, and the problem cleared up again. Finding a good pharmacist and great medicine may be time-consuming, but the effect is definitely worth the trouble."

Alternative Medicine and Alternative Therapies

Today there is a great deal of interest worldwide in alternative medicine and treatments that were until recently considered unorthodox or out of line with traditional Western medicine. Because the theory behind these treatments may sound offbeat, and because it is sometimes difficult to test the procedures and results scientifically, Western medical doctors in general have been reluctant to consider them as valid, and insurance companies have been unwilling to pay for them.

But as people search for "gentler" alternatives to use either alone or in conjunction with conventional medicine, governments have begun to respond. In the U.S., the National Institutes of Health has started to fund studies in alternative medicine in an effort to determine the therapeutic value of these forms of treatment. In Japan, oriental medicine, or *tōyō igaku* 東洋医学 (literally, "Eastern medicine," as opposed to conventional or Western medicine *seiyō igaku* 西洋医学), has made a strong comeback in recent years, after having been gradually displaced by Western-style medicine after the Meiji Restoration in 1868. Since Eastern medicine is said to have few side effects, it is thought to be a milder, less disruptive way to diagnose and treat, and more and more doctors are starting to advocate it as a complement to Western medicine. In recent years universities have also set up research facilities with outpatient departments.

Eastern medicine can be effective in relieving chilling, flushing, headaches, and pain in the shoulders, back, knees, etc. It is especially good for patients whose illnesses cannot be clearly diagnosed, but who continue to suffer from sluggishness, lack of appetite, upset stomach, etc. In general it is not considered effective against cancer, malignant tumors, typhus, dysentery, tuberculosis, syphilis, bacterial diseases causing high fever, etc.

Available in Japan are all kinds of alternative therapies, such as acupuncture *hari* 鍼, moxibustion *kyū* 灸, acupressure or *shiatsu* 指圧, herbal medicine *kanpō* 漢方, and orthopedic procedures such as *sekkotsu* 接骨 and chiropractic treatment. However, some of the more esoteric practices familiar to Westerners, such as biofeedback, hypnosis, and homoeopathy, may be harder to locate. Various alternative therapy practitioners who welcome English speakers often advertise in magazines like *The Tokyo Journal*, *Kansai Time Out*, and *Tokyo Whole Life Pages* (see page 353). Check these out for Ayurveda, rolfing, *reiki*, and many others.

Before You Use an Alternative Clinic

■ Before you consult a practitioner, first check with a medical doctor to make sure your condition has been diagnosed accurately. If you are pregnant, speak to your obstetrician before using any kind of alternative therapy.

■ If possible, get your medical doctor and alternative medicine practitioner to collaborate on your care.

■ Become as well-informed as possible about your therapy. Ask questions, and if you have any doubts, get a second opinion.

The Theory Behind the Practice

The ancient Chinese were the first to note points of increased sensitivity on the skin of people experiencing impairment of a body organ or function. It was found that, according to the organ involved (for example, the liver, heart, or lungs), a series of electrically charged hypersensitive points, or *tsubo* ツボ or 壺, could be identified on the skin, and a line or meridian (*keiraku* けいらく) drawn to connect these points. Fourteen pathways, or meridians, were identified, which connect points on the skin with internal organs.

It is thought that a person's vital energy or life force, or *qi* 气 in Chinese and *ki* 気 in Japanese, flows along these meridians. When a person is healthy, the energy flows along freely, but if there is an abnormal functioning in an internal organ, or an abnormal external stimulation such as stress, an imbalance in the flow of energy is created which adversely affects the health. The energy itself is considered to be a balance of two opposite forces called yin and yang (*in* 陰 and *yō* 陽 in Japanese), and an imbalance between these two forces causes illness or disease.

The oriental medicine practitioner uses four different examining methods *shishin* 四診 to diagnose any imbalances. In *bōshin* 望診, or visual examination, the face, nails, and tongue are examined for abnormalities. *Bunshin* 聞診 involves the examination of the sound of the patient's voice, and of the odor of the phlegm and stool. These days, blood tests may also be used. *Monshin* 問診 refers to the taking of a complete personal history, which may include questions about dreams, sensations in response to hot and cold, etc. Finally, *sesshin* 切診 involves taking six pulses at the wrist and abdominal palpation.

The patient's symptoms are then grouped together into a pattern known as *shō* 証. There are eight principal patterns composed of polar opposites, but a patient may present any number of variations. It takes a skilled practitioner to identify the pattern and the organ involved, and to decide on the appropriate treatment.

The eight principal patterns are:

Yin/yang: A negative pattern *inshō* 陰証 as opposed to *yōshō* 陽証, or positive pattern.

Deficiency/excess: A pattern of weak movement, tiredness, lack of appetite, etc. (*kyoshō* 虚証) as opposed to *jitsushō* 実証, which is characterized by ponderous, heavy movement, coarse respiration, etc.

Interior/exterior: An interior disharmony *rishō* 裏証 usually found with a chronic condition, as opposed to an acute illness *hyōshō* 表証 with an aversion to heat or cold.

Cold/hot: A pattern of slow, deliberate movement, a pale face, and fear of cold *kanshō* 寒証, as opposed to quick agitated movements, delirium, and fever *netsushō* 熱証.

Yin patterns of disharmony are usually interior, deficient, and cold patterns, whereas yang patterns are exterior, excessive, and hot. Other variations of patterns identified may involve either excesses or deficiencies in *qi (kitaishō* 気滞証), blood (*ketsutaishō* 血滞証), or water (*suitaishō* 水滞証). Each *shō* has a specific treatment, such as herbal medicine and/or acupuncture.

Japanese Herbal Medicine *kanpō yaku* 漢方薬

Introduced in the sixth and seventh centuries, *kanpō* (literally, "Chinese medicine") was slowly modified and adapted to Japan's climate and environment. The majority of the medications are of plant origin, with just a few being animal or mineral. The prominent theoretical base used in Japan is the Koiho school *koihō-ha* 古方派. The main differences between today's *kanpō* in Japan and oriental medicine in China are that Japan uses fewer drugs (100 to 200, compared to as many as 500 in China); smaller doses are prescribed in Japan; and prescriptions vary between the two countries.

Kanpō therapy has become increasingly popular in Japan in recent years because it has relatively few side effects in comparison with Western medications. *Kanpō* is prescribed not only for the affected part but also to strengthen other areas of the body that may be weakened by the illness. In Japan *kanpō* is particularly popular for allergic skin rashes, infertility treatment, poor digestion, premenopausal symptoms, circulatory ailments, respiratory ailments (colds, bronchitis, bronchial asthma), ENT ailments (vertigo, chronic sinusitis), orthopedic ailments (arthritis, low back pain, sciatica), kidney and urinary tract ailments (chronic cystitis, benign prostatic enlargement), nervous disorders (habitual migraines, insomnia, depression, post-stroke disabilities), and chronic viral hepatitis. However, *kanpō* is not very effective for acute febrile illnesses. In the U.S. *kanpō* has also been prescribed for patients with AIDS to control nausea and to improve appetite.

Since 1976 certain Japanese *kanpō* medications have been covered by public health insurance when prescribed by regular medical doctors. *Kanpō* specialists may be medical doctors or pharmacists who have studied oriental medicine independently, with a research group, or with a learned teacher. In 1988 the Japanese Oriental Medicine Society was approved as part of the Japan Medical Association, and a system was established to qualify doctors specializing in oriental medicine. Hospitals may have separate research facilities for Eastern medicine (*toyō igaku kenkyū-jo* 東洋医学研究所), where *kanpō* may be prescribed along with acupuncture. Other hospitals may have a separate outpatient department (*toyō igaku-ka* 東洋医学科), and in other cases a single outpatient doctor, such as a dermatologist, will prescribe *kanpō*.

At the Oriental Medicine Clinic

Following the theories of Eastern medicine, a detailed history will be taken, and physical exam *shishin* 四診 performed, in order to make a diagnosis according to your pattern, or *shō* 証. Give the doctor a complete medical history including any medications (prescription or nonprescription) you are presently taking, to prevent over-medication, since some Western medications contain the same ingredients as *kanpō*. Depending on your symptoms, medications may need to be taken over a long period of time for the full effect. You may find that your formula will be altered several times until the optimal combination is found. Make sure to keep a note of the prescribed formulas, their effectiveness, and any side effects, so you have a record of your treatment.

Alternative Healing

Clinics and Hospitals with Medical Doctors Prescribing Oriental Medicine

Note that insurance does not cover all treatments. *Kanpō* is covered in its powdered form and for some types in its crude form. (Traditionally, medicines were prescribed in crude form *shōyaku* 生薬. These medicines receive the minimum amount of processing and are prescribed in large quantities. They are usually brewed up with hot water, like tea. The more convenient powdered medicine *ekisu zai* エキス剤, which is processed and freeze dried, has recently become very popular.) An appointment, along with Japanese ability or a translator, is usually necessary.

Nihon Kanpo Research Institute Shibuya Clinic
Nihon Kanpo Igaku Kenkyujo Shibuya Shinryojo
日本漢方医学研究所付属渋谷診療所
Shin Taiso Bldg. 2, 4 Fl., 2-10-7 Dogenzaka
Shibuya-ku, Tokyo
03-3464-6431 (Pub. Ins., Eng.)

Tokyo Metropolitan Otsuka Hospital
(Toshima-ku, Tokyo; see page 344)

Tokyo Women's Medical College Oriental Medicine Research Center
Tokyo Joshi Idai Toyo Igaku Kenkyujo
東京女子医大付属東洋医学研究
Shinjuku NS Bldg. 4 Fl., 2-4-1 Nishi-Shinjuku
Shinjuku-ku, Tokyo
03-3340-0821 (Pub. Ins.)

Kitasato Institute Oriental Medicine Research Center
Toyo Igaku Kenkyusho
東洋医学研究所 (北里研究所)
5-9-1, Shirokane, Minato-ku, Tokyo
03-3444-6161 (Eng.)

Yokohama Pia City Toyo Clinic
Yokohama Pia Shiti Toyo Shinryojo
横浜ぴあシティ東洋診療所
Pia City 5 Fl., 1-1 Sakuragicho, Naka-ku
Yokohama-shi
045-212-1640 (Pub. Ins., Eng.)

Kan'ichi Clinic
Kan'ichi Shinryojo 漢一診療所
3-21-11 Kirigaoka, Midori-ku, Yokohama-shi
045-923-0150

Nihon Kanpo Research Institute Nagoya Clinic
Nihon Kanpo Igaku Kenkyujo Nagoya Shinryojo
日本漢方医学研究所付属名古屋診療所
Kawamoto Bldg., 4-11-39 Osu, Naka-ku
Nagoya-shi
052-242-1332 (Pub. Ins.)

Hosono Clinic
Hosono Shinryojo 細野診療所
54 Miyanomae-cho, Shishigatanikami
Sakyo-ku, Kyoto-shi
075-761-2156 (Eng.)

Dr. Ken Chen's Physical Clinic
Chen Naika I'in 陳内科医院
2-6-2 Kitano-cho, Chuo-ku, Kobe-shi
078-242-4600 (Pub. Ins., Eng.)
Mainly internal medicine. Japanese insurance does not apply to oriental treatments.

Kinki University Oriental Medicine Research Clinic
Kinki Daigaku Toyo Igaku Kenkyujo Fuzoku Shinryojo
近畿大学東洋医学研究所附属診療所
377-2 Ono Higashi, Sayama-shi, Osaka-fu
0723-66-0221 (Eng.)

Harada Clinic
Harada Naika 原田内科
2-22-8 Tsutsumi, Jonan-ku, Fukuoka-shi
092-863-1211 (Pub. Ins., Eng.)

Kariyushikai Heart Life Hospital
Kariyushikai Hato Raifu Byoin
かりゆし会ハートライフ病院
Izu 208, Aza Nakagusuku-son, Nakagami-gun, Okinawa-ken
098-895-3255 (Pub. Ins.)

Oriental Medicine Pharmacies

Another source for *kanpō* is pharmacies with a pharmacist or *kanpō* specialist who is available for consultation and who will suggest appropriate medication. Note that health insurance will not cover this medication. About 150 ready-made formulas are available in drugstores. Ready-made formulas are particularly popular for soothing indigestion and for hangovers.

Mimi Pharmacy 美美薬局
(Shibuya-ku, Tokyo; see page 255)
03-3463-6419; 9:00 A.M.–11:00 P.M.
Pharmacist Mariko Fujisawa has studied abroad and has a deep interest in oriental medicine. Phone for an appointment for *kanpō* consultation and treatment. Open all year.

Nagai Pharmacy 永井薬局
1-8-10 Azabu-Juban, Minato-ku, Tokyo
03-3583-3889; 10:00 A.M.–7:00 P.M.; closed Tues.
Traditional Chinese and Japanese medicine.

Seishundo Pharmacy 青春堂薬局
7-20-1-111 Arakawa, Arakawa-ku, Tokyo
(In front of Keisei Machiya Station)
03-3803-0646; 10:00 A.M.–7:00 P.M.; closed Sat. afternoon and Sun.
Can introduce a doctor able to prescribe *kanpō* under Japanese health insurance.

Koseido Pharmacy 更生堂薬局
150 Yamashita-cho, Naka-ku, Yokohama-shi
045-662-8383; 10:00 A.M.–9:00 P.M.; closed Wed.
Kanpō prepared in Yokohama's Chinatown.

Kintetsu Abeno Department Store 近鉄阿倍野デパート
1-1-43 Abenosuji, Abeno-ku, Osaka-shi
06-624-1111; 11:00 A.M.–7:00 P.M. Closed Tues. and Thurs.
Individual consultation possible.

Dai Oh Kampo 大王漢方
1-3-2 Motomachi-dori, Chuo-ku, Kobe-shi
078-333-6965
One of the largest *kanpō* pharmacies in Kobe.

(All except the Mimi Pharmacy speak only Japanese.)

Your Oriental Medicine Formula

There are four basic classifications of medications. A formula containing as many as ten or more ingredients is prescribed for one illness. Depending on your symptoms, more than one formula may be recommended.

Happyozai Formula 発表剤
To encourage sweating.
Examples: *Keishitō* 桂枝湯, containing cinnamon *keishi* 桂枝, peony root *shakuyaku* 芍薬, red date *taiso* 大そ, and licorice *kanzō* 甘草. For patients in a weakened condition with headache, fever, or the beginning of a cold. *Maōtō* 麻黄湯, containing ephedra *maō* 麻黄, apricot *kyōnin* 杏仁, cinnamon, and licorice. For patients who are strong but suffer from fever, chills, etc. Also for rheumatoid arthritis, asthma, and children's stuffy nose. *Kakkontō* 葛根湯, containing *kuzu* root *kakkon* 葛根, ephedra, and

red date. For patients who do not sweat and who have symptoms of cold and fever. Also for infections like conjunctivitis.

Kizai Formula 気剤
To help release pent-up feelings, and return mood to normal.
Examples: cinnamon prescribed alone as a tranquilizer. Also *hangeikō bokutō* 半夏厚朴湯 containing, among other things, roots from the sweet potato and magnolia families. Prescribed for nervous stomach, morning sickness, and insomnia.

Shazai Formula 寫剤

Has a cathartic effect.

Example: rhubarb *daiō* 大黄, prescribed for constipation or as a diuretic. This medication also works as an antibacterial, an anticoagulant, an anti-inflammatory, and a stimulant for body's natural production of interferon.

Hozai Formula 補剤

Enhances absorption of nutrients and builds up body strength.

Example: ginseng *Chōsen ninjin* 朝鮮人参, prescribed for of ailments such as fatigue, stress, low male hormones, prevention of stomach ulcers, etc.

Acupuncture *hari* 鍼

Acupuncture is an ancient technique introduced to Japan in the sixth century and is popularly regarded as an effective means of medical treatment and health maintenance. Used to anesthetize and to relieve pain, it is also effective in controlling weight and in alleviating depression, insomnia, constipation, menstrual disorders, and some sexual problems. Some people have a weekly acupuncture session for fine-tuning and health maintenance. In the U.S. it is also used for treatment of drug addiction and chronic fatigue syndrome. Those in the racing world might be interested to know that it has also been used successfully to cure fatigue and prevent intestinal problems in racehorses.

Treatment consists of inserting fine needles along the meridians at certain *tsubo*, or electrically-charged sensitive points. It may sometimes be prescribed in combination with *kanpō* therapy. In Japan most practitioners use fine disposable needles ranging from 3–9 centimeters (1.2–3.5 inches) in length, which are thrown away after one use. However, if you intend to go frequently, you may want to invest in your own set of needles (either gold, silver, or stainless steel), which will be labeled with your name and sterilized between treatments.

Needles are inserted to an appropriate depth and then either removed immediately or left in place for a short time, and sometimes even twirled and moved up and down. The doctor may leave some tiny intradermal needles two millimeters long in place. Don't worry, the doctor hasn't forgotten them; they will be removed at the next treatment a few days later. Because the needles are so fine, you should feel little or no pain, although this seems to depend on the individual. After initial treatment there is sometimes an aggravation of symptoms before distinct signs of improvement are seen. The type and the frequency of treatment depend on the patient's condition. Acupuncture is not usually done on children, although children's skin may be stroked with a needle.

Japanese public health insurance covers treatment if a medical doctor has prescribed it and your acupuncturist accepts the insurance. Doctors may prescribe acupuncture as well as moxibustion for chronic conditions such as neuralgia, arthritis, and lumbago. Fees vary, but without insurance you can expect to pay between ¥5,000 and ¥10,000 per visit.

A qualified acupuncturist is known as a *harikyū-shi* 鍼灸師. Study ranges from courses at technical colleges to graduate programs. The college curriculum usually offers a major in combined study of acupuncture and moxibustion therapy, or sometimes a double major in acupuncture and shiatsu/massage. Since 1993, all new graduates have been required to take national licensing exams.

Moxibustion *kyū* 灸

Moxibustion is another Eastern medical practice, in which small amounts of the oriental plant *mogusa* (*artemisia vulgaris*), or moxa, is burned at the patient's *tsubo* points.

Moxa is said to increase the body's powers of resistance, stimulate the flow of energy, and aid in preventing illness. A good quality moxa—which is fine, pale yellow, and pleasant to the touch—is preferable, since it burns well and at an even rate. The moxa is usually formed into cone shapes of various sizes. The technique and amount of moxa used depends on the type of symptom. The longest-acting stimulus is produced by the direct combustion method—small moxas, about the size of a grain of rice, are placed on the skin at the correct *tsubo*, ignited with an incense stick, and then allowed to burn all the way down to the skin until a blister is formed. This may be repeated several times in one session. This method can be rather painful, depending on the size of the blisters that are formed. In the indirect combustion method, a small slice of ginger or garlic is placed between the moxa and the skin. Since this produces only moderate heat and doesn't burn the skin, it is a popular method. Large moxas, the size of the thumb, are also sometimes used, but are removed as soon as the skin senses heat. Moxa may also be administered in the end of a needle during acupuncture treatment, so that heat passes directly to deep tissues in order to relieve muscle pain and referred pain from the internal organs.

Moxibustion is usually administered by an acupuncturist, but you can also try it yourself. Ready-made moxa in several sizes are available in drugstores, as are sticks and cones made in China. For additional explanation, see "Further Reading."

Japan Acupuncture and Moxibustion Therapists Association
Nihon Shinkyu Shikai
03-3985-6771 (in Japanese)
Call for information on acupuncture and moxibustion therapists in your area. They have no information on the languages spoken by individual therapists or offices.

Edward's Acupuncture Clinic
Co-op Sangenjaya 3 Fl.
2-17-12 Sangenjaya, Setagaya-ku, Tokyo
03-3418-8989, also fax
Also shiatsu, amma, and Western massage. Edward Obaidey is a columnist on oriental medicine for *The Japan Times*.

Soma Acupuncture House
Soma Shinkyuin 相馬鍼灸院
3-9-26 Sakurajosui, Setagaya-ku, Tokyo

03-3329-3955 (Eng.)
Also shiatsu.

Okabe Clinic
Okabe Shinkyu Naika 岡部鍼灸内科
1-14-9 Jinnan, Shibuya-ku, Tokyo
03-3461-2426 (Pub. Ins., Eng.)
Also *kanpō*, internal medicine. Japanese insurance only for Western medicine. Can fill out foreign insurance forms.

Kuroda Acupuncture Clinic
Kuroda Hari Chiryoin 黒田鍼治寮院
Takenaka Mansion 1-C, 3-8-15 Minami-Aoyama
Minato-ku, Tokyo
03-3408-8304

Meiji College of Oriental Medicine Clinic
Meiji Shinkyu Daigaku Ekimae Clinic
明治鍼灸大学付属京都駅前鍼灸センター
579-11 Higashi-Shiokojicho, Shin-machi

Higashi-Iru, Kizuyabashi-dori, Shimogyo-ku
Kyoto-shi (in front of Kyoto Station)
075-361-8998 (Eng.)
Note also that the American branch of the college, at 1426 Fillmore Street, San Francisco, CA,
offers a master's program.

Shimada Clinic
Shimada Seijutsusho 嶋田施術所
Suminoue Court 207, 1-4-50 Suminoe
Suminoe-ku, Osaka-shi
06-675-6418
Also offers shiatsu and massage.

Shiatsu 指圧 and Amma Massage 按摩マッサージ

Amma massage is a traditional oriental technique that was introduced to Japan at the same time as acupuncture. It was considered a major medical treatment until the nine-teenth century, when Western medicine and French-style massage techniques were introduced.

Like acupuncture, amma massage is based on the theory of the meridian system. Begin-ning at the center of the body and moving outward, specific *tsubo* and joints are rubbed lightly (*keisatsu* 軽擦), kneaded softly (*junetsu* 柔練), tapped (*koda* 小太), or squeezed (*annetsu* 圧練) to help restore the organs to proper functioning.

Sometimes called acupressure, shiatsu is a newer therapy based on amma massage and judo hand techniques. In shiatsu, which literally means "finger pressure," a practitioner applies varying amounts of pressure to specific *tsubo*. The amount of pressure used, duration of each push, and speed of the hand movements are all determined on the basis of whether body functions are judged to be hyperactive (*jisshō*) or sluggish (*kyoshō*).

There are several different types of shiatsu, each with a different emphasis. The Namikoshi-style, developed by Tokujiro Namikoshi, is the traditional school and is based on Western physiology. Namikoshi established the Japan Shiatsu Institute (Nihon Shiatsu Senmon Gakko; see page 283) in 1940. It was through his leadership that shiatsu was recognized by the Ministry of Health and Welfare in 1964 as being independent from other forms of massage. Other types include Zen Shiatsu, developed by Shizuto Matsu-naga, which proposes a more complex network of meridians, and Tsubo Therapy, which is more closely related to acupuncture. Each school of thought encourages people to learn self-shiatsu, so that they can treat themselves and their own families. The basic philosophy behind shiatsu is to restore the normal functioning of the body, rather than to treat symptoms.

Shiatsu can be helpful in relieving weariness, sluggishness, stiff shoulders, insomnia, pains in the hips and back, and poor circulation in the hands and feet. In the U.S., the therapy is being tried with children with attention deficit disorder in the hope that it will improve their concentration.

After going through the diagnostic procedure and determining the patient's condition, the patient is usually asked to remain seated, and therapy is started. Later the patient will be asked to lie down on the side, front, or back. Techniques may vary, but pressure is exerted on the *tsubo* with the therapist's fingers, thumbs, and palms. The most widely used method is to apply pressure gently and gradually, and then gradually release. One application takes from three to five seconds. A combination of sedation, tonification, and manipulation techniques is usually used. It takes about fifty minutes for a total body shiatsu, with ten additional minutes necessary if there are specific problems. Depending on your physical condition, sensations may range from very comfortable to slightly painful.

If a medical doctor prescribes therapy for neuralgia, rheumatism, "neck and arm syndrome" (*keiwan shōkōgun*), stiff and painful shoulders, or lumbago, Japanese public insurance will cover a percentage of the cost of treatment (if your therapist accepts the insurance). Without insurance, expect to pay between ¥4,000 and ¥10,000.

Therapists usually study in a three-year program that offers a major in combined study of amma massage and shiatsu. They may also have done further study in acupuncture. Since 1993, all new graduates have been required to take the national licensing exam. Since there are different schools of shiatsu, theories and techniques may vary. Some practitioners believe that feeling pain helps to relieve pain.

Kimura Shiatsu Institute 木村指圧
1-48-19-713 Sasazuka, Shibuya-ku, Tokyo
03-3485-4515 (Eng.)
Shiatsu classes and treatment.

Japan Shiatsu Institute
Nihon Shiatsu Senmon Gakko
日本指圧専門学校
2-15-6 Koishikawa, Bunkyo-ku, Tokyo
03-3813-7354 (college)
03-3813-7481 (clinic)
Appointment necessary. Also offers a 2-month shiatsu course for beginners.

Namikoshi Shiatsu Clinic 浪越指圧
Dai 7 Seiko 3 Fl., 5-5-9 Akasaka
Minato-ku, Tokyo
03-3583-9326 (Eng.; by appointment)

Namikoshi Shiatsu Clinic 浪越指圧
Sugahara Bldg. 3 Fl., 3-2-26 Sakae-cho
Kawaguchi-shi, Saitama-ken
0482-56-7830

Namikoshi Shiatsu Yurakucho Center
浪越指圧有楽町センター
Tokyo Kotsukaikan 3 Fl., 2-10-1 Yuraku-cho
Chiyoda-ku, Tokyo
03-3211-8008 (Eng.)

Rikobian Shiatsu
Iwataso 1 Fl., 37 Rendaino-cho
Murasakinomiya Nishi-cho, Kita-ku, Kyoto-shi
075-491-2144 (Eng.)

Tanaka Shiatsu Clinic
田中指圧クリニック
Lion's Mansion Nakayama 101, 4-18-3
Naka Yamate-dori, Chuo-ku, Kobe-shi
078-242-3734

Sekkotsu Therapy 接骨
This is a traditional bonesetting therapy that was developed along with the martial arts, particularly judo. A therapist, or *seikotsu-shi* 整骨師 or, more technically, *judo seifuku-shi* 柔道整復師, uses his hands to diagnose and treat sprains, dislocations, bruises, and even simple fractures. Focusing on the muscles rather than the placement of nerves and bones, the therapist uses a combination of massage techniques to treat the injury. Although therapists cannot take X-rays, prescribe medicine, or do any kind of surgery, they must complete at least a three-year study program and pass a national licensing exam. They can treat simple fractures and dislocations; however, you may want to have these

diagnosed by a medical doctor before you visit a clinic (known alternatively as *sekkotsu-in* 接骨院 or *seikotsu-in* 整骨院). *Honetsugi* is the old term for *sekkotsui*, and practitioners who advertise themselves as *honetsugi* probably don't have a license.

Although the main focus of *sekkotsu* therapy used to be judo-related injuries, the treatment is also beneficial for such problems as lower back pain, whiplash, and golf-related injuries. Public health insurance may cover part of the treatment—look for the sign 各種保険労災取扱 (*kakushu hoken rōsai toriatsukai*), indicating that insurance is accepted, but note that you will still need your insurer's prior approaval for insurance coverage). Otherwise, expect to pay about ¥5,000 per visit. Wear loose clothing. The massage may range from relaxing to very painful (especially with initial treatments). As healing takes place, less and less pain should be felt with each treatment.

Uchiike Shinkyu Seikotsu-in
内池鍼灸整骨院
B2 Fl. Plazio Bldg., 2-7-13 Kita-Aoyama
Minato-ku, Tokyo
03-5411-0115
Also acupuncture.

Saito Seikotsu-in 斎藤整骨院
3-40-14 Eifuku, Suginami-ku, Tokyo
03-3321-9321 (Eng.)

Miki Seikotsu-in 三木整骨院
1-1-3 Kamirenjaku, Mitaka-shi, Tokyo
0422-53-6474

Matsumoto Seikotsu Shinkyu-in
松本整骨鍼灸院
595 Ubaganishi-cho, Senbon Higashi Iru
Kamidachiuri-dori, Kamigyo-ku, Kyoto-shi
075-414-0458 (J. only)
Also acupuncture and moxibustion.

Hasegawa Hari Kyu Seikotsu-in
長谷川はり灸整骨院
4-jo 10-2-3 Shinkawa, Kita-ku, Sapporo-shi
Hokkaido
011-762-1230
Also acupuncture, moxibustion and massage.

Chiropractic カイロプラクティック

Chiropractors (*kairodokutā* カイロドクター) do spinal manipulations or "adjustments" consisting of short hard taps on specific problem areas and/or pushing on the vertebrae, on the basis of a theory that most back pain occurs because of problems in the way the spine moves. This type of therapy is relatively new in Japan and encompasses various schools of thought, ranging from the traditional one using manipulations only to correct back pain, to a "broad scope" school that recommends treatment for a wide range of diseases. *Seitai* 整体 and *sōtai* 操体 are original Japanese therapies developed to balance the body, so you may see them advertised too.

Since chiropractic has not been approved by the Ministry of Health and Welfare as a medical treatment, it is not covered by Japanese health insurance and there is no system of licensing. Presently over 10,000 persons in Japan are advertising as chiropractors, but until March 1998, which saw the first graduating class of doctors of Western chiropractic in Japan (through the Royal Melbourne Institute of Technology), only sixty actually had the equivalent of the doctoral degrees in the field that would be expected in the West. Since these sixty all studied abroad, most can speak English. Chiropractors in the U.S. must complete four years of postgraduate study and pass state and national exams.

The Chiropractic Council of Japan is a group of internationally qualified chiropractors practicing in Japan. To find CCJ members, contact the AMDA Centers or the CCJ chairman, Dr. Kawanishi (below). The CCJ web site also has a list in Japanese (http: www.asahi-net.or.jp/~na8m-endu/). The following are all CCJ members.

Akasaka Chiropractic Kenkyujo (Research Center)
赤坂カイロプラクティック 研究所
La Casa Kobayashi Bldg. 3 Fl., 3-18-3 Akasaka
Minato-ku, Tokyo
03-3589-1905 (Eng.)

Koike Chiropractic Center
小池カイロプラクティック
2-2-10-601 Kita-Otsuka, Toshima-ku, Tokyo
03-3915-5515 (Eng.)
699-12 Gumisawa, Gotenba-shi, Shizuoka-ken
0550-88-1115 (Eng.)
Mon.–Thurs. in Tokyo; Fri. and Sat. in Gotenba

Shiokawa Chiropractic Office
塩川カイロプラクティック
No. 1 Toyo Bldg. 7 Fl., 1-2-10 Nihonbashi Honcho
Chuo-ku, Tokyo
03-3241-3216 (Eng.)

Holistic Health Otani Clinic
ホリスティックヘルス研究所
1-8-8 Yakumo, Meguro-ku, Tokyo
03-5701-7713 (Eng.)
Also acupuncture and shiatsu.

Holistic Chiropractic Center
ホリスティックカイロセンター
3-6-19 Motoazabu, Minato-ku, Tokyo
03-3402-1654 (Eng.)
U.S.-qualified. Also bioenergy therapy.

Shinsaibashi Chiropractic Center
Yozo Kawanishi, D.C., C.C.S.P.
心斎橋カイロプラクティックセンター内
Minami Daiwa Bldg. 6 Fl. #702, 3-6-25
Minami-Senba, Chuo-ku, Osaka-shi
06-245-6511 (Eng.)

Kobe Oriental Medicine Center
Kobe Toyo Igaku Center, Shingo Fukinbara, D.C.
神戸東洋医学センター
Kobe Yamate Hanshin Bldg. 5 Fl., 5-1-1 Naka-Yamatedori, Chuo-ku, Kobe
078-371-3203 (Eng.)

Hara Chiropractic Office
原カイロプラクティック
Shin Nishio Bldg. 5 Fl., Bukkoji Sagaru
Omiyadori, Shimogyo-ku, Kyoto-shi
075-812-0093 (Eng.)
Also *sekkotsu*.

Aromatherapy *hōkōryōhō* 芳香療法

Aromatherapy was only recently introduced to Japan, so no system for licensing therapists has yet been established. Aromatherapy cannot be prescribed legally as a medical treatment. Instead it is used mainly in beauty treatments and for stress relief. Also, some oriental medicine practitioners are combining it with their therapies, and some midwives are using it for women in labor.

Essential oils are available in Japan, either at stores or by mail order, should you be armed with a do-it-yourself text and like to give aromatherapy a try.

A professional journal called *Aromatopia*, published in Japanese by Fragrance Journal, Ltd. (Japan) will give you the latest news on the subject.

Alexandra Nishiki
0422-46-0868, fax 0422-48-0850
Uses essential oils, natural products, electrical stimulation, and lymphatic drainage to rejuvenate the skin. Two-hour sessions; appoint-ment necessary.

Joan Matthews
5-15-15 Kamiuma, Setagaya-ku, Tokyo
03-3418-6493, also fax

Certified British aromatherapist. Also massage. Specializes in stress-related problems. Also offers courses in various aspects of aromatherapy.

TEC Company
Four Seasons Bldg. B-1, 3-5-2 Oyamadai
Setagaya-ku, Tokyo
03-5706-2811 (J. only), fax 03-5706-5561 (in Eng.)
Provides imported essential oils to salons around Japan and can direct you to these salons. Also can send oils through the mail; order by phone or fax.

Natural Life Chiryoshitsu—Anjoux
Natural Life 治療室アンジュ
Sosei Bldg. 3 Fl., 1-9-7 Ebisu-Nishi, Shibuya-ku
Tokyo
03-3496-6453 (Eng.)
Shiatsu combined with a new type of aromatherapy based on the precepts of oriental medicine. Reservations necessary for any treatment

except 10-minute massage. Also acupuncture and moxibustion.

Green Flask Store
グリーン・フラスコ
Thanks Nature 2 Fl., 2-3-12 Jiyugaoka
Meguro-ku, Tokyo
03-5729-4682
03-3707-6290 (Seta branch store)
Essential oils store; also aromatherapy school.

Culpeper House
3-6-20 Kita-Aoyama, Minato-ku, Tokyo
03-3486-8763 (Eng.)
Large selection of oils; also has stores in Ginza, Kamakura, and Fukuoka.

Grace House Kitayama
43-1, Rendaino-cho, Murasakino-Nishi
Kita-ku, Kyoto-shi
075-493-8002, also fax (Eng.)
Also essential oils mail-order service.

Qigong   *kikō*   気功

Qigong, pronounced chee-gung or chee-kung, and known as *kikō* in Japan, refers to a variety of Chinese health exercises used to strengthen and balance the body. Ancient Chinese metaphysics states that the whole universe and everything in it is a manifestation of *qi*, or energy, in an infinite variety of formation and flow. In the human body, *qi*, as bio-electromagnetic current, circulates through all the organs and limbs. The state of one's health is determined by the condition of *qi* balance. Qigong refers to ways of training to access and enhance the generation, circulation, strength, and refinement of *qi*.

When healers or medical practitioners discharge their *qi* through their hands into patients to effect healing, they are performing *wai*, or external, qigong (*gaikikō* in Japanese). This is not used very much in Japan. When individuals work on self-healing or maintenance of their health, the method is called *nei*, or internal, qigong (*naikikō* in Japanese).

There are thousands of qigong exercises used by the various schools and systems in the fields of martial arts, self-healing, health maintenance, and oriental medicine. When you attend qigong exercise classes in Japan you will be doing a pattern of forceful exercises interspersed with quiet relaxation. Look for qigong classes at local culture centers and Chinese martial arts groups.

The Art of Light
03-3396-5608
A school of traditional tai chi/qigong and related arts. Traditional teachings of Yang Family and Chungnan schools. Twenty-eight years of instruction experience. Fluent English and small classes. Kichijoji (Tokyo) area, near stations.

Nihon Kiko Kyokai 日本気功協会
Ichigaya K.T. Biru 5 Fl., 4-7-16 Kudan Minami
Chiyoda-ku, Tokyo
03-3261-7871 (J. only)
Arranges classes, ranging from beginners to advanced, throughout Tokyo. Call for schedule.

Shaolin Qigong (Greg Winder)
Traditional Chinese energy-moving exercises, slow and gentle, for health and self-defense. Beginners welcome. Classes at the International Yoga Center (below), Temple University 03-5441-9800 (ask for Ginny), and Yoyogi Park. 0425-98-1672, fax 0425-98-1072

International Yoga Center (see below)

Kansai Kiko Kyokai 関西気功協会
4-32 Kitazonomachi, Takatsuki-shi, Osaka-fu
0726-85-6790 (J. only), fax 0726-85-6791
Information on qigong classes in Western Japan that emphasize health maintenance.

Yoga ヨガ

The style of the exercises may differ with the teacher and the school.

International Yoga Center
Fukumura Ogikubo Bldg., 5-30-6 Ogikubo
Suginami-ku, Tokyo
03-5397-2741
Classes in English in various types of yoga, and in qigong, tai chi, and African dance.

The Yoga Circle
Azabu Kumin Center 麻布区民センター
5-16-45 Roppongi, Minato-ku, Tokyo
also Aoyama Bell Commons
2-14-6 Kita-Aoyama, Minato-ku, Tokyo
03-3582-3505, fax 03-3586-7848 (Rajay)

Regular and prenatal yoga, both taught in English by Rajay Mahtani, certified BKS Iyengar instructor.

Tokyo Yoga Center
1-26-12-906 Shinjuku, Shinjuku-ku, Tokyo
03-3354-4701
Private lessons in English or Japanese.

Osaka Yoga School 大阪ヨガスクール
4-7-15 Minami Senba, Chuo-ku, Osaka-shi
06-252-0396 (Eng.)
Instruction in Japanese.

Tai Chi *taikyokuken* 太極拳

Tai chi, or tai chi chuan (also taiji quan), is a comprehensive, multipurpose training system of self-healing, self-defense, and self-development, with a history of over seven hundred years. Based on traditional Chinese medical theory, it is a part of the qigong group of exercises. The exercises are more complicated and less repetitive than those used in basic qigong, with the most famous being the set pattern of slow movements that you see people performing in parks under the trees. By performing the specially designed static/moving forms and using regulated breathing techniques, combined with concentrated effort, proper attitude, and regular training, the sincere practitioner will accrue many benefits. These include a strengthened immune system, improved all-around health, posture, and general appearance, and a harmonization of mind and body that will allow a lighter and more relaxed outlook on life.

There are numerous schools of tai chi chuan, and hundreds of groups, but few provide comprehensive instruction in authentic teaching. Most schools offer short-forms, or simplified tai chi, as opposed to the original, long-form tai chi chuan. Check out the information at local culture centers and Chinese martial arts schools.

The Art of Light
(Kichijoji, Tokyo; see page 286)

Yomeiji Style Tai Chi Association
03-3367-8044 (J. only)

List of centers nationwide offering classes.

Shin Taikyokuken
075-213-3204
Classes in Kyoto, Osaka, and Takarazuka.

Balneotherapy *yoku-ryōhō* 浴療法

Hot Springs onsen-ryōhō 温泉療法

Bathing in Japan is a daily ritual, not just to clean the body but also to relieve stress, relax, and—especially in winter—warm the body before sleeping. With its thousand-year history starting with the public baths offered at temples during the Nara period, bathing is a traditional method of health maintenance.

In Japan, for a warm water spring to be considered a spa *onsen* 温泉, the water must be over twenty-five degrees centigrade, and the concentration of minerals in the water must be richer than normal. Since Japan was formed by volcanos, there are hot springs everywhere, even a few in Tokyo. In other countries, especially in Europe, to "take a cure at a thermal bath" means both bathing and drinking the water. In Japan, balneotherapy extends only to bathing; imbibing the water is not the usual custom. This may be explained by historical and cultural differences, but scientifically speaking Japanese hot springs are high in temperature, but low in mineral content. Drinking the water would have little medicinal effect.

Because Japanese natural hot springs tend to be very hot (seventy percent are over forty-two degrees centigrade), if you have any of the following conditions, it is suggested that you not bathe: any acute disease, especially with a fever; active tuberculosis; chronic ulcers (stomach, etc.); severe heart disease; respiratory insufficiency (like emphysema); kidney insufficiency; hemorrhagic disease; severe anemia; or pregnancy, (especially during the first or third trimester).

If you have high blood pressure, it's important to avoid any dramatic temperature changes, so these suggestions apply even when you're bathing at home.

■ If the water temperature is 42° C. or less, a relaxing bath will act as a stress reliever and actually lower blood pressure. Temperatures above 42° C. can raise your pressure.

■ Although it is a wonderful feeling, bathing in water up to your neck, as in a traditional bath, puts added strain on your heart. Water should reach only to chest level.

■ Stepping out of a bath or hot spring into a considerably colder room or environment can raise your blood pressure.

■ Just as drinking and driving don't mix, drinking and bathing don't either. Every year people die of heart attacks or strokes on trips to hot springs, after combining their bathing with heavy consumption of alcohol.

Note that proper bathing etiquette must be observed at public baths and hot springs. First wash your body briefly at the row of faucets, and rinse well. Now you're ready to enter the bath for a short soak. Get out again and get down to some serious scrubbing. Look for the tools for the job in your local stores—large scrubbing brushes, luxurious loofahs, and nylon gloves and towels. Once you're squeaky clean, you can relax in the tub for as long as you like.

Hot springs provide welcome respite from the stress of living in Japan. The mineral-rich waters may also provide relief from illnesses ranging from rheumatism to dermatitis. You may find people sitting under a waterfall letting the waters crash down upon their back and shoulders—they are not just cooling off, but using the water to massage aching shoulders, backs, and inflamed joints and tendons. Sand baths also make for an interesting change—enjoy being buried up to your neck in sand and feel the minerals in the sand working on that rheumatism, lumbago, and neuralgia. The area around Ibusuki in Southern Kyushu is famous for this kind of bath.

The type of bath or mineral content of the water can be selected according to the relief desired. See also "Further Reading."

Soft-Water Spas *tanjun-sen* 単純泉
With their comparatively low mineral content, these hot springs are considered good for relaxation and for rehabilitation after a stroke or a broken bone.

For bleaching and softening the skin, diabetes, gout, drug addiction, bronchial problems, and gallstones.

Sulfur Springs *iōsen* 硫黄泉
For acne and complexion, but not for delicate skin. May tarnish jewelry.

Carbon-Dioxated Spas *tansan-sen* 炭酸泉
Rich in carbon dioxide, these waters are bubbly and help to stimulate the circulation. For rheumatism, heart disease, and impotence. Drink the water to aid digestion.

Sulfate Spas *ryūsan'en-sen* 硫酸塩泉
For chronic rheumatism, sprains, and burns.

Salt Spas *ensen* 塩泉
For arthritis, infertility, and circulation.

Sodium-Bicarbonate Spas *jūsō-sen* 重曹泉

Public Baths *sentō* 銭湯

The old custom of visiting the neighborhood public bath to scrub, soothe away the day's tensions, and catch up on the latest local news is rapidly disappearing as nearly all apartments and houses now include a cramped one-person *o-furo* bathtub. The *o-furo* is much more convenient and, of course, private, but sad to say the friendly custom of going to the public bath is dying out. Try to find one of the ones left in your own neighborhood.

Spa Resorts and Health Programs

The word *kuahausu* クアハウス is taken from the German word "*Kurhaus*," used to denote hot spring resorts that are utilized for the treatment and cure of various conditions (illnesses) in Germany. In Japan, too, the ministry of Health and Welfare has evaluated hot spring resorts nationwide as to the mineral content of the water, facilities provided, and qualifications of the personnel. If a resort gains the ministry's approval, it is designated as a health-promotion facility, and you will see a certificate marked *kōsei daijin nintei onsen riyō-gata kenkō zōshin shisetsu* 厚生大臣認定温泉利用型健康増進施設 prominently displayed near the reception desk. To date, twenty-two resorts have received this designation.

In Japan, the word "kur" appears in the name of many resorts, although one organization, Nihon Kuahaus Kyokai 日本クアハウス協会, has obtained the copyright on the word "*kuahausu.*" This group has about forty member resorts nationwide, fifteen of which have gained ministry approval as actual health resorts. Each resort has a variety of baths and a weight room, and over half of them also have swimming pools and coed baths. You can easily pass the day at a resort like this, all for one modest fee.

The Japan Kurhaus Association
Nihon Kuahausu Kyokai
日本クアハウス協会
03-3255-2277, fax 03-3255-7722 (J. or Eng.)
Information/list of member resorts.

Kuahausu Katsuura Parkland
クアハウス勝浦パークランド
377 Kaikake, Katsuura-shi, Chiba-ken
0470-76-0911

Heiwajima Kuahausu 平和島クアハウス
1-1-1 Heiwajima, Ota-ku, Tokyo
03-3768-9121

Kuahausu Kikusuikan クアハウス菊水館

439-1 Mine, Kawazu-cho, Kamo-gun, Shizuoka-ken
0558-32-1018

Kuahausu Shirahama クアハウス白浜
3102 Shirahama-cho, Nishimuro-gun
Wakayama-ken
0739-42-4175

Kuahausu Iwataki クアハウス岩滝
470 Aza-Iwataki, Iwataki-cho, Yosa-gun
Kyoto-fu
0772-46-3500

Kuahausu Imabari クアハウス今治
36 Yunoura, Imabari-shi, Ehime-ken
0898-47-0606

Special Baths at Home nyūyokuzai iriburo 入浴剤入り風呂

Traditionally the Japanese have added ingredients to their bath tubs to enjoy a relaxing aroma, bring a bit of nature into the home or sometimes, mark the passing of the seasons. For example, the citron bath is usually taken on December 22, the winter solstice, to ensure good health on the longest night of the year. On Children's Day (May 5) the leaves of the *shobu* are used. Commercial bath salts which try to re-create the aroma and effects of famous hot springs are sold in supermarkets and drugstores.

Special baths that you can prepare at home are listed below. Other additives include milk, salt, and daikon leaves. Doctors and *kanpō* pharmacists sometimes prescribe *kanpō* medications, particularly to patients with skin diseases or skin allergies. These medications have to be boiled for an hour and strained, before the resulting tea is added to the bath.

Rice wine bath *sakeyu* 酒湯
Add 200–300 cc of saké to your tub; promotes circulation and sweating.

Iris leaf bath *shōbu yu* 菖蒲湯
Cut leaves in half and add to very hot water; stimulates the skin and improves circulation.

Garlic bath *ninniku yu* ニンニク湯
Cut up a bulb, wrap it in cheesecloth and add it to bath water. Good for allergic dermatitis. Rinse well.

Peach leaf bath *momo no ha yu* 桃の葉湯
Brew 110 g of leaves; add liquid to bath. Good for rashes.

Loquat leaf bath *biwa no ha yu* ビワの葉湯
Crumble 15–20 dried leaves into a piece of cheesecloth; add to water. Good for arthritis and lower back pain.

Citron bath *yuzu yu* 柚子湯
Add 2–3 *yuzu* (or citron) to the bath, or simply wrap peel in cheesecloth and float it in the water. Good for lower back pain, rheumatism, and anemia.

Pine needle bath *matsu no ha yu* 松の葉湯
Brew 200–300 g of ground fresh pine needles in hot water; let stand, and then add to bath. Good for chronic aches and pains and stress relief.

15

Are You Eating a Healthy, Balanced Diet?

*If you total **80** points or more, you're eating healthily (according to Japanese nutritionists).*

1. *Do you eat a little of everything on the dinner table, with no strong likes or dislikes?* **6**

2. *Do you usually eat dinner with your family, happily conversing?* **6**

3. *Do you not let between-meal snacks affect your appetite?* **6**

4. *Is at least half your meal homemade, with a wide variety of vegetables?* **6**

5. *Do you eat at least thirty different kinds of food a day?* **6**

6. *Do you eat carrots, winter squash, spinach, nira, green pepper, komatsuna and shungiku?* **6**

7. *Do you eat various root vegetables like potatoes and taro satoimo?* **6**

8. *Do you eat konbu, wakame, and shiitake every day?* **4**

9. *Do you eat meat and vegetable stew (nikujaga) regularly?* **4**

10. *Do you clean out, disinfect, and adjust your refrigerator temperature monthly?* **3**

11. *Do you take care not to add too much sugar to coffee and tea, and to reduce your intake of sweetened drinks?* **4**

12. *Do you eat some kind of soybean product (about 100 g) daily?* **6**

13. *Do you read labels when buying food products?* **6**

14. *Do you have miso soup every day?* **6**

15. *Do you alternate meat and fish dishes?* **6**

16. *Do you have an egg a day, and at least 200 cc of milk?* **6**

17. *Do you eat sardines (iwashi), mackerel (saba), and pacific saury (sanma) frequently?* **4**

18. *Do you eat an appropriate amount (about 200 g) of fruit daily?* **3**

19. *Do you eat seasonal foods (fresh fruit and vegetables)?* **2**

20. *Are you careful not to overeat salty foods?* **4**

Your first reaction on walking into a Japanese supermarket may well be total confusion. Rows and rows of packaged products with names and instructions written in Japanese, vegetables and some fruits that you've never seen before, fish of every size and color (many with the head still attached), and in the meat department everything cut up in small pieces and cuts identified by Chinese characters. Even if you've eaten Japanese food before, you may be more familiar with such "festive" dishes as *sukiyaki* and *shabu-shabu*, than with everyday fare like *nattō* (fermented soybeans) or ground chicken. Some flavors like *miso* or even green tea may not appeal the first time you try them, but allow yourself two or three chances before you decide you don't like something. Experimenting with new flavors, textures or even colors (especially black seaweeds such as *nori* or *hijiki*), will definitely be worth it, enriching your stay in Japan.

In recent years, dietary guidelines in various countries have been revised to encourage people to eat more vegetables, fruits, and grains, and to include less fat in the diet, in order to help prevent adult-onset diseases. The well-balanced and healthy Japanese diet has a long history and although it has recently become more Westernized to include more meat and dairy products, its basic components of rice, soup, a protein source such as fish, and two or three small vegetable side dishes remain unchanged. Traditionally the diet revolves around a "five tastes, five colors" theory. The tastes are sweet, sour, salty, bitter, and spicy, and the colors are white, red, yellow, green, and black, indicating respectively rice (energy); fish, meat, beans (protein); root vegetables like potatoes (vitamins, fiber); green vegetables (vitamins, fiber); and seaweed and mushrooms (minerals). Incorporating all these colors into your meals is fun and healthy. The traditional Japanese diet, low in saturated fat and high in fish oils, is said to contribute to Japan's relatively low incidence of arteriosclerosis as compared with other developed countries, although its high salt content may contribute to the greater incidence of high blood pressure and stomach cancer.

Incorporating Japanese Foods into Your Diet

Fruit kudamono 果物

Imports and the use of greenhouses now make abundant fruits available year round. Here are some that may be new to you. Apricots *anzu* 杏 and loquats *biwa* 枇杷 are high in vitamin A and fiber. Kiwi fruits, originally from New Zealand but now grown in Japan, and the Japanese persimmon *kaki* 柿 are both high in vitamin C and fiber. Although it has only half the vitamin C of a navel orange (35 mg compared with 60 mg), the mandarin orange *mikan* みかん is available everywhere and inexpensive throughout fall and into winter. However, the Japanese pear *nashi* なし, a favorite of many, unfortunately is not nutritionally remarkable in any way.

Saburaka Orchard
20-19 Nishikawaraishi-cho, Kure, Hiroshima
0823-22-0962 (hours irregular)
Order superb-tasting mikan which are completely chemical-free (late November or early December) as well as *deko pon* and *amanatsu*, two other delicious citrus fruits (March and April).

Vegetables yasai 野菜

Explore your local supermarket and enrich your dinner table with the wide variety of exotic vegetables on offer year round (remember to wash them well before eating). The following common Japanese vegetables are high in vitamin content, but comparatively low in price:

Shungiku 春菊 or Kikuna 菊菜
(Edible chrysanthemum)
Distinctive flavor. Boil lightly; serve in *sukiyaki* and other *o-nabe* dishes. High in vitamins A, C, and B2 and fiber.

Chingensai チンゲンサイ
Chinese-style green leafy vegetable used in stir-fry dishes. High in vitamin A and calcium.

Komatsuna 小松菜
Very similar to spinach, except that it doesn't have reddish colored roots. Lightly stir-fry in oil to enhance the body's absorption of vitamin A. High in calcium and fiber.

Nira にら
A kind of leek with a strong smell and medicinal properties; a common ingredient in Chinese dumplings (*gyōza*). Lightly stir-fry, or mix with scrambled eggs, etc. High in vitamins A and B2.

Daikon 大根
Giant white radish is usually grated finely and used as a condiment, but it is also cut into matchsticks and added to salads, or sliced thick and slowly simmered. Said to aid in digestion of fatty foods. Leaves are used in soup, or salted to make pickles. The root is high in fiber; the green leaves are high in vitamin A and calcium.

Kinoko きのこ
A great variety of mushrooms rich in vitamins and fiber are available, such as *shiitake* しいたけ, *maitake* まいたけ, *enoki* (*take*) えのき(たけ), *shimeji* しめじ, *nameko* なめこ, and the expensive *matsutake* 松茸 (available only for a short time in autumn).

To learn more about mushroom cultivation, visit the Mushroom Hall (Kinoko Kaikan), 8-1 Hirai-cho, Kiryu-shi, Gunma-ken (0277-22-0591).

Gobo ゴボウ
Edible burdock root is used medicinally in Europe and China; Japan is the only nation that eats it as food. Delicious stir-fried with carrots. High in fiber, potassium, and zinc.

Moroheiya モロヘイヤ
Originating in the Middle East, *moroheiya* is increasingly seen on Japanese supermarket shelves. Rich in vitamins A, B1, B2, and C, as well as in iron, calcium, and carotene, *moroheiya* is good in scrambled eggs, fried, or chopped fine and mixed with *nattō* and bacon bits.

Spinach *hōrensō* ほうれんそう, with its red roots, in Japan is mild in flavor and delicious, so a favorite with all. It's high in iron, vitamins A and B2, and fiber. (Carrots and broccoli are also high in Vitamin A.)

Fish sakana 魚

Although tests are not yet conclusive, making fish a regular part of your diet appears to lower the risk of coronary artery disease, and may prevent senility. This is thought to be due to the substances in fish oils called omega 3-fatty acids, which may lower blood triglyceride levels, help with blood circulation, repair damaged tissue, and lower blood pressure. The two most common omega 3 acids are EPA (eicosapentaenoic acid) and DHA (docosapentaenoic acid). In Japan, the latest fad is to supplement all kinds of food, from baby formula to chewing gum, with DHA and EPA. However, to make sure you're getting enough, check out your local fish counter—fatty, cold-water fish such as pacific saury *sanma* さんま, mackerel *saba* 鯖, bluefin tuna *hon maguro* ほんマグロ, and sardines *iwashi* 鰯, are not only high in protein, iron, and vitamins B1 and B2, but are also particularly high in these acids.

So that you don't lose any of the fish oil, fish should be either eaten raw, or wrapped in foil and steamed or baked. Unsaturated fatty acids are easily oxidated, so either eat fish fresh as soon as you arrive home from the market, or wrap the fish well and refrigerate it to avoid exposing it to the air.

White-fleshed fish like sea bream *tai* 鯛 and flatfish *karei* 鰈 do not have the fish oils, but are a good source of protein and are low in fat. Shellfish like the many different types of clams available and *kaki* かき oysters, are a source of iron and calcium.

If you grill fish, watch it carefully. It is thought that charred fish skin may contribute to the high rate of stomach cancer among Japanese.

Watch out for imitation fish products like imitation crab, scallops, and squid fillets. These are made from fish paste *surimi*, and many are so well reproduced that the only giveaway is their inexpensive price. These products are much higher in sodium than the real thing; this also applies to *surimi*-based products such as *kamaboko* and *chikuwa*. Keep an eye out for suspiciously cheap salmon roe *ikura* and herring roe *kazunoko*— they're probably made from salad oil and gelatin.

Seaweed *kaisō* 海草

Salt-water plants are used in soups, salads, and side dishes and are an important source of iodine, so cases of goiter are rare in Japan. Since table salt is not supplemented with iodine the way it is in some countries, try slipping some seaweed into your green salad. All varieties of seaweed are completely without calories, making them excellent diet foods. Some are particularly high in nutrients. When dried and reconstituted, *wakame* わかめ (in the dry foods section of the supermarket) is a good source of fiber, magnesium, zinc, and copper; when fresh (at the fish counter) it is high in vitamin A and calcium. Kelp *konbu* 昆布 is high in calcium and vitamin B1. Because of its high iodine content, kelp should be eaten with care, since it can cause symptoms that mimic hyperthyroidism in some people. *Hijiki* ひじき is high in iron, fiber, and calcium, and green laver *yakinori* 焼きのり (also referred to as simply *nori*) is rich in vitamin A and calcium.

Rice *o-kome* お米

Short-grained rice, or the Japonica variety, is the basic staple of the Japanese diet. Once cooked it is called not *o-kome* but *gohan* 御飯, *meshi* 飯, or *raisu* ライス. The three most popular brands are *sasanishiki*, *koshihikari*, and *akita komachi*. Although the basic appearance is the same, gourmets can tell the variety of seed and even the growing area by the taste and texture. Rice is also used to make saké and a delicate vinegar used in cooking.

The market is slowly opening to such imported rice products as long-grain rice. Since the Japanese import about half of their food supply, they have traditionally felt that they should keep their production of rice as self-sufficient as possible (since it is their main source of energy), and have feared that opening their markets to lower-priced imports would cause domestic production to fall.

White Rice *hakumai* 白米

White rice, which has had its husks removed and is well polished, is the most common type sold in Japan. Vitamins and nutrients are not added, so it's all right to wash the rice well (until no cloudiness remains in the water) before cooking. For extra nutritive value, additives such as vitamins, extra fiber, vitamin E, and wheat germ oil are available in the rice corner of most supermarkets. Some people add a small portion of barley *mugi* 麦 and cook it together with the raw rice, to provide extra nutrients. Note that preparation differs according to product, so check the packet carefully for directions.

Brown Rice *genmai* 玄米

Brown rice, or any partially polished rice that has a germ, is higher in fat and will become rancid faster, and so should be kept refrigerated or frozen. Brown rice has a different appearance and flavor, and contains more fiber and nutrients than white. Try mixing a portion of *genmai* (about a third or less of the total), in with your white rice and cook normally in your ricecooker. The finished product is a bit chewier than normal, but there's little difference in taste. If your ricecooker doesn't have a setting for 100 percent *genmai*, use a pressure cooker, but be sure to follow the directions in the manual carefully.

Rice-Germ Rice *haiga-mai* 胚芽米

Another nutritious alternative is *haiga-mai*, which is incompletely polished rice that retains the germ and extra nutrients. Since washing may allow nutrients to escape, soak the rice for an hour, then scoop the scum from the top of the water and prepare as you would polished rice. Partially polished rice called half-milled rice *hantsuki-mai* 半つき米 or under-milled rice *shichibutsuki-mai* 七分つき米 can probably be ordered from a rice store, but you will need to experiment with preparation times. Also available is sticky, glutinous rice *mochigome* 餅米, which is steamed and used mainly in sweets. This is a traditional food at the New Year's, and unfortunately each year several people, particularly the elderly, die from choking on the gooey cakes. The fire department regularly warns people to chew *mochigome* well and eat it slowly.

What's in Your Rice? (per 200 cc bowl of cooked rice)

	calories	protein (gm)	phosphorus (mg)	B1 (mg)	B2 (mg)
white rice	148	2.6	30	0.03	0.01
haiga-mai	147	2.9	30	0.03	0.01
genmai	153	3.3	30	0.03	0.01
RDA (Recommended Daily Allowance)		63	800	1.5	1.7

Soybean Products *daizu-rui* 大豆類

Soybeans, often referred to as "meat from the field," are the only vegetable source that is a complete protein, containing all nine essential amino acids, making it comparable to meat or dairy products as a protein source. Soybeans also contain important plant chemicals called isoflavones. Recent research indicates that isoflavones have directly or indirectly lowered blood cholestrol levels, inhibited bone reabsorption, and so prevented osteoporosis and relieved menopause symtoms. They are even sometimes said to help prevent cancer. Most traditional soy foods, like tofu and soy milk, provide between 30 to 40 mg of isoflavones per serving, although no recommended daily allowance has yet been set. Other products, depending on how they are processed, have less. Only soy sauce and soybean oil have no isoflavones. Some products are high in fiber (see the table on page 298). Soybeans are a readily absorbed source of calcium, and contain copper and magnesium as well as B vitamins.

Mature soybeans *daizu* 大豆 that are soaked and then boiled in a lightly seasoned broth make a welcome addition to any meal. *Edamame* 枝豆 are green soybeans, picked before fully mature, then boiled in the pod and lightly salted. They're perfect with a cool beer on a hot summer night. *Kinako* powder きな粉 is usually sweetened with sugar, then used with *mochi* or other Japanese desserts. *Nattō* 納豆 (fermented soybeans) has a very distinctive smell and flavor—try it rolled in rice and *nori* (*nattō-maki*) to get used to the flavor of this very nutritious food. Soybean sprouts *daizu moyashi* 大豆もやし are an essential part of any stir-fry recipe; to preserve their fiber, it's best to eat them nearly raw. Other soybean products include a variety of tofu 豆腐 (soybean curd), miso 味噌, *okara* おから (the soybean pulp by-product of tofu), soy milk *tōnyū* 豆乳, and soy milk skin *yuba* 湯葉, which is usually sold dry and can be eaten in that form or steamed, boiled, or fried.

Traditional seasonings made of soybeans are soy sauce and *miso*. Soy sauce (しょうゆ, 醤油) is made from soybeans, wheat, and water. Tamari soy sauce is made almost entirely from soybeans, with very little wheat. This produces a product with a good flavor, but little fragrance. *Tamari* has a slightly higher protein content than regular soy sauce, but in any case soy sauce in general has little nutritional value. See also Salt section (page 301).

Miso, or fermented soybean paste, is used not only to flavor *miso* soups *misoshiru* 味噌汁, but in numerous other dishes as well. It is a traditional source of protein for the Japanese, and combined with rice is a nearly complete protein. Like soy sauce, though, it has a high salt content, and Japanese are now being encouraged to use it in foods only once or twice a day. Low-salt miso *gen'en miso* 減塩 味噌 is also available.

Soybean products including tofu, fried tofu, and soy milk can be bought at your neighborhood tofu store. An old Japanese adage says that the newspaper delivery man, the baker, and the tofu maker are the first three people up in the morning; making tofu is a very time-consuming process. These products are usually made fresh on the day that you buy them, and contain no preservatives. So unlike those that are packaged and sold in the supermarket, they are edible for only a day or two. Flavors, especially of the deep-fried products, vary, so you may want to try a few shops before deciding on your favorite. If you like to drink soy milk with no sugar or other preservatives added, you can take your own container to the store and have it filled. Tofu that has been deep fried (*usuage; atsuage*) should be placed in a colander and rinsed under boiling water before it is eaten, to remove excess oils and improve the taste.

What's in Your Beans?

	serving (g)	calories	protein (g)	iron (mg)	B1 (mg)	B2 (mg)	Ca (mg)	fiber (g)
boiled soybeans	50g	90	8	1.0	0.11	0.04	35	0
boiled *edamame*	50g	70	5.7	0.85	0.14	0.07	13.5	8
kinako	60g	262	21	5.5	0.46	0.16	0	3.3
nattō	50g	100	8.25	1.65	0.04	0.28	0	2.5
uncooked *moyashi*	75g	41	4	0.53	0.1	0.08	60	
RDA (Recommended Daily Allowance)			63	10	1.5	1.7	60	

Noodles menrui めん類

Check out the wide variety of noodles in Japan, which make for quick nutritious lunches.

Ramen ラーメン

This dish of Chinese-style noodles in broth is very popular, but relatively high in calories, fat, and salt, and low in everything else, so although *rāmen* may fill you up, it is not a very nutritious food to eat regularly. To lower the salt intake, try leaving most of the broth.

Soba そば

Soba buckwheat noodles are far more nutritious than wheat flour–based *udon* noodles. Serve with a *dashi*-based dipping sauce, and condiments such as *nori* seaweed, and chopped green onions; flavor with *wasabi*. High in vitamin B1, protein, and iron.

Tea

The leaves of the tea plant, Camellia sinensis, are processed in various ways to produce green tea *ocha* お茶, black tea *kōcha* 紅茶, and Chinese-style tea *oolong cha* ウーロン茶. The benefits of tea have been recognized for hundreds of years and in Japan you have a particularly good opportunity to test out the myriad medicinal properties of tea. The many kinds of tea sold in dispensing machines make a thirst-quenching alternative to high-calorie soft drinks when you're on the go. Herbal teas made from Chinese herbs are also widely available. Green tea contains the astringent catechin, which has significant antioxidation properties, and is said to help reduce the risk of some cancers, and to kill germs that are suspected of causing ulcers or cancers. The American Medical Association has stated that catechin can help lower blood cholesterol and decrease the risk of stroke in men. Tea leaves must be brewed for at least three minutes to allow the catechin to be released. Unfortunately, canned teas contain only about half as much catechin as a freshly brewed cup. Tea leaves also contain some vitamins and fluoride, but most of these are lost in the brewing process. To make a healthy late-night snack with tea, pour a cup of *ocha* over a bowl of leftover rice; add salmon flakes and strips of *nori*.

Green Tea *ocha* お茶 (36 mg caffeine per cup)
No meal is complete without a cup of tea. Tea leaves are first sterilized with steam which stops fermentation from occurring and prevents the leaves from changing color. They are then rolled, dried, and packaged. The price and the taste reflect the different grades of tea:

■ *Matcha* 抹茶 Top-grade, ground into powder for tea ceremony, brewed at a lower temperature. (After boiling the water, wait 5 or 10 minutes until the water has cooled to 60–80°C before preparing.)

■ *Gyokuro* 玉露 Top-grade, mild flavor, best brewed at a lower temperature.

■ *Sencha* 煎茶 Common-grade, slightly astringent, brewed at a lower temperature.

■ *Bancha* 番茶 Low-grade, mildly astringent, brewed at a higher temperature (90–100°C). (Brewed in the same way as English tea.)

■ *Hoji-cha* ほうじ茶 Low-grade, fragrant, best brewed at a higher temperature.

■ *Genmai-cha* 玄米茶 Green tea mixed with popped, unpolished rice kernels.

English Tea *kōcha* 紅茶 (110 mg caffeine per cup)

Leaves turn black in the fermentation process.

Oolong Tea *ūroncha* ウーロン茶 (55 mg caffeine per cup)
Oolong tea is semi-oxidized so the leaves are partly brown and partly green, producing a distinctive flavor.

(For the sake of comparison, drip coffee has 60 mg to 180 mg caffeine per cup, and a 12-oz. Coke has 46 mg.)

Barley Tea *mugi-cha* 麦茶
Roasted barley tea is said to be the perfect drink for the warm summer months, since it is thirst-quenching, but contains no calories or caffeine, and can even be given to small children.

Other Varieties
There are other types of drinks also called *cha*, or tea, such as *sakura-cha* 桜茶, a brew made from cherry blossoms. *Kobu-cha* 昆布茶, or kelp tea, is very high in salt and should be avoided if you are on a salt-restricted diet. *Soba-cha* そば茶, roasted buckwheat tea, is another flavorful alternative to *mugi-cha*.

Flavorings ajitsuke 味つけ

Most Japanese foods are flavored delicately with soy sauce *shōyu*, *miso*, saké 酒, *mirin* みりん (a heavily sweetened rice wine), and a delicate rice vinegar *su* 酢. Japanese soup stock, called *dashi*, is used in most soups and stewed dishes. Made from dried kelp *konbu* 昆布, and dried bonito flakes *katsuobushi* かつお節 (which look like wood shavings), this lightly flavored, delicious broth gives Japanese foods its delicate taste. However, the broth prevents many foods from being considered strictly vegetarian, because of its fish base. Rather than any strong spices that might block out the taste of the natural ingredients, the following seasonings and spices are used:

Horseradish *wasabi* わさび
Hot green paste used to flavor sushi; also used as a condiment with noodle or rice dishes.

Ginger *shōga* しょうが
Used as flavoring in many dishes; also sliced and marinated in vinegar and used as a garnish for sushi and other dishes.

Sesame Seeds *irigoma* いり胡麻
Sprinkled on various rice and noodle dishes for added flavor and nutrition. Partially grind for full nutritional value.

Japanese Pepper *sanshō* 山椒
Sprinkled on broiled eel, teriyaki, etc.

Red Pepper *tōgarashi* 唐辛子
For making pickles and seasoning.

Shichimi Togarashi 七味唐辛子
"Seven-spice red pepper." Fiery powder of seven spices sprinkled on noodles and other dishes.

Shiso しそ, 紫蘇
Green leaf of beefsteak plant for garnish; also chopped and added to various dishes as flavoring, or fried whole in tempura.

Kaiware Daikon かいわれ大根 **Mitsuba** みつば, 三菜
Radish sprouts *kaiware daikon* are a source of magnesium and zinc, and trefoil *mitsuba* has vitamin A. They are both used as garnishes and subtle flavorings.

Citron *yuzu* ゆず
The peel may be chopped fine to add flavor to many dishes, or the juice used in *ponzu* sauce.

Traditionally, ginger, garlic, horseradish, and other spices have been termed *yakumi* (medicinal spices) and thought to kill germs in the foods they flavor.

See also discussion of soy sauce, under Soybean Products, page 297.

Special Concerns

Bread *pan* パン

Bread made with whole grains may be difficult to find anywhere other than Kinokuniya Supermarket, but a number of the mail-order companies listed on page 309 feature a variety of home-made breads in their catalogs. Yeast, called *kōbo* 酵母 or *īsuto* イースト, is sold in any supermarket, and a variety of flours are available from health food stores if you'd like to make your own bread.

Warabe-mura
342 Takanosu, Kamonocho, Minokamo-shi
Gifu-ken
0574-54-1355, fax 0574-54-2253
About ten different kinds of bread, such as pain de paysan, pain de complet, pita bread, and Egyptian bread supposedly made from a 3,000-year-old recipe are available from this mail-order company (also see page 309).

Nova Bakery
3-3-5 Nakamaru, Kitamoto-shi, Saitama-ken
0485-92-6491 fax 0485-93-0536 (J. only)
No eggs or milk are used in Nova's chemical-free,

additive-free bread; 8 kinds in all including whole wheat and whole rye; whole wheat flour also available; delivery nationwide. Chemical and additive-free breads.

Levain Bakery
3-32-10 Kikunodai, Chofu-shi, Tokyo
0424-81-1341 (also fax; J. only)
This bakery supplies bread made without sugar or eggs to many health stores. Also delivery nationwide; call for pamphlet and order by fax. Has a popular store near Yoyogi-Hachiman Station (03-3468-9669).

Milk *gyūnyū* 牛乳

Understanding what's what in regard to Japanese milk and milk products can be difficult, due to the wide range available. There are four basic types of milk available here and all are homogenized. Most are treated by a flash pasteurization method, of heating to 120–140°C for two to five seconds. Also available at a slightly higher price is milk that has been pasteurized at 62°C for thirty minutes *teion sakkin gyūnyū* 低温殺菌牛乳, which is said to have an improved flavor.

For the most part, milk is not supplemented with vitamins A or D as it is in other countries.

Whole Milk

The butterfat content of whole milk, around 3.5 percent, is noted in large figures on the container. Its shelf life is about 7 days; date of packaging is printed on the top of the carton. It is not fortified with any vitamins. "Long-life milk" *rongu raifu gyūnyū* ロングライフ牛乳 has a shelf life of sixty days; it is marked *jōon hozon kanō hin* 常温保存可能品, and does not need to be refrigerated until it has been opened.

Processed Milk

Kakōnyū 加工乳 contains milk and milk product additives such as non-fat milk powder, non-fat condensed milk, and cream, but has no non-milk additives. Low-fat milk *tei shibō nyū* 低脂肪乳 contains about 1–2 percent butterfat; strangely, the only additive is the fat. (In Japan, the fat is first completely removed, and then the appropriate percentage is actually put back.)

Skim Milk

Skim milk *mushibō* 無脂肪 and nonfat ノンフ ァット milks are difficult to find, but be on the lookout for powdered skim milk containing 1 percent butterfat from Yukijirishi Company.

Milk Beverages

Milk beverages *nyū inryō* 乳飲料 may contain additional milk products and a reduced percentage of butterfat, but also non-milk additives such as sugar, riboflavin, vitamins C and E, iron, or flavorings. The iron in iron-enriched milk is not readily available, since much of it binds with the calcium in the milk. This category also includes lactobacillus drinks *nyūsankin inryō* 乳酸菌飲料, the most well known of which is Calpis.

Resources

Tomo Rakuno Farm 東毛酪農
741-1 Matsunoki, Ichinoi-aza, Nitta-machi, Nitta-gun, Gunma-ken
0276-57-0111 (J. only)
Milk pasteurized at low temperatures, and additive-free cheese, tofu, yogurt, and icecream. Become a member and make a monthly order, or call and they'll refer you to the nearest health store which carries their products (Kanto area).

Salt shio 塩

Although the Japanese diet is generally very healthy, it does contain a large amount of hidden sodium in the forms of salt and soy sauce. For example, broiled fish is usually lightly salted before it is cooked; *tsukemono*, Japanese-style pickles, are usually prepared in salt; and *miso*, used as a soup base, has a high salt content. One teaspoon of regular soy sauce contains 900 mg of sodium and a great many Japanese foods are seasoned with this flavoring. For your own cooking, you can buy low-salt soy sauce, called *gen'en shōyu* 減塩しょうゆ. This contains just half, or 450 mg, the sodium of regular soy sauce per teaspoon. But don't confuse this with *usukuchi* うすくち soy sauce, which is lighter in color but actually has as much as or more salt than regular soy sauce. In health food stores, such as Natural House, you may find a series of soy products containing less salt.

Other products containing reduced amounts of salt, such as low-salt *miso*, will be labeled *enbun hikaeme* 塩分ひかえめ or *gen'en* 減塩. Salted fish, such as salmon, is labeled *amashio* 甘塩 "least salty";*chūkara* 中辛 "medium salty"; and *ōkara* 大辛 "saltiest."

In Japan, the recommended salt intake per day is 10 g or less, while people with high blood pressure are limited to 6 g or less. In the U.S., intake is in the 2–4 gram (2000 mg to 4000 mg) range, with 2 grams or less often recommended for hypertensive patients. A glance at the sodium content of the common Japanese dishes below shows how easy it is in Japan to have a very high salt intake without even realizing it:

Ramen 5.8 g (per serving) **Curry Rice** 4.0 g **Katsudon** (pork cutlet on rice) 6.7 g
Unagi (broiled eel) 5.7 g **Sukiyaki** 5.0 g

Sugar Substitutes

The main artificial sugar substitute used in Japan is aspartame, known as PAL. Note that it breaks down when heated, so it can't be used for cooking. Other nutritive sweeteners are available, such as those containing maltose, lactose and fructose, stevioside (a natural sweetener made from plants), and erythritol (derived from dextrose). The nutritive sweeteners don't promote tooth decay, and some, like the lactose and fructose types, are said to be good for the intestinal tract by stimulating the production of lactobacillus bacteria. Products with reduced sugar are marked *teitō* 低糖, while sugar-free products are labeled *mutō* 無糖. For information on managing diabetes, see page 186.

Diet Foods

Look out for such low-fat (*tei-shibō* 低脂肪 or ローファット) foods as yogurt, milk, cheese, and margarine. Low-calorie salad dressings are marked as non-oil ノンオイル, or with a fraction showing the calories cut. Remember, though, that these products are usually higher in salt and sugar than regular dressings.

There is not a particularly wide variety of products available, but Nissin Foods has just produced a low-calorie instant ramen meal that has only 178 calories and is made without oil for the noodles, which is selling better than the company expected, so more low-calorie and low-fat items may be developed for the Japanese market.

Calcium カルシウム

Women aged twenty-five to fifty need about 900 mg of calcium to prevent osteoporosis. This is equivalent to 720 cc or three eight-ounce glasses of whole, low-fat or skim milk. U.S. recommendations for pregnant or nursing women and for teenage girls are 1200 mg, while those for postmenopausal women are 1500 mg. Japanese recommendations are somewhat lower. If your diet doesn't offer sufficient calcium, several calcium-enriched drinks and "The Calcium," a cookie providing 600 mg of calcium, are available. You can always sprinkle 10 gm of *shirasuboshi* シラス干し, or small white dried fish, on your rice to supply 52 mg of calcium (but also note that this also adds 1000 mg of salt).

Vitamin D works with calcium to maintain muscle function and enhance bone formation and maintainence by aiding the absorption of calcium. Milk and milk products are usually not fortified with vitamin D, so you'll need to find other sources. Food sources include egg yolks, liver, tuna, herring, sardines, and salmon. Vitamin D can also be synthesized in the skin by exposure to the sun. Thirty minutes of exposure, without sunscreen, three times a week will provide an adequate supply of vitamin D.

When planning your diet, note that animal sources of calcium are more easily absorbed than vegetable, with the exception of soybeans. Remember too that dietary sources are better than supplements.

Foods with Calcium Equal to 1 American Cup (240 cc) of Milk

1 1/2 cups of ice cream; 1 cup of yogurt; 2 cups of cottage cheese; 1 cup of greens such as *komatsuna* or *shungiku*; 3/4 cup of homemade macaroni and cheese; 9 oz of tofu, or *okara*; 1 1/2 oz of cheddar cheese; 2 1/2 cups of cooked soybeans; 6 to 7 sardines (small, with bones); 5 oz of canned salmon (with bones).

Fiber sen'i shitsu 繊維質

From being a cure for cancer and an aid in reducing cholesterol levels, a lot of astounding claims have been made in recent years concerning the magical properties of a high-fiber diet. However, a rational approach is encouraged by nutritionists: eat in moderation a variety of high-fiber foods, such as whole grain bread, pasta, cereals, fruit, and vegetables, to ensure that you have a daily intake of 15 to 35 g. Remember that there are a number of different types of fiber so relying on pasta every meal for your fiber intake is not enough.

Japanese foods high in fiber are seaweeds such as *konbu*, *hijiki*, and *wakame*; soybeans including *okara* and soy flour *kinako* (きなこ, 黄粉) vegetables such as burdock *gobo*, dried gourd shavings *kanpyo*, and dried white-radish shavings *kiriboshi daikon*; devil's-tongue jelly *konnyaku* こんにゃく, and agar-agar *kanten* かんてん, mushrooms such as *enoki*, *kikurage* (Jew's ear), and dried *shiitake*. Kiwi fruit, apples, and oatmeal are also good sources. Recently drinks like "Fiber Mini" have become popular. However, since they contain only one type of fiber, you shouldn't rely on this source alone.

Iron tetsubun 鉄分

The recommended daily allowance of iron is 8–12 mg; pregnant women and nursing mothers need 15–20 mg daily. Iron derived from animal sources is generally better absorbed than that derived from plant sources. Oatmeal is also available at any supermarket.

Japanese foods high in iron include chicken hearts or livers *yakitori* and seafood such as short-necked clams *asari*, oysters *kaki*, lean tuna *hon maguro*, semi-dried whitebait *shirasuboshi*, and Japanese sea bass *suzuki*. Plant sources include *hijiki* seaweed, tofu, dried tofu *kōya-dōfu*, spinach *hōrensō*, and *komatsuna* greens. Plant sources of iron should be combined with vegetables and fruits high in vitamin C, or with a small amount of meat, to facilitate absorption. Remember that too much green tea, black tea, coffee, milk, or antacids can interfere with absorption.

Vitamins

In general, foods aren't supplemented with vitamins in Japan, reflecting the Japanese hesitancy to put additives in food and drink. Sometimes foods may be supplemented, but not with the same things as in your own country. For example, baby food may have added calcium or vitamin C, but rarely iron.

The Foreign Buyer's Club (see the endpapers and page 309) is a source for a wide range of vitamin tablets. The Japanese prefer vitamin drinks, sold in abundance in drug stores and convenience stores. These can be divided into two categories: medicinal and soft drinks. Although they both contain the vitamin B complex, the medicinal type can only be sold in drug stores and must have a full label listing ingredients and quantities. The soft-drink type usually have reduced quantities, although this is rarely clear from the label. Prices can go up to ¥4,000 for drinks enriched with royal jelly and ginseng and other exotic ingredients. Almost all these drinks contain caffeine and alcohol, and so are not recommended for children or drivers.

The word *nikochin-san* ニコチン酸 on the label does not stand for nicotine, but rather nicotinic acid, which is usually shortened to niacin, or vitamin B3. New jellied health drinks used in place of food, like "Calorie Mate" (containing dietary fiber, vitamins, and calories), are selling well among young women.

Japanese Tips for Preventing Adult-Onset Diseases

■ Eat tofu with *konbu* and other seaweeds for good thyroid function.

■ Add *wakame* seaweed (high in potassium) to *miso* soup to offset the effects of sodium.

■ Eat grated radish with *o-mochi* (rice cakes) and other hard-to-digest foods, to improve digestion.

■ Combine proteins—for example, eating bonito flakes (*katsuobushi*) with tofu, or eggs with *nattō*—for maximum nutritional benefit.

■ Eat grated radish with fish (including intestines or bones) to get full nutritional benefit.

■ Use rapeseed oil *nataneyu* 菜種油 or other vegetable oils like corn or safflower oil, all of which are low in saturated fats. Avoid margarine, as well as oil made from cottonseed oil *menkayu* 綿花油, which has a higher fat saturation.

■ Foods high in cholesterol include any kind of fish eggs, such as salmon roe *ikura* イクラ or salted cod roe t*arako* たらこ, squid *ika* いか (including dried, roasted *surume* するめ), and of course shrimp *ebi* えび. *Sukiyaki* すきやき and *shabu shabu* しゃぶしゃぶ cuts of beef, although delicious, may contain added marbled fat as a tenderizer.

■ Studies have shown that drinking more than three cups of coffee a day can raise your cholesterol.

■ Being overweight is a contributing factor in hypertension, heart disease, and diabetes, the three main adult-onset conditions.

Children's Nutrition

Baby Formulas

Of course, breast-feeding is still the method of choice, but many brands of powdered formula for babies are available, such as Meiji, Morinaga, Snow Brand, Nestle, and SMA, which have all been tested and approved by the Ministry of Health and Welfare. Special formulas *tokushu miruku* 特殊ミルク are sold for babies with problems such as allergies and metabolic disorders. In particular, Meiji has a complete series of formulas for babies with allergies to lactose, milk, soy products, etc. Most companies also make a "follow-up" enriched milk to be used together with baby food from nine months until babies are weaned to regular milk. Canned liquid baby formula has not been approved by the government, and so is not available here.

Baby Foods

Traditionally, one of the rites of passage to being a "good mother" in Japan was striving to prepare nutritional bite-sized portions of food *rinyū shoku* 離乳食 for your six-month-old child. The relaxation of apron strings and the changing status of women has led to the introduction of many brands of prepared baby food, including Wakodo, Meiji, Morinaga, Snow Brand, Kewpie, and Gerber. Japanese mothers prefer freeze-dried to bottled, so most products are sold in packets. Baby food manufacturers also provide free cookbooks, showing how to supplement baby food with vegetables, etc., for the mother who likes the "homemade" touch.

Neighbors or friends who are of an older generation will easily be able to give you advice about how to use local ingredients to make delicious baby food. A recent issue of a Japanese mother's magazine gave the following time-saving tips to simplify preparation. (Baby food grinders should be available at large department stores.)

■ Wrap up small bits of vegetables like squash or carrots, together with a bit of water, in plastic wrap, soften the mixture in the microwave, then squeeze the wrap with your fingers until mushy.

■ Cook carrots, chicken, white-fleshed fish, or spinach, and cut or form small portions into a stick shape, wrap in plastic, and freeze. While still frozen, grate with a fine grater. Similarly, grate freeze-dried tofu blocks (*kōya-dōfu* 高野豆腐 or *kōri-dōfu* 氷豆腐) into a fine powder that can be added to any food to give it added nutrition.

■ To make foods gel together, use a naturally sticky food like yogurt, banana, or *nattō*, or the thickening agent "Toromichan."

■ To prevent choking, mix cornstarch with any kind of minced meat before cooking it in boiling water; it will come out soft and ready to eat.

■ To make small portions of rice porridge *okayu* おかゆ, after you rinse your own raw rice and ready it for cooking, place a small glass or ceramic dish with an infant's portion of uncooked rice and extra water (you'll need to experiment with quantities) into the ricecooker right on top of the rice and water, close the lid, and cook as you would normally. Your child's porridge will be ready with your rice at the end of the cooking cycle.

Vitamins for Children

Vitamins for children are expensive and do not generally include an iron supplement. Order a supply from your own country or from the Foreign Buyers' Club (see the endpapers and page 309) or try adding Nestle's Milo (which supplies eight nutrients) to milk. Teenage girls may need iron supplements. Consider giving vitamin D supplements to your children to prevent rickets, especially if you live in "snow country" which gets little sun in winter, since vitamin D is produced in the body from exposure to the sun, and is not usually supplemented in the milk. See also Fluoride, page 270.

Shopping Tips

If you're a new arrival in Japan or still get confused in the supermarket, Carolyn R. Krouse's *A Guide to Food Buying in Japan* (Charles E. Tuttle Books, 1986) is a must. Although it's a bit dated, it does explain in detail how to read package labels.

Reading packages for nutritive information is difficult in Japan because everything is listed for 100 g, rather than by serving size. If you don't plan to eat 100 g of something at one sitting, you'll need a calculator, plus a good idea of how much you will eat to figure out the nutritive value of the food. For example, you'd need to eat 50 sheets of dried *nori* seaweed to receive the nutrients listed for 100 g.

The date of manufacture is listed as *seizō nengappi* 製造年月日. Note that the Japanese calendar is often used, rather than the Western—for example, Heisei 12 and not 2000. The expiration date is *shōmi kigen* 賞味期限. Easily perishable products are marked with a use-by date *shiyō kigen* 使用期限. The expiration date on goods with a longer shelf life is indicated with *hinshitsu hoji kikan* 品質保持期間. The following may also be helpful in deciphering labels:

ingredient	*genzairyō*	原材料
preservative	*bōfuzai*	防腐剤
(artificial) coloring	*(gōsei) chakushokuryō*	(合成)着色料
(artificial) preservative	*(gōsei) hozonryō*	(合成)保存料
(artificial) flavoring	*(gōsei) chakkōryo*	(合成)着香料
monosodium glutamate	*kagaku chōmiryō*	化学調味料
how/where to store	*hozon hōhō*	保存方法
refrigerate	*yōreizō*	要冷蔵
refrigerate after opening	*kaisengo yō reizō*	開栓後要冷蔵
weight of contents	*naiyōryō*	内容量
caution after opening	*shiyō-ue no chūi*	使用上の注意

For an illustrated, bilingual explanation of Japanese packaging labels, check out:

Read labels carefully, particularly those of hamburger, which may be made from a mixture of pork, beef, and chicken. In general, products labeled "ham" are pork, but watch out for pressed ham *puresu hamu* プレスハム, which may contain a combination of pork, beef, mutton, goat, and chicken. When buying ham, look for top quality *tokkyū* 特級, superior *jōkyū* 上級, and regular *hyōjun* 標準.

The Ministry of Health and Welfare stamps its seal of approval on products that have had their nutritional value changed in some way, for example by the addition of vitamins or calcium. You'll see the stamp on products like baby formula or low-salt foods.

JSD stands for Japan Special Labeling Diet, indicating that the Japan Nutritional Products Association (Nihon Eiyo Shokuhin Kyokai) 日本栄養食品協会 has tested the product and given it its stamp of approval. The nutritional value of 100 g serving should also listed be on the package.

Ordering out from Restaurants *demae* 出前

Depending on where you live, many neighborhood restaurants will deliver dishes to your home without an added delivery charge. If you have a favorite restaurant in your neighborhood, ask whether you can order by phone, and take a menu home with you. You'll need to be able to give your name, address, and what you want to order in Japanese (this is also good practice for calling an ambulance). Meal prices may be slightly higher than in the restaurant and there is usually a minimum order of two meals or items. Don't forget to wash the dishes and set them outside your door to be picked up the following day.

See "References and Further Readings" for a natural foods restaurant guide and a book that gives calorie counts and nutritional breakdown of foods on the menu in the major chain restaurants around Japan.

Meal Delivery Services

Meal delivery services are available for those who for some reason don't have time to plan a meal and shop. The companies listed below offer a menu for the week (usually with two choices of a main dish) and the company delivers daily just the quantity of food you need to make a meal in a short period of time. Some companies cater to the elderly and people with specific health problems such as diabetes and hypertension, while others cater to working wives. You need to understand enough Japanese to order the weekly menus and understand the recipes.

Taihei Company
7-8-10 Matsue, Koto-ku, Tokyo
0120-144-910 (toll-free)
Taihei operates a chain of 400 stores nationwide, and caters to diabetics, those suffering from high blood pressure, and dieters. Order from the two-week menu and ingredients will be delivered to your door along with cooking manuals to ensure the dish is prepared correctly. Daily supply is usually under ¥2,000.

Princess Company
5-24-19 Miyamae, Suginami-ku, Tokyo
03-3335-5775

This company operates nationwide and delivers two frozen pre-cooked meals at a time—just pop in the microwave. For diabetics, dieters, the elderly, and those with kidney problems. Various monthly plans up to ¥50,000; membership fee ¥5,000.

Life Elegance ライフエレガンス
4-25-5 Mukohara, Higashi-Yamato-shi, Tokyo

0120-1213-64 (toll-free)
Regular and special diet menus that require a minimum of preparation. It's necessary to order at least two servings, but daily deliveries ensure freshness (Tokyo and surrounding prefectures only).

Health Foods and Organic Produce

Organic farm produce is recently becoming popular, although it does not yet account for one percent of domestic agriculture production. The hot and humid climate, typhoons, and insect population make the growing of organic produce a major challenge in Japan: this is reflected in prices, which are generally higher than those of regular vegetables.

Guidelines established in 1993 list the following catagories for produce:

■ Organic produce *yūki munōyakusan* 有機無農薬産
This term means that the crops have been cultivated in a field that has been free from chemicals for more than three years. Such fields are usually fertilized with compost.
■ Produce cultivated without use of farm chemicals *yūki saibai* 有機栽培
■ Produce grown with reduced amounts of chemicals *tei-nōyaku yūki* 低農薬有機 or 少農薬 *sho-nōyaku.*

There is still concern among consumers that some produce being labeled and sold as organic does not really qualify, since no independent verification organization has been established yet. Consumer groups are also lobbying for clear labeling of imported organic produce that has been irradiated or genetically engineered. Japan has not yet approved domestic production of genetically-engineered products, and Japanese consumers in general are wary of possible side effects of unknown allergens or toxins.

Health Food Stores

Anew Natural Group
アニュ　ナチユラルグループ
0120-032070 (toll-free; J. only)
This chain has over twenty years of experience and over 600 stores nationwide. Almost 1,000 different products, most additive-free.

Gruppe
5-27-5 Ogikubo, Suginami-ku, Tokyo
03-3393-1224 (J. only)
Wide range of macrobiotic food; check out the natural food restaurant on the second floor.

Lisely
1-28-3 Takadanobaba, Shinjuku-ku, Tokyo

03-3232-6527 (J. only)
Wide range of natural food; also herbs and natural cosmetics.

Natural House
3-6-18 Kita Aoyama, Minato-ku, Tokyo
03-3498-2277 (J. only)
Wide range of products including organically-grown vegetables, fresh and prepared foods, and the company's own brand of vitamins and low-calorie sweeteners. Also stocks natural cosmetics. Twenty stores nationwide; call to find the branch nearest you.

Osawa Japan (Higashi-Kitazawa Store)
11-5 Oyama-cho, Shibuya-ku, Tokyo
03-3465-5021 (store; J. only)
0492-55-7236 (mail order; J. only)
(Osawa Macrobiotic Center 03-3469-7631)
Organic vegetables, bread, etc. Mail-order service also available for nonperishable goods.

Nagamoto Kyodai Shokai
Hobbit Mura Bldg. 1F, 3-15-3 Nishi-Ogi-Minami Suginami-ku, Tokyo
03-3331-3599 (J. only)
Wide range of excellent quality organic food.

Shizen Shokuhin Center
自然食品センター
1-10-6 Jinnan, Shibuya-ku, Tokyo
03-3461-7988 (J. only), fax 03-3780-0359
Branch stores (all J. only):
03-3932-5211 (Itabashi-ku)
045-901-5111 (Yokohama)
0720-38-5211 (Osaka)
092-831-5211 (Fukuoka)
Catalog service and 4 stores selling Tenmi brand

natural food products, diet products, natural cosmetics, and herbal medicine. Also on same premises, Tenmi, one of the oldest natural food restaurants in Tokyo.

Seishoku Kyokai
2-1-1 Awaji-cho, Chuo-ku, Osaka-shi
06-941-7506 (J. only)
Macrobiotic center for Kansai area. Cooking classes, macrobiotic products, and monthly magazine.

Resources

Global Village
Mail-order ecology goods, etc. (see the endpapers).

Global Village's The Fair Trade Company Shop
3-7-2 Jiyugaoka, Meguro-ku Tokyo
11:00 A.M.–8:00 P.M. Closed Wed.
03-5701-3361 (Eng.)
Organic foods, ecological fashions, in-shop seminars, and more.

Food Delivery Services

A number of companies now offer mail-order services and will send catalogs on request.

Tengu Natural Foods
Umehara 50-2, Hidaka-shi, Saitama-ken
0429-85-8751, fax 0429-85-8752 (Eng.)
Just reading through their catalog is enough to make your mouth water. Many of their products are organic, but this doesn't mean that they're boring. They have bagels, pita bread, cashews, flour tortillas, etc., etc. Place order by mail, fax or phone, in English or Japanese and they'll deliver anywhere in Japan. Pay at your local post office after delivery.

Foreign Buyers Club
Check out FBC's mouth-watering catalog, which features 25,000 top-selling items of more than 40,000 food and sundry items imported from the U.S. (see the endpapers for details).

Warabe-mura
A wealth of fascinating food—from everyday basics such as homemade soy sauce, soy milk, olives, sauerkraut, and sesame oil to the more esoteric such as lotus candy, mugwort soba, and

pickled plum vinegar. Get together with your friends—orders over ¥20,000 are delivered free. Check out the English catalog and free fun English newsletter with simple cooking tips and hot news from the macrobiotic world, discussion of food and environmental issues
To contact, see page 300.

Shojiki-mura
1-2-41 Ningyo, Konosu-shi, Saitama-ken
0120-42-1351 (J. only)
Organic vegetables, rice, eggs, milk, soy sauce, ham, sausage, bread, etc. Membership fee (about ¥3,000) and yearly fee (¥1,000). Can also order from catalog; delivery nationwide.

Polan Hiroba
Tokyo 0428-24-7200; Nagoya 0568-34-0775;
Osaka 06-866-1456 (all J. only)
Over 700 items including organic vegetables, natural yeast bread, eggs, etc. Membership fee (about ¥5,000) and yearly fee (¥5,000). Weekly arrangement whereby members are sent ¥1,000-

worth of whatever vegetables are in season. Other items can also be ordered via 24-hour phone service.

Yamagishi-ism
5010 Takanoo-cho, Tsu-shi, Mie-ken
0592-30-8011 (J. only)
Organic vegetables, eggs, milk, bread, meats, natural seasonings, *hechima* (loofah) water, etc. No membership fee; pay in advance; delivery nationwide.

Ninjin Club
2-11-7 Tokugawa, Higashi-ku, Nagoya-shi
052-931-4010 (J. only)
Vegetables, beans, bread, fish, and natural soap delivered nationwide. Membership fee ¥5,000; monthly fee ¥400.

Imran Trading Company
8-6-18 Fukami-nishi, Yamato-shi, Kanagawa-ken
0462-77-6844, fax 0462-60-0475 (Eng.)

Over 700 different imported groceries for South Asian cooking available at its five stores and through its mail-order service. Also halal meat, spices, curries, etc. Refundable membership fee. Send for English catalog. Delivery nationwide.

Co-op
Seikatsu Kyodo Kumiai
生活協同組合 (usually shortened to Seikyo)
For this great food delivery service, you must form a group (usually at least three) or join an existing group, and take turns in receiving the produce which is delivered together (most companies require you to be at home when the delivery is made). You need enough Japanese to look over their weekly catalog and to be able to separate your order when it arrives. Refundable membership fee; minimum order per month. Seikyo delivery day is a good opportunity to make friends with your Japanese neighbors.

Zen Macrobiotic Diet

With careful planning, most vegetarian diets are healthful, but one very restricted diet called the Zen Macrobiotic Diet, can be very inadequate nutritionally. Developed by a Japanese, George Ohsawa, who first coined the term "macrobiotic," it encompasses both a diet and and a way of life. This diet has ten stages; as the follower progresses from the beginning stage (–3) to the highest (+7), desserts, fruits and salads, animal foods, soup, and vegetables are eliminated in that order, and are replaced by cereal grains, so that at the highest level only brown rice and tea or water are consumed. At its upper stages the diet is very unbalanced, and when combined with the liquid restriction it can pose serious health problems. Infants, children and pregnant mothers—all of whose nutritional needs are greater—are at particular risk from the restrictions.

Holistic Health Retreats

For a list of places to stay nationwide that offer healthy vegetarian cuisine amid beautiful surroundings and at reasonable prices, send ¥250 plus postage to Global Village (see the endpapers).

Nutritional Counseling

If you need help in planning your diet, the following offer nutritional counseling.

Edward Fujimoto
Tokyo Adventist Hospital
Suginami-ku, see page 344.
Bilingual, U.S.-certified specialist in health promotion offers preventive care and nutritional counseling for weight control, specific disease diets, and sports nutrition.

Can Do Harajuku
(Shibuya-ku, Tokyo; retreat in Hakone. See page 244.)

Ohara Clinic
Dai Ichi Iwata Bldg. 6 Fl., 1-1-5 Hatagaya
Shibuya-ku, Tokyo
03-3299-0017 (J. only)
Hideo Makuuchi, a lecturer in medical nutrition, gives diet counseling on Wednesdays. Rather than a macrobiotic diet, a balanced basic diet is advocated. Phone for appointment. Insurance not accepted, but the fee for two sessions is reasonable.

Kobe Kaisei Hospital
(Kobe, see page 348)
Nutrition counseling from registered dietician (usually with referral from doctor).

Cooking Classes

Check at your local community center for details of cooking classes—as most classes are demonstration-style, Japanese ability may not be too important. Tokyo Union Church (03-3400-0942; Mon.–Fri. 11:00 A.M.–1:00 P.M.) offers classes through its women's groups.

Konishi Japanese Home Cooking Class
3-1-7-1405 Meguro, Meguro-ku, Tokyo
03-3714-8859
Kiyoko Konishi has been teaching foreigners the art of Japanese cookery for 30 years. She is also the author of several best-selling cookbooks.

Yuka Cooking Studio
4-8-19 Hachiman-cho, Nada-ku, Kobe-shi
078-802-4199
Japanese cooking lessons in English with Tomoko Ota. Also special classes for people suffering from diabetes, high blood pressure, etc., taught in Japanese by registered dietician.

"A Taste of Culture" Cooking Class
3-8-16 Yoga, Setagaya-ku, Tokyo
03-5716-5751
Courses in homestyle, vegetarian, and seasonal dishes, taught by long-time resident and author Elizabeth Andoh.

Food Poisoning

In Japan, freshness of food and beauty of presentation seem to be integrally linked with hygiene in the kitchen or the factory. Restaurants, markets, and factories are strictly monitored, and there is generally no need to worry about the cleanliness or safety of the food you buy.

But there are cases of food poisoning reported each year, and because of the increase in centralization of food processing for school lunches and fast-food restaurants, the actual number of people affected in each incident tends to increase yearly. Cases have also been blamed on imported food products prepared under less stringent sanitation standards.

In Japan, food poisoning is usually divided into two main categories, in which the causes are known and unknown, with the known subdivided into natural poisons and bacteria. Unknown causes accounted for 14 percent of the incidents reported in 1996.

Natural poisons are those found in plants and animals, and are usually limited to poisonings from mushrooms and blowfish. In the case of mushrooms, the culprit is not the commercially packaged produce sold in stores, but rather the enthusiast's custom of eating wild mushrooms in season. This caused one death and 181 illnesses in 1996. The famous blowfish, or puffer fish *fugu* ふぐ was responsible for three deaths and 47 injuries. *Fugu* needs to be prepared by licensed chefs to ensure that the poison found in the internal organs has been properly removed before eating. As long as you eat your *fugu* at a restaurant, you will be able to enjoy it without having to worry about being rushed to the hospital in respiratory failure.

The heat and humidity of July through October make ideal breeding grounds for bacteria and contribute to the vast majority of incidents reported. Salmonella usually occurs in eggs and dairy products with many cases occuring from eating homemade mayonnaise that was not properly refrigerated. The now infamous strain of E. coli-0157 (known familiarly in Japan just by its numbers), usually causes diarrhea and vomiting, but can sometimes affect the kidneys and be lethal. The source is usually fecally-contaminated meat which was also undercooked, but in the summer of 1997, in Japan the exact source which caused 12 deaths and 9000 illnesses is still not known. Cases of seafood and salted pickles being contaminated with V. parehaemolytic bacteria have also been reported.

Prevention of food poisoning usually involves common-sense measures of keeping your kitchen utensils (knives, cutting boards, and counters etc.) clean, washing your hands frequently, keeping cold foods cold (below 40°F or 6°C) and hot foods hot (above 140°F or 60°C), and not allowing foods to be out of their proper storage environment for more than two hours. Prepared foods should generally be eaten quickly, since even if food is contaminated, the bacteria takes time to mulitiply sufficiently to cause symptoms of illness.

In Japan, the Anisaki's parasite is rare but can sometimes contaminate raw fish. It can cause stomach pain, and needs to be removed with an endoscope by a doctor.

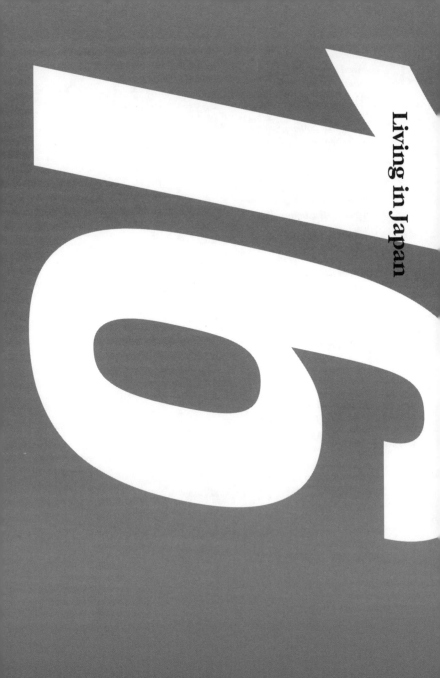

Living in Japan

*"I left my kerosene
heater on in a small
closed room while I was
making dinner in the
kitchen. When I
returned, thick black
smoke was pouring out
of the heater. I learned
never to leave a heater
unattended again."*

*"The night we moved
into our new house, the
gas mysteriously shut off.
My husband wasn't
home and having no
idea of what to do, I
went to my neighbor's.
He immediately called
the gas company on his
cellular phone and
walked outside with me
to my gas meter. Bracing
the phone with his
shoulder, holding a
flashlight in his left
hand, and following the
instructions of the gas
company over his
telephone, he had our
gas back on in five
minutes."*

Before You Leave

All members of the family should get a complete physical examination, including dental and vision checkups, while you are still in your home country, so that you can get any current problems taken care of before your departure. Adults should have a tetanus booster if you have not had one within the last ten years. No vaccines are required for entry to Japan. Check your insurance coverage to see if it covers medical care in a foreign country (see "Health Insurance").

What to Bring

■ Copies of recent physical examinations. Even if you aren't receiving treatment, such records will give an idea of your normal, healthy state, in the event that you do become ill while in Japan.

■ Vaccination records for children. Physical exam and vaccination records are required to enter school.

■ Records of allergy shots.

■ Copies of eyeglass prescriptions and an extra pair of glasses or contact lenses.

■ Copies of any X-rays.

■ An extra pair of dentures.

■ Certified copies of your birth certificate and any marriage license or divorce records. This information is necessary in cases of change in legal status (for example, for the birth of a child).

■ Supply of hard-to-find health care products such as birth control products.

■ Supply of medications that you are now taking to keep you going until you can see a new doctor (see "All About Drugs and Drugstores").

■ Copies of prescriptions. Foreign prescriptions cannot be filled here, but they may be useful to show your new doctor.

■ A general family medical encyclopedia, a baby health guide, etc.

■ Phone number of your family doctor, in case you should ever need his advice.

"When I first came to Japan I was frustrated at having to book tennis courts a month in advance and having to share mountainsides and ski slopes with half the population of Japan. Then I discovered my local sports club which offers all kinds of enticing group courses like stick fighting and a chance to use the tennis courts, squash courts, and pool without having to fight my way through the crowds."

Sports and Exercise

It is practically impossible to live in Japan without participating in some sort of sports or exercise. Even if it is only running to catch the train or climbing all those stairs in railroad stations, exercise is a part of the Japanese life-style.

Sports have long been popular in Japan, especially organized team sports in schools and universities. But the last thirty years or so have seen a burst of participation in recreational sports by the ordinary person. Because the government realizes the benefits of having a healthy population—particularly in terms of keeping health care costs down for the increasing number of elderly citizens—it now actively promotes exercise and fitness at all age levels to increase stamina, reduce stress, help control adult-onset diseases like high blood pressure, heart disease, or diabetes, and help prevent mental deterioration. "Walk 10,000 steps (about 6.2 kilometers) a day," is just one of the catchphrases with which the government promotes exercise for the sake of good health. Women and the elderly have become noticeably more active in recent years.

Opportunities for getting exercise and participating in sports are numerous and varied. If you really want to start moving, with just a little effort you can find a sport or activity to fit your physical level and interest. Golf, swimming, tennis, neighborhood ball games, cycling, and many other activities are sure to be available in your city. A little Japanese language ability or a helpful Japanese-speaking friend may be necessary to make the first contacts.

Radio Exercises

Start your day along with millions of Japanese by tuning in to NHK Radio 1 at 6:30 in the morning to join in a ten-minute set pattern of bends and stretches (*rajio taisō* ラジオ体操) that have been loosening people's kinks since 1928. The program is repeated at 8:40, 12:00 noon, and 3:00 p.m. on NHK Radio 2, so you can soon memorize the basic patterns. A book of the exercises NHKテレビラジオ体操1997 (*NHK terebi rajio taisō 1997*) sold at your local bookstore, contains clear pictures of the exercises, as well as those used in the NHK television exercise programs. This is a really easy way to start getting into the habit of daily exercise.

Hiking and Mountain Climbing

If your tastes run to hiking and mountain climbing, you are definitely in the right country. Since Japan is basically one long mountain range, the choice of paths is varied, and the scenery glorious.

If you want company while you hike, check your city, ward, or prefecture newspaper for details of outings. Many prefectures have international group newsletters which may have announcements of excursions. Contact also:

International Adventure Club—Kanto
03-5370-4230
http://www2.gol.com/users/adventure
Hiking and skiing excursions all around Japan.

International Outdoor Club—Kansai
http://www.ioc-kansai.com/
Planned outdoor activities: hiking, water, etc.

See monthly announcements in the magazine *Kansai Time Out.*

Friends of the Earth-Japan
2 Fl., 3-17-24 Mejiro, Toshima-ku, Tokyo
03-3951-1081, fax 03-3951-1084
http://www.vcom.or.jp/~foe-j/
Ecology-oriented day hikes from Tokyo.

Resource

Chiyoda Hoken Center
Chiyoda Shibuya Bldg. 2 Fl., 2-14-18 Shibuya
Shibuya-ku, Tokyo
03-5466-8687, fax 03-5453-1932 (Contact:
Hirobumi Amano)

Offers mountain climbing insurance (*sangaku hoken* 山岳保険) covering search and rescue, hospitalization, and death benefits. Mountain rescue services are not free in Japan.

For information on sports injuries, see pages 194–96.

Neighborhood Sports and Exercise Circles

Jazz dance, karate, yoga, table tennis, aerobics, aikido, tai chi, round dancing, rhythm exercise, and Japanese folk dancing are just a few examples of the different circles you may find in your area. If you can't read your community newsletter, tell a neighbor what you're looking for and ask him or her to let you know what is on offer.

Fitness Clubs *supōtsu kurabu* スポーツクラブ

Joining a private fitness club is a relatively expensive way to exercise, but it may be more convenient for you, especially if you choose one near your home or workplace. These clubs vary in what they offer, but may include a pool, weight-lifting equipment, racketball and squash courts, health or diet counseling services, and aerobics classes. Some, on the other hand, may have only a swimming pool.

To find a fitness club located near you, call in Japanese:

Central Sports
03-5543-1800 (175 clubs all over Japan)

United Sports Club XAX
03-3561-9595 (more than 100 clubs in Japan)

Tipness
03-3464-3531 (8 clubs in Tokyo, 3 in Osaka)

Levene Sporting World
03-3720-4110 (6 in Tokyo, 1 in Chiba, 1 in Kanagawa, and 1 in Osaka)

Nautilus Health Club
03-3405-1177 (Akasaka)
http://www.sumitomo-rd.com/nautilus/
(for nationwide clubs)

The following clubs have been particularly recommended:

Do Sports Plaza
Sumitomo Sankaku Bldg. Bekkan
2-6-1 Nishi-Shinjuku, Shinjuku-ku, Tokyo
03-3344-1971
Squash courts, pool, weights, sauna

Tokyu Sports Oasis (in Hygeia Health Plaza)
2-44-1 Kabukicho, Shinjuku-ku, Tokyo
03-3200-0109, (toll-free) 0120-61-0109
Dance studio, aerobics, weight machines, pool.

Takaido Swim
3-8-20 Takaido-Higashi, Suginami-ku, Tokyo
03-3333-0007
Maternity swimming/aerobics.

Keio Sports Club
4-11 Mejirodai, Hachioji-shi, Tokyo
0426-67-7311
Gym, swimming, aerobics.

Den-en Athletics Club
2-3-5 Miyazaki, Miyamae-ku, Kawasaki-shi
044-854-3771
Pool, exercise room, sauna; reasonable prices.

Higashi Tokorozawa Sports Club
1-10-5 Higashi-Tokorozawa, Tokorozawa-shi
Saitama-ken
0429-44-2344
Swimming, ballet, gymnastics.

Be Healthy Plaza
2-7 Tsurumi-Chuo, Tsurumi-ku, Yokohama-shi
045-521-9393 (Keikyu Tsurumi Station)
Aerobics, pool, maternity swimming, jazz dance.

Oak Three
506-1 Mizuno, Sayama-shi, Saitama-ken
0429-56-0093
Pool, aerobics, machines.

Hello Sports Plaza Kyoto
561 Komanocho, Marutamachi-Sagaru
Nakasuji-dori, Kamigyo-ku, Kyoto-shi
075-252-0086
Pool, weights, jazz dance, sauna.

For yoga classes, see page 287.

Martial Arts budō 武道

The various methods of self-defense include not only defensive and offensive tactics, but also spiritual training. These popular sports (or arts) are taught in physical education classes at schools and colleges as well as in company clubs and at many local private and public sports facilities. Kendo 剣道, the way of the sword (actually a hollow bamboo rod) and judo 柔道 and aikido 合気道 (both unarmed techniques whereby the attacker's strength and momentum are used to deflect an attack) have become popular worldwide and have their own international competitions. Karate 空手, which literally means "empty hand," is actually an import from China and is also considered a martial art.

Martial arts schools *dōjō* 道場 are listed in the yellow pages under *dōjō* or under the individual arts. Classes are also held at public sports facilities and in neighborhood circles.

For information on tai chi, and qigong (in Japanese, known as *kikō*) see "Alternative Healing."

International Aikido Federation
03-3203-9236

All Japan Judo Federation
03-3818-4171
03-3818-4172 (International Section; classes for foreigners)

Japan Karate Association
03-3440-1415

Tokyo Kendo Federation
03-3211-5967

All Japan Kendo Federation
03-3211-5804

The following magazines print announcements of various sporting activities. You can find them in English-language bookstores, or call for subscription information.

Sports World Japan
03-5691-0564

Kansai Time Out
078-232-4516/4517

Everyday Life and Health

Whether you're in Japan for a short-term contract or have a Japanese spouse and plan to stay a lifetime, the following tips, information, and suggestions should help you maintain a healthy life-style in Japan.

Tatami

Traditional flooring, or *tatami*, provides a breathable, cushiony surface for sleeping and sitting. *Tatami* mats actually consist of a 6-centimeter (2.4-inch) base (*toko*) of straw covered with a soft surface (*omote*) of woven rush. *Tatami* is said to act as a type of filter, absorbing carbon dioxide. Each mat can also absorb up to 500 cubic centimeters of water when humidity is high, so *tatami* rooms should be aired frequently, and wet clothes should not be allowed to drip onto the mats. Manufacturers recommend airing *tatami* in the sun twice a year to prolong its life. Rugs shouldn't be placed on top of *tatami*, since this prevents the regular circulation of air and moisture exchange. It also allows dust to build up under the rug, encouraging dust mites, which can cause allergies.

Tatami can be vacuumed with the grain and/or wiped with a slightly damp cloth. New *tatami* mats have been treated, so they should be wiped with a dry cloth. Mats that have been burned by the sun can be treated with a vinegar and hot water solution to restore the surface.

Futon

At night *futon*, or bedding, is taken out of the *oshi-ire*, or large storage closets, and spread out on the floor. In the morning, this bedding is then folded and stored back in the closet. Most *futon* are filled with cotton batting. If 100 percent cotton is used, the *futon* tend to be heavy and difficult to handle, so now a mixture of 30 percent synthetic fiber and 70 percent cotton is used (although they may still be marked as 100 percent cotton). More people are starting to use wool-filled *futon*. Although these are also more expensive and don't look as thick as the cotton ones, they are warmer, lighter weight, and don't need airing as often. Using a sponge mat underneath your futon provides a very comfortable way to sleep, and offers a bit more support for your back.

Futon need to be aired at least once a week for about two hours on a sunny day to prevent them from becoming damp. If left outside too long, the cotton fibers will expand too much, becoming brittle and easily damaged. When outside, the *futon* should be covered by at least a sheet to protect the outer shell from the direct rays of the sun. Contrary to popular belief, cotton-filled *futon* shouldn't be beaten, as this will break the fibers and decrease the bedding's life. Instead, brush lightly to get rid of any dust. Polyester-filled comforters can be beaten to make them fluffy again.

For people that either don't have the time, place, or the sun to air a *futon*, *futon* dryers (*futon kansōki* 布団乾燥機) are available. These will usually dry out a *futon* in one or two hours, depending on the brand. If you don't have the inclination to put your *futon* away every day, you should at least move them to a different area of the room to allow the *tatami* underneath to dry out. If you have *futon* that aren't regularly used, store them in special *futon* bags or wrap them in a sheet to keep dust off and air them periodically to prevent mildew and a musty odor.

Bathrooms and Toilets

Unless you live in the far north of Japan, fill your bathtub with water in the morning to allow it to reach room temperature so you'll need less gas to heat it in the evening. Filling your tub in the morning will also allow you to have a large amount of clean water on hand in case of an earthquake or fire. Many Japanese reuse their bathwater for cleaning or washing clothes. If you have small children, be sure to keep a cover on the tub when you aren't using it, to prevent accidental drowning. Cover the tub while the water is heating too, to conserve the heat.

Many homes have Western-style toilets now, but public toilets in train stations and parks are usually the squat style. These are very hygienic since there's no contact, but if you have a heart condition, your doctor may recommend that you avoid this type.

Electricity and Gas

Electricity supplied to homes is 100 volts. Your local electric power company is responsible for service problems such as fixing short circuits and extending special wiring. For help, call the service number written at the bottom of your bill.

There are thirteen types of city gas used in different regions of the country. It is very dangerous to use gas appliances that are not made for the type of gas used, since this may cause fire or poisoning from incomplete combustion. Appliances can be adjusted by your gas company for a fee.

Micon-meters are gas meters with an incorporated IC microcomputer, which can check for gas leaks and shut the gas off in an earthquake. For more detailed explanations—of how to reset the meter, for example, after an earthquake—refer to the English manual that your gas company can provide upon request. Also available from the gas company are incomplete combustion detectors *gasu more keihoki*, which emit a buzzing sound if a gas leak is detected. Some gas heaters also have a safety device, or *anzen sōchi*, which turns the appliance off if incomplete combustion occurs. When using your range or kitchen water heater, be sure to switch the ventilation fan on. If you use a heater without an outside flue, make sure that you open the windows periodically. Some pilot lights are lit by battery. If you're having problems, it may be that the battery needs to be changed.

Finally, if you think you smell gas, shut off all appliances, close your gas valves and also the main valve near your gas meter, and call the gas company. They'll answer calls twenty-fours hours a day. Give them your service number written on the bill. Don't turn on any electric switches, even the overhead ventilation fan, since this could cause sparks that can ignite the gas. Instead, open your windows.

■ *Gasu more desu. Tasukete kudasai!*
There's a gas leak! Please help me!

■ *Watashi no shiyō bango wa _____ desu.*
My customer service number is _____ .

Fires

The Japanese are well aware of the havoc that fire can wreak, as Japanese homes have traditionally been made of wood and built very close together. Even today in some parts of Japan, the tradition continues of volunteers walking around the neighborhood in the evening, banging two sticks together and shouting the warning "*matchi ippon, kaji no moto*" (it only takes one match to start a fire).

Most years arson ranks as the top cause of fires, followed by kitchen fires, careless smoking, bonfires, and children playing with matches. The fire department recommends that each home should have a fire extinguisher (*shōkaki* 消火器) and ideally a smoke detector (*kasai hōchiki* 火災報知器). Remember that the size you buy will determine the size of the fire that can be extinguished. (Usual sizes range from one kilogram to six kilograms; refills are also available.)

In Japan, prosecution under the law for a fire can be brought about by either civil or criminal law. Surprisingly, the criminal law definition is rather broad and parents of children who were playing with fire (particularly those under seven or eight years of age) may be accused of negligence and in extremes cases, even carelessness. A landlord's insurance coverage may be inadequate, so if a fire starts in a rented apartment and destroys the building, the court may find the tenant responsible and require that he reimburse the owner for the damages incurred. If a death occurs, although it's not always legally necessary, the responsible party will probably pay monetary compensation (*baishō kin* 賠償金) to the deceased's family members. When renting a home or apartment, check what kind of insurance is required. If the landlord is adequately insured, you will only need to have "tenant insurance," which will cover your personal items as well as any water damage caused while the fire is being extinguished.

Pollution *kōgai* 公害

Accompanying the industrialization process in Japan, as in other parts of the world, was the dark shadow of pollution. People's health first began to be affected in the fifties and sixties when economic growth gave rise not only to improved living standards, but also to severe environmental pollution. In four infamous incidents, pollution caused permanent physical damage and even death, and the victims began to seek legal recourse in the courts. Minamata disease, caused by eating fish contaminated by mercury discharged by chemical companies, occurred in both Minamata in Kumamoto Prefecture and in Niigata in Niigata Prefecture. *Itai itai* disease was caused by cadmium discharged by a mining and smelting plant in Toyama Prefecture's Fuchu. Respiratory problems including asthma, were caused by air pollution, the most famous case occurring in Yokkaichi in Mie Prefecture.

The court cases concerning these acts of pollution helped lead to the enactment of the Basic Law for Environmental Pollution Control (*kōgai taisaku kihon hō* 公害対策基本法) in 1970, which set maximum permissible levels for six catagories; air, water, soil, noise and/or vibration, land sinkage, and foul odors. In addition, the Japanese government will compensate citizens who have developed chronic diseases due to pollution—usually asthma sufferers. Benefits include medical care allowances, compensation allowances, compensation payments to survivors, and funeral expenses. Polluting companies are fined and pay fees proportional to the amount of pollutants released.

As a result of this legislation, pollution has decreased, although it hasn't disappeared completely. While the number of complaints in the six main areas is gradually declining, other complaints relating to, for instance, complaints about animals (especially barking dogs), management of vacant lots, and illegal dumping of waste have been increasing. If you have any complaints about pollution, report them to the Pollution Control Section *kankyō kōgai hokenka* 環境公害保健課 of your city office.

Air Pollution

The progress that has been made in cleaning up industries has been offset by the growing number of motor vehicles. The air in large cities is regularly tested at monitoring stations for sulfur dioxide, carbon monoxide, nitrogen dioxide, suspended particulate matter, and photochemical oxidants—which are the elements that act as precipitators of smog. Sulfur dioxide and carbon monoxide levels have decreased remarkably, but the level of nitrogen dioxide, a pollutant linked directly to car exhaust, remains high. In the "total emission–regulated area" which includes the cities of Tokyo, Yokohama, and Osaka, the yearly average level of nitrogen dioxide in the air exceeds the daily recommended standard of between 0.04 and 0.06 (or less) parts per million, as measured at ninety percent of the automobile exhaust measurement offices. Lower-emission vehicles are encouraged, but their influence on air quality remains to been seen.

Photochemical smog—which causes irritation of the eyes, nose, and throat and respiratory disturbances—has decreased considerably. When excessive amounts of photochemical oxidants are detected in the air, smog warnings (*kōkagaku sumoggu chūi* 光化学スモッグ注意) are issued, warning people to stay indoors if possible, with their windows and doors closed, and factories are requested to reduce their emissions.

Cutting Exposure to Pollution

■ If you have asthma or other respiratory problems, check at the city office to see which areas of the city have a higher incidence of air pollution or smog before selecting a house. If possible, choose a home near a wooded area.

■ Exercise outdoors early in the morning when the air is relatively clean, and avoid major thoroughfares, where levels are higher.

Water Pollution

Although water quality testing standards are generally being met, water may sometimes taste unpleasant or have a musty smell. Many people complain that the permissible levels for toxic substances are inadequate since they don't take into account many of the newer manmade chemicals used in manufacturing, agricultural insecticides, and herbicides. In addition, sewage treatment facilities have not kept pace with urbanization, particularly in the newer bedroom communities on the outskirts of large cities.

Given people's general anxiety about water quality, sales of water filters (*jōsuiki* 浄

水器), domestic and imported bottled mineral water, and electric (voltage) alkali ion water energizers (*ion seisuiki* イオン整水器) have increased sharply in the past few years. A wide variety of filters are available, most of which will remove the chlorine smell from the water, but not all of which remove the musty odor caused by algae, etc. Changing the filter's cartridge more frequently may give the best results. Some of the more expensive filters also remove chemicals and carcinogenic agents such as trihalomethane, which forms when chlorine added at the filtration plant combines with organic materials already in the water. (It is interesting to note that trihalomethane is almost completely removed, and chlorinated organic solvents are reduced by half, simply by boiling the water.) Filters also remove most of the purifying agents, so filtered water should either be used immediately or simply discarded, since bacteria can easily grow in it.

If you are planning to buy bottled water, consider whether you want it for mineral content or for safety. Japanese tapwater averages about 67 milligrams of minerals, which is actually more than most domestic brands of bottled water. Bottled water from natural springs is usually untreated, and so tends to contain more bacteria per milliliter than the public water supply. In view of the expense and the growing problem of disposal of the plastic bottles, boiling the tapwater in a pot without a cover (to allow impurities to escape with the steam) may be a more economical way to ensure that your water is safe. The Global Village (see the endpapers) has water test kits for sale, leaflets on water filters, and details on how to improve your water.

Product Liability

The government is still in the process of establishing standards for health care products and cosmetics, and controls on advertisements leave a lot to be desired. Mail-order brochures are filled with wonderful devices to dramatically improve your eyesight and exotic potions to cure all your ills. Remember that if you buy these products there probably isn't a money-back guarantee if you're not satisfied.

Safety Marks

Written warnings sometimes seen on product packaging include the terms *kiken* 危険 (danger), *mazeruna* まぜるな (don't mix), *kanensei* 可燃性 (flammable), and *chūi* 注意 (caution).

■ JIS Mark

Given to industrial and household products meeting the criteria set by Japan Industrial Standards.

■ JAS Mark

Given to ham, canned food, processed food, plywood, and other products meeting criteria set by Japan Agricultural Standards.

The following marks on product packaging mean that restitution will be made if use of the product results in bodily injury or property damage:

■ SG Mark

Given to baby and children's products, furniture, sporting goods, and recreational products that meet safety standards of the Product Safety Association.

■ ST Mark

Given to toys that meet the safety standards of the Japan Toy Association.

■ SF Mark

Given to fireworks that meet the safety standards of the Japan Fireworks Association.

Earthquakes

Japan is one of the most seismologically active areas in the world, thanks to the pushing and shoving of three major plates located right under Japan's doorstep. Numerous earthquakes occur annually, although most are small and cause little, if any, damage. While you can't stop nature from taking its course, you can be prepared with equipment and supplies. Participate in neighborhood drills, know your designated evacuation site *hinan basho* 避難場所, and visit your city office for disaster instructions, so that you're mentally prepared to face an emergency situation.

Tips on Preparing for an Earthquake

■ Prepare a three-day emergency supply of drinking water (three liters of water per day per person); a three-day supply of canned or dehydrated food; a first-aid kit (see page 51); personal medications; a transistor radio, a flashlight, towels, socks, etc.; candles and matches; copies of your passport, bankbook, etc. Ready-made kits *saigaihin* 災害品 are sold in large department stores, sometimes in fireproof bags.

■ Keep a fire extinguisher on hand and learn how to use it correctly.
■ Secure any furniture which might fall over in an earthquake. Remove all heavy or potentially dangerous objects from shelves.
■ Discuss with your family where you will all gather; make sure you know the evacuation site at your children's school and the procedure for picking up your children.

What to Do in an Earthquake

Major earthquakes are usually over within one minute. Stay calm and remember the following:

■ Turn off the gas in your house or apartment, including that used for stoves or other cooking appliances, as soon as the quake starts.
■ Open a door to the outside, for possible use as an emergency exit, as soon as the quake starts. Door frames can jam during an earthquake and trap you inside.

■ Seek shelter under a door frame, table or desk, to protect yourself from falling objects.
■ If you are indoors, stay there. The second floor of a wooden house is generally safer than the first. Remember that the upper floors of a tall building will shake more violently than the lower floors. Going outside increases your chance of injury from falling objects. If you are

already outside, immediately seek shelter or proceed to an open area.

■ Most elevators stop automatically at the nearest floor. Get off immediately when the door opens.

■ Keep away from narrow alleyways, concrete –block walls, and embankments, since falling objects and broken glass are major causes of injury.

■ If you are driving, immediately stop your car on the left-hand side of the street and turn off the engine. Driving will be banned in all restricted areas.

■ If you are on a train, chances are it will stop abruptly, so hold on tight and follow the directions of the conductor. If you need to evacuate, keep away from hanging electric wires.

■ If the quake was very large and you do not feel safe in your own house, proceed to designated evacuation areas as soon as the quake is over.

■ Listen carefully to the radio or television for information and instructions.

Travel in Japan

Japan is an extremely safe place to travel, with few of the hazards of traveling that you would find in many other Asian countries. However, if you're in the Okinawa area, watch out for the *habu*, a large, extremely poisonous snake which causes several deaths each year. The *mamushi* is the only poisonous snake on the mainland, and although many people are bitten by it each year, very few die.

Please note that emergency care is available at Narita and Kansai international airports, the Travelers' Rest Centers at Tokyo, Nagoya, Kyoto, Osaka, Shin-Osaka, Tennoji, Hiroshima, and Okayama stations (center hours may be limited), and on Mount Fuji (seventh station, Yamanashi Prefecture–side; open only 1 July–27 August).

Travel in Asia

In order for the body to develop full immunity to a disease, two or more injections of the same vaccine have to be given, with a time lapse of a month between injections, so plan ahead before your trip. Immunizations available in Japan for overseas travel include rabies, hepatitis A, hepatitis B, Japanese encephalitis, cholera, and yellow fever. Note that you may need a series of shots against certain diseases—the rabies vaccination, for instance, is three shots given over a period of time. Your travel agent may have a list of clinics where these inoculations are available. Vaccination against yellow fever is given only by appointment at designated quarantine offices. Chloroquine or mefloquine tablets for the prevention of malaria are not offered at quarantine stations here, but are available through the International Clinic and the Tokyo Medical and Surgical Clinic, or can be sent from home. The International Clinic is perhaps the only place in Japan offering vaccinations against typhoid fever and meningitis.

Parasites such as amoebas are endemic in many countries, and infection may involve hospitalization of a week to ten days in Japan. If you find yourself ill upon your return, consult the quarantine office at the airport or call your local public health center to find a hospital with a tropical disease specialist, as doctors without experience or the proper laboratory facilities to diagnose a tropical disease may have difficulty treating you.

Resources

Japanese Quarantine Association
Nihon Keneki Eisei Kyokai
日本検疫衛生協会
Tokyo Clinic: Daiichi Tekko Bldg. 5 Fl.
1-8-2 Marunouchi, Chiyoda-ku, Tokyo
03-3201-0848/1308
Yokohama Clinic: Sangyo Boeki Center Bldg. 3 Fl.
2 Yamashita-cho, Naka-ku, Yokohama-shi
045-671-7041/7042
Travel vaccines and childhood immunizations. Appointment necessary only for yellow fever. Forms in Japanese and English.

Tokyo Medical and Surgical Clinic
(see page 33)

The International Clinic (Tokyo; see page 33)

Osaka City General Hospital
Osaka Shiritsu Sogo Iryo Center
大阪市立総合医療センター
2-12-22 Miyakojima-Hondori, Miyakojima-ku
Osaka-shi
06-929-1221
Immunization against typhus, rabies, cholera, hepatitis A, hepatitis B, influenza, smallpox, TB, and childhood diseases.

Japan Baptist Hospital (page 347)

The International Travelers' Hotline
1-404-332-4565, fax 1-404-332-4559
Prerecorded information available 24 hours a day from push-button phones.
http://www.cdc.gov/travel/travel.html

For health information related to international travel, see "References and Further Reading," page 356.

Death and Dying

"When my Japanese father-in-law was in the final stages of lung cancer, my husband refused to let me say anything about his real diagnosis. As he got weaker, he tried to talk about death, but everyone around him kept telling him not to worry and to save his strength for getting well. One of the final comments he made to the family was, 'I have some money in an envelope in my dresser. Please use it to buy Jane some black clothes. We can't have her looking untidy at the funeral.' I'm sure he would have welcomed discussing his impending death with someone."

Japanese Attitudes Toward Death

Traditionally, terminally ill patients were rarely told outright about their impending death. However, the situation in Japan is changing as more and more patients and their families are starting to demand detailed information about their conditions and to expect a caring and supportive environment during their last days.

On the other hand, in many cases, the doctor still only tells a few members of the family anything about the patient's real condition, and both doctor and family avoid discussing the subject with the patient. When one of the people involved is a foreigner with different beliefs about death and dying, there is ample room for confusion and awkwardness. An awareness that this is a transitional period may help in understanding a situation in which a doctor bluntly tells a foreign patient that there is no hope and promptly leaves the room. Medical professionals realize that other cultures may be more forthright in discussing death and dying, but the accompanying emotional and psychologically supportive manners are not yet completely understood or mastered. Medical schools are just starting to introduce into the curriculum studies on how terminal care differs from regular curative medical treatment. For more on Japanese attitudes toward death, see the two etiquette books listed on page 356.

Hospice Care *kanwa kea* 緩和ケア

Most Japanese today die in the hospital. Although dying at home used to be common, the custom now is to be treated by a physician right up until the very end of life.

The idea of hospice care, which encompasses an honest dialogue with the patient about impending death, making the person as physically comfortable as possible, and giving spiritual, mental, and social support and encouragement in the last days of life, is a relatively new concept in Japan. For various cultural and philosophical reasons, the idea has been difficult to accept, and few independent hospice facilities have been established. Instead some hospitals, including university medical centers, are starting to experiment with care for the terminally ill in special hospice units. As of January 1998, more than thirty such hospice care units *kanwa kea byōtō* 緩和ケア病棟 were registered with prefectural governments. Typical patients are those who have less than six months to live regardless of the medical care they are given, those who are in great pain, those who have difficulty breathing, and those who can no longer move freely.

A hospice volunteer worker explains,"You might think a hospice would be a dark and depressing place. But it isn't—the rooms are light and cheerful. There's less of the hustle and bustle that you associate with ordinary hospital wards. The staff have more time to sit, listen, and talk with the patients and their families about their relationships with each other, their beliefs about death, and what meaning their lives have held for them."

Hospice care is covered under public health insurance plans.

For the names of hospices around Japan other than those included in the following list, call the Hospice Care Research Group (see the following), in Japanese.

Salvation Army Kiyose Hospital
Kyuseigun Kiyose Byoin
救世軍清瀬病院
Kiyose-shi, Tokyo
0424-91-1411

Tokyo Adventist Hospital (see page 344)

Peace House
ピースハウス病院

Nakai-machi, Kanagawa-ken
0465-81-8900

Japan Baptist Hospital
(Kyoto-shi; see page 347)

Kobe Adventist Hospital (see page 348)

Yodogawa Christian Hospital
(Osaka-shi; see page 348)

Pain Control

Pain control is an integral aspect of care for the dying, but pain medication is not given generously, even for cancer patients. Surveys have shown that most doctors at cancer and general hospitals agree that not enough painkillers are used and that medical schools fail to teach enough about pain control. Despite the increased interest shown in the management of pain by the medical profession, the amount of pain medication prescribed is still only a fraction of that used per person in many Western countries. Hospices, however, consider pain control to be one of their major functions, and give pain-relieving morphine orally, rectally, by infuser, or in whatever combination is best suited to the patient's needs. Other pain control methods such as breathing, relaxation, visualization, and acupuncture are also practiced. If you are not satisfied with the medication provided by your doctor, call the following organizations for names of doctors across the country who understand the importance of pain control.

Hospice Care Research Group
Hosupisu Kea Kenkyukai
ホスピスケア研究会
3-18-34-601 Minami-Ikebukuro, Toshima-ku, Tokyo
03-3984-3291 (J. only), fax 03-3984-3292

Newhope Hospice Institute
1-3-45 Motomachi, Suite 5 Kiyose-shi, Tokyo
0424-91-2462, fax 0424-91-2406
Interdisciplinary research institute for hospice care, meets every 2nd Saturday in Tokyo. Seminars on hospice care, as well as international seminars at various overseas settings.

Home Care for the Terminally Ill

For those who would like to stay in their own homes during their last days, care is rather difficult to arrange because it requires finding a doctor who is willing to visit, in order to supervise care and medications. You can ask local doctors near you if they would be willing to visit your home and prescribe drugs as necessary, but there are still too few who are willing. To encourage home care, the government has slightly increased health insurance payments to doctors to cover examinations and treatments done in the home. Private home-care firms can assist in giving physical care. Contact the Elderly Services Providers Association (see page 225) for reputable firms in your area. This care is not covered by public insurance, and is expensive. Your city or ward office may also have suggestions.

Home Hospice Care

Nakajima Clinic and Hospice, Med. Corp.
1-3-45 Motomachi, Kiyose-shi, Tokyo
0424-95-6727, fax 0424-95-6729

Medical Director Dr. Michiko Nakajima is a pioneer in the use of morphine for pain control in Japan. 24-hour medical attention at home by a team of MDs, RNs, and chaplains.

Living Wills/Advanced Directives *ribingu uiru, adobansu deirekuteibu, jizen shiji* リビング ウイル，アドバンス デイレクテイブ，事前指示

A living will expresses a person's wishes regarding the type of medical treatment he or she wants (or doesn't want) at the end of life. Traditionally, the Japanese patient has trusted the doctor to give the necessary appropriate care, and has not participated in planning that care. The idea of someone's preparing for death by writing a living will while still healthy is gradually becoming known in Japan, but the living will itself is not legally binding, and the doctor still has the final say as to the type of treatment given. It is suggested that all members of the immediate family sign the living will when it is written, to show that they support the wishes expressed by the patient. It is also imperative that the doctor be told that the patient has written a living will. The patient will not be asked upon admittance to the hospital, so it will be the responsibility of the patient or the patient's family to describe and give a copy of the will to the doctor.

Japan Hospice Living Will Society
1-4-26-102 Okubo, Shinjuku-ku, Tokyo
03-5273-8055 (J. only), fax 03-3205-6767
This group distributes forms for making a living will stating the members' wishes with regard to medical treatment deemed necessary to prolong his or her life in incurable cases. The society safeguards one copy of that will. Also promotes terminal care in hospices, in an effort to maintain quality of life until death.

Children and Death

Make-A-Wish (Japan)
Sogo-Hanzomon Bldg. 7 Fl, 1-7 Kojimachi, Chiyoda-ku, Tokyo
03-3221-8388
Affiliate of the largest wish-granting organization in the world for children with life-threatening illnesses. Sponsors various activities to make these children's wishes come true.

Prenatal and Infant Death Support Group
03-3442-0950 (Stephanie Fukui)

0425-93-0376 (Patricia Iida)
For support and help in the event of a miscarriage, stillbirth, Sudden Infant Death Syndrome (SIDS), neonatal death, or death of a child up to two years old, in English or Japanese.

Family House
03-3639-2146
Inexpensive lodgings for family members of hospitalized children, short- and/or long-term. Call in Japanese for nearest lodging nationwide.

Death in Japan *shi* 死

In Japan, a death is usually followed by two or three days of religious rituals and services, after which the body is cremated and inte red in an old or a new family grave *o-haka* お墓. A funeral home *sōgisha* 葬儀社 takes charge of all the details. Traditionally, the wake *o-tsuya* お通夜 and religious service were held in the home, with neighbors and family helping. However, as houses have become smaller, services are increasingly held in rented halls, temples, or at the crematorium under the direction of the funeral home. In addition, the choice of observances has widened to include light and sound shows, new types of coffins, and fancier or more individualized gravestones.

In a set package price ranging anywhere between ¥400,000 and ¥1,200,000 or more, items would include:

■ Casket: from ¥130,000–¥300,000 or more, depending on the shape and material, and the person's body length and weight.

■ Crematorium: ¥80,000–¥230,000 in Tokyo; much cheaper outside Tokyo.

■ Hearse: ¥58,000–¥65,000, based on type.

■ Urn: ¥25,000 (economy-style) to millions of yen (for a work of art).

■ Funeral home assistants: ¥20,000 per day per person.

■ Gratuity to workers at the crematorium: ¥30,000 –¥60,000.

■ Flowers: ¥150,000–¥400,000.

■ Miscellaneous expenses: costs associated with heating, tents, video equipment, lunch, buses, rental cars, hearse mileage, etc.

Prices can vary greatly, depending on location, type of funeral, and family preferences. It goes without saying that the family must make clear, at the beginning of the negotiations, just how much it wants to spend. The funeral home takes care of practically everything, and saves both time and worry during that stressful time.

Most funerals in Japan are conducted in the Buddhist tradition, but Shinto rites can also be followed; *mushūkyō* funerals with no particular religious focus are also possible. A Christian funeral service at the church of the deceased is one of the least expensive of organized religious funerals.

Immediately Following Death

The patient must be pronounced legally dead by a doctor before anything else can be done. Do not move the body. If the patient has died in a hospital, the hospital will be responsible for providing a death certificate *shibō shindansho* 死亡診断書, which the attending physician will sign. If the person has died outside the hospital, the doctor of the deceased must be notified. If the deceased's doctor cannot come to view the body, or if you do not know the doctor of the deceased, call the police at 110 (not 119) and they will arrange for a medical examiner to examine the body and issue a death certificate. If there is no obvious reason for the death or if the cause of death is in question, an autopsy *shitaikaibō* 死体解剖 will be performed.

In the meantime, inform the embassy or consulate of the death, giving the passport number and other personal information of the deceased, together with the name and whereabouts of the next of kin. Embassy staff will advise on procedures to be followed, although helpfulness varies among embassies. If necessary, contact the next of kin to decide how to dispose of the body. (The embassy may wish to make this call.) Contact the spiritual adviser of the deceased, if appropriate. No matter how good your own Japanese language ability is, it may be useful to ask a Japanese friend to help with communication and cultural considerations. Contact the lawyer and the employer of the deceased.

Whether a person dies in the hospital or at home, according to custom, family or friends are expected to stay with the body until it can be removed to a funeral home or crematorium (even if the body is held overnight at the hospital).

A family member or person close to the deceased must take the death certificate, together with the deceased's Alien Registration Certificate, to the city or ward office and fill out a Notice of Death form *shibō todoke* 死亡届. Without this form, cremation or burial of ashes in the grave cannot take place.

Where appropriate, the spiritual adviser of the deceased can help with appropriate funeral and burial preparations as well as giving emotional and spiritual support to family and mourners. Contact the Jewish Community of Japan 03-3400-2559, the Japan Muslim Association 03-3370-3476, or the Kobe Islamic Mosque 078-231-6060 for assistance with a funeral and disposal of a body. A number of companies familiar with Christian burial rites are included in the list below. For more detailed descriptions of the cultural practices surrounding death and funerals, see "References and Further Reading."

Final Arrangements

Funeral arrangements can be made through the ward or city office using public facilities, or through a private funeral or mortuary service company. The following mortuary service companies are accustomed to taking care of foreigners:

International Mortuary Systems
048-261-3302
Western embalming; shipping; works with embassies; 24 hours nationwide.

Iisuta Shikitensha
078-753-0162
Christian funerals only.

Japan Ceremony Service Network
0120-25-1251
Embalming, shipping, 24 hours nationwide.

Santoku Funeral Parlor
03-3551-2047
Shipping and embalming.

Toso Company
03-3400-2670
Shipping, embalming, all kinds of funeral services.

Nazare Kikaku
03-3310-6733
Christian funeral director, pre-planning consultations, respect for the family's preferences, shipping.

Yokohama Mortuary Systems
044-366-4444
Western embalming, shipping.

Embalming *shitaibōfu* 死体防腐

Embalming is not a traditional custom in Japan. Since Buddhism was introduced in the eighth century, cremation has become the usual method of disposing of the body. However, if cremation has to be postponed until family members arrive from overseas, for example, the body may be embalmed. Although Jews and Muslims expressly forbid it for cultural or religious reasons, embalming may be necessary or expected in the case of a death that occurs overseas. Embalming is best done within twelve hours of death, although dry ice can be used to preserve the body for a time. Funeral companies which undertake embalming, as well as those that do Western-type embalming (which prepares the body for viewing) are listed above. American citizens can also request through the U.S. embassy that embalming be done at Yokota Air Force Base. The police may have information regarding hospitals in your area that offer Japanese-style embalming (these are usually university hospitals).

Alternatives

Other options for short-term preservation include dry ice and refrigeration. The funeral home can provide dry ice for preserving the body for a couple of days (crucial during the summer months) while preparations are completed. If a longer storage period is needed, and the patient has died in a large hospital, the hospital morgue's refrigeration facilities may be available for a daily charge. If the patient has died elsewhere, refrigeration facilities may be more difficult to arrange and may depend on hospital policy, space availability, and circumstances of death. St. Luke's International Hospital (03-3541-5151) sometimes provides this service. The police or your ward or city office may be able to help.

Shipping a Body

Whether you decide to send a body home or not will depend on your religious and cultural beliefs, personal sentiments, and also financial situation.

Before a body can be shipped from Japan, several points need to be taken into account. First, check the legal status of the deceased and make sure that the country to which the body is being shipped will accept it. You may also need to arrange for a funeral company in the home country to accept delivery. You must be sure to comply with the regulations on packing procedures and the completion of legal documents required by the Japanese government, the airline, and the home country. The specialists in funeral services and shipping listed on the previous page will complete these formalities for you if necessary. As expenses should be paid before the body leaves Japan, you should count on a minimum outlay of ¥1,000,000. Note that the embassy of the deceased will not be responsible for providing these funds, but may assist you in getting funds transferred more quickly to Japan.

Expenses will include:

■ Professional services of the funeral home.

■ Casket—wooden, metal, or a combination. (Save on shipping charges by choosing a simple wooden one; a fancier one can be purchased in the home country.)

■ Tin-lined wooden shipping container, required by Japanese law (about ¥300,000).

■ Overland shipment charges within Japan. Charged by the kilometer, these can add up

quickly.

■ Airline charges by weight or a combination of weight and cubic measurement (an average weight would be 150 kilograms—figure on ¥1,900 per kilogram to New York, and ¥2,600 per kilogram to London).

■ Consumption tax.

■ Airline cargo commission fees (about ¥40,000).

Burial in Japan

Not only is cremation of the body and internment of the ashes in an urn a long-standing Buddhist practice, it is also a highly practical idea today, given the scarcity of burial space in crowded modern Japan. Although the arrival in Japan of foreigners with different burial practices necessitated the establishment of several foreigners' cemeteries, these are now almost or completely full, so it can be very difficult to bury a body in Japan today. These organizations managing individual cemeteries consider applications on a case-by-case basis.

Kobe International Cemetery and Osaka Foreign Cemetery
078-881-9533 (Contact: Philip A. Campanella)

Foreigners' Cemetery in Yokohama
045-622-1311 (J. only)

Cremation kasō 火葬

After the Notice of Death form is submitted *shibō todoke* 死亡届, a cremation permit *kasō kyokasho* 火葬許可証 allowing the body to be cremated can be issued. Cremation cannot take place until at least twenty-four hours after the death. City or ward office employees will explain what cremation facilities are available in your area.

If you decide to use city-run facilities, those outside Tokyo may be especially inexpensive (for example, ¥7,000 for residents aged twelve or over, and ¥3,500 for a child under twelve). Non-residents might pay ¥30,000 and ¥15,000, respectively, for the basic cremation. In comparison Tokyo prices may range from ¥80,000 to ¥230,000 depending on the type chosen—greater heat is faster and more expensive. All other services (room rentals, hearse, urn for the ashes, and other funeral equipment) are extra. If you decide to use a funeral company, the ward or city office, or the embassy or consulate, can suggest some in your area.

Finding a Final Resting Place for Ashes

After cremation the mourners assist in placing the ashes and remaining bone fragments in an urn *kotsu tsubo*, and the urn is sealed. The urn can then be carried or shipped back to the home country with relative ease. Embassies will provide a certificate making customs clearance easier.

If you need a burial plot, remember that the price varies greatly according to location. A new cemetery in the northern part of Saitama Prefecture sells two-meter–square plots for ¥220,000 and charges a yearly maintenance fee of ¥5,000. On the other hand, a similar plot in a cemetery closer to Tokyo may go for over ¥700,000, with an annual maintenance fee of ¥10,000. Expenses for building the small burial chamber can multiply the price several times.

Other suggested locations for a final resting place for ashes include the cemetery at the temple or the burial chamber of the church of the deceased.

Natural Funerals

Natural funerals, whereby the ashes are scattered at a memorable outdoor site or over the sea in accordance with the wishes of the deceased, are now legal in Japan. Following the cremation, you can take the urn containing the deceased's ashes and then scatter the ashes at a convenient time and with as much or as little ceremony as is fitting. This type of funeral is not considered a desecration or abandonment of the corpse or a health hazard, provided that the ceremonies accompanying the burial are of a respectful nature.

Legalities and Last Business

■ Report the death within seven days to the city or ward office in the town in which the deceased lived.

■ Return the Alien Registration Card (if applicable) of the deceased to the issuing ward or city office within fourteen days of the death.

■ Return the passport of the deceased to the appropriate embassy for cancellation.

■ Contact the company of the deceased (if applicable) for assistance with Employees' Health Insurance, death benefits, and funeral expense assistance *sōsaihi* 葬祭費 procedures (see page 73).

■ If the deceased was enrolled in the national insurance system, contact the insurance desk at the ward or city office for help with death benefits and funeral expense (see page 77).

Grief Counseling

See resources in Mental Health Chapter.

Compassionate Friends
03-5481-5020 (Contact: Graham Harris)
An international grief support group which meets in the Tokyo area when there is a need. Can send literature in English and put you in touch with American or British organizations.

Be Prepared

Although death and dying are probably not on your list of most fascinating conversation subjects, every year foreigners do die in Japan. (It is not just the elderly who need be concerned—not long ago, for example, two young foreign nationals died while climbing Mount Fuji.) Taking a little time to consider these eventualities will make it easier for your family and friends if the situation should ever arise.

If you are ever diagnosed with a terminal disease, consider where and how you want to live the last days of your life and whether your health insurance will cover your plans. If you die in Japan, what kind of funeral and burial would you want? Write down your wishes and give copies to your spouse, your family, or a close friend, and place it in your personnel file at work. Consider making a Living Will. See also Organ Donations, pages 208–209.

Regional Resources • References • Glossary • Index

The following resources are by no means the only ones available in your area. Your first stop after moving to a new area should be to register at your ward or city office and collect all the helpful information available. Don't forget to go to the health insurance and/or public health department counters as well, to pick up health-related brochures. Make a point of getting maps of your city and prefecture, even if they are in Japanese, as these often note hospitals and clinics. If the city office does not give you a free map, you can buy one at your local bookstore. By bike or car, locate the nearest large hospital and night/weekend emergency clinic, so that you are prepared if an emergency strikes. "Choosing a Caregiver and Using the System."

Resources are grouped together under the headings of Japan's eight regions and arranged in order from north to south. Resources covered include:

A. Organizations: Prefectural (pref.), city, or international (int'l) organizations which offer informational services, including hospital and clinic information, or general counseling to foreigners. Most have English-speaking staff.

B. Publications: Publications containing health information for the local area. May provide names of hospitals, clinics, English-speaking emergency clinics, public health centers, and/or sports facilities. Ask for such publications at the above organizations and at prefectural, city and ward offices.

C. Emergency Numbers: Organizations that provide telephone numbers for facilities offering emergency medical care during evenings, weekends, and holidays.

D. Web Sites: Some prefectures and cities have begun to put hospital information in English on their Internet web sites. A few URLs to try are: [http://www.pref.*the name of the pref*.jp] or [http://www.city.*the name of the city*.jp].

E. Major Hospitals: A few representative large hospitals in the area, listed alphabetically by prefecture. Most specialties are offered at the following types of hospitals, but always call ahead to check if your condition can be treated. **Medical University**: Ika Daigaku; **City**: Shiritsu; **National**: Kokuritsu; **Red Cross**: Sekijuji. **(T)** denotes a prefectural trauma center, where trauma specialists are on duty 24 hours a day. If the English name is listed, the hospital is mentioned elsewhere in this book. The name in **( )** denotes the shorter name by which the hospital is known locally. For specialty hospitals and clinics, look in the index under "Hospitals" or "Clinics," or turn to the relevant chapter or section of the book. For more extensive lists of local hospitals, ask at your city or ward office.

Hokkaido: Comparatively clean air. Does not have a rainy season. Less mold. Fewer allergens than in the rest of Japan. The best place to live if you have asthma.

A. Plaza i: 011-211-3678 Daily 9:00 A.M–5:30 P.M.

B. *Handbook for Daily Life* (Sapporo City)

C. Hokkaido Kenko Zukuri Zaidan: 011-232-5500 (J. only), during office hours. Will provide emergency info. tel. numbers in your area. **Dentists**: 011-511-7774 (J. only), 7:00 P.M.–7:00

A.M. **Sapporo Night Emergency Center:** 011-641-4316 (J. only) Daily 7:00 P.M.–7:00 A.M.

Asahikawa Sekijuji Byoin (T)
旭川赤十字病院
Akebono 1-jo, 1-chome, Asahikawa-shi
0166-22-8111

Hokkaido Daigaku Igakubu Fuzoku Byoin
(Hokudai Byoin)
北海道大学医学部附属病院
Nishi 5, Kita 14-jo, Kita-ku, Sapporo-shi
011-716-1161 http://soi/met/hokudai/ac/jp

Nikko Kinen Byoin 日鋼記念病院
1-5-13 Shintomi-cho, Muroran-shi
0143-24-1331

Sapporo Medical University Hospital
Sapporo Ika Daigaku Fuzoku Byoin
札幌医科大学付属病院
Nishi 16-291, Minami 1-jo, Chuo-ku
Sapporo-shi 011-611-2111

Shiritsu Hakodate Byoin (T)
市立函館病院
2-33 Yayoi-cho, Hakodate-shi
0138-23-8651

Shiritsu Kushiro Sogo Byoin (T)
市立釧路総合病院
1-12 Shunkodai, Kushiro-shi 0154-41-6121

Tohoku Region: Aomori, Iwate, Miyagi, Akita, Yamagata, Fukushima. Short summers and long winters. Lots of snow on the Japan Sea side. Great for skiers, not good for those with seasonal depression. Aomori is largely free from the rainy season.

A. Aomori Foundation for Advancing Int'l Relations: 0177-35-2221 Mon.–Fri. 8:30 A.M. –5:00 P.M.; **Coordinator for Int'l Relations, Mutsu City:** 0175-22-1111 (ext. 224) Mon.–Fri. 9:00 A.M.– 5:00 P.M.; **Akita Int'l Assoc.:** 0188-64-1181 Mon.–Fri. 9:00 A.M.–6:00 P.M.; **Miyagi Int'l Assoc.:** 022-275-3796 Mon.–Fri. 8:30 A.M. –5:15 P.M.; **Sendai Int'l Center** (Koryu Corner): 022-265-2471 Daily 9:00 A.M.–8:00 P.M.; **Sendai English Hotline:** 022-224-1919 Daily except 2nd Sun. 9:00 A.M.–8:00 P.M.; **Yamagata Information Services for Foreigners** (Pref.): 0236-24-9960 Mon.–Fri. 10:00 A.M.–5:00 P.M. (before

2:00 P.M. is better); **Fukushima Int'l Assoc.:** 0245-24-1315 Mon.–Fri. 10:00 A.M.–5:00 P.M.

B. *Health Guide to Aomori* (Pref.); *Life in Akita* (Pref.); *Hello Miyagi* (Pref.); *Sendai Hospitals and Clinics*; *Yamagata Living Guidebook*; *Guidebook for Living in Fukushima*; *A List of Medical Inst. (Hospitals) that Offer Medical Services in Foreign Languages* (Fukushima Pref.)

C. Sendai Emergency Treatment Information Center: 022-234-5099 (J. only)
7:30 P.M.– 6:00 A.M.

■ **AOMORI-KEN**
Aomori Kenritsu Chuo Byoin (T)
青森県立中央病院
2-1-1 Higashi-Tsukurimichi, Aomori-shi
0177-26-8111

Aomori Shimin Byoin
(Shimin Byoin) 青森市民病院
1-14-20 Katsuta, Aomori-shi
0177-34-2171

Hachinohe Sekijuji Byoin
(Sekijuji Byoin) 八戸赤十字病院
2 Nakaakedo, Tamonoki, Hachinohe-shi
0178-27-3111

Hirosaki Daigaku Igakubu Fuzoku Byoin
弘前大学医学部附属病院
53 Hon-cho, Hirosaki-shi
0172-33-5111 http://www.hirosaki-u.ac.jp

■ **IWATE-KEN**
Iwate Ika Daigaku Igakubu Fuzoku Byoin (T)
岩手医科大学医学部附属病院
19-1 Uchimaru, Morioka-shi
0196-51-5111 http://www.iwate-met.ac.jp

Morioka Sekijuji Byoin
(Nisseki Byoin) 盛岡赤十字病院
6-1-1 Sanbon-Yanagi, Morioka-shi
0196-37-3111

■ **MIYAGI-KEN**
Ishinomaki Sekijuji Byoin
(Nisseki Byoin) 石巻赤十字病院
1-7-10 Yoshino-cho, Ishinomaki-shi
0225-95-4131

Kokuritsu Sendai Byoin (T)
(Kokuritsu Byoin) 国立仙台病院
2-8-8 Miyagino, Miyagino-ku, Sendai-shi
022-293-1111

Sendai Sekijuji Byoin
(Nisseki Byoin) 仙台赤十字病院
2-43-3 Yagiyama-Honcho, Taihaku-ku, Sendai-shi
022-243-1111

Sendai Shiritsu Byoin Kyukyu Center (T)
仙台市立病院救急センター
3-1 Shimizukoji, Wakabayashi-ku, Sendai-shi
022-266-7111

Tohoku Daigaku Fuzoku Byoin
(Tohoku Idai Byoin)
東北大学医学部附属病院
1-1 Seiryo-machi, Aoba-ku, Sendai-shi
022-717-7000

■ **AKITA-KEN**
Akita Daigaku Igakubu Fuzoku Byoin
秋田大学医学部附属病院
1-1-1, Hondo, Akita-shi 0188-34-1111

Akita Sekijuji Byoin (T)
秋田赤十字病院
222-1 Naeshirozawa, Aza, Saruta, Kami-Kitade
Akita-shi 018-829-5000

■ **YAMAGATA-KEN**
Tsuruoka Shiritsu Sonai Byoin
(Sonai Byoin) 鶴岡市立荘内病院
2-1 Baba-cho, Tsuruoka-shi 0235-22-1515

Yamagata Daigaku Igakubu Fuzoku Byoin
山形大学医学部附属病院
2-2-2 Iida-Nishi, Yamagata-shi
0236-33-1122 http://www.id.yamagata-u.ac.jp/

Yamagata Kenritsu Chuo Byoin (T)
(Chuo Byoin) 山形県立中央病院
7-17 Sakura-cho, Yamagata-shi
0236-23-4011

Yamagata Shiritsu Byoin Saiseikan
(Shiritsu Byoin) 山形市立病院済生館
1-3-26 Nanoka-machi, Yamagata-shi
0236-25-5555

■ **FUKUSHIMA-KEN**
Fukushima Kenritsu Aizu Sogo Byoin
福島県立会津総合病院

10-75 Shiromae, Aizuwakamatsu-shi
0242-27-2151

**Fukushima Kenritsu Ika Daigaku Igakubu
Fuzoku Byoin** (Fukushima Dai Byoin)
福島県立医科大学医学部附属病院
1 Hikarigaoka, Fukushima-shi
0245-48-2111
http://www.fmu.ac.jp/welcome-s.html

Iwaki Shiritsu Sogo Iwaki Kyoritsu Byoin (T)
(Kyoritsu Byoin)
いわき市立総合磐城共立病院
16 Kusehara, Mimaya-machi, Uchigo, Iwaki-shi
0246-26-3151

Ota Sogo Byoin Fuzoku Ota Kinen Byoin (T)
太田総合病院附属太田記念病院
5-25 Naka-machi, Koriyama-shi 0249-25-0088

Kanto Region: Ibaraki, Tochigi, Gunma, Saitama, Chiba, Tokyo, Kanagawa. Chiba, Saitama and Kanagawa have the lowest number of hospital beds per 100,000 population, of any prefectures in Japan. The Tokyo-Yokohama metropolitan area has the greatest concentration of hospitals and health care personnel in the country. Tokyo has 109 dentists per 100,000 people vs. 49.7 for Saitama Prefecture.

A. Ibaraki Int'l Assoc. (Pref.): 029-244-3811 Mon.–Fri. 9:00 A.M.–5:00 P.M., 2nd and 4th Sat. 11:00 A.M. –3:00 P.M.; **Tochigi Int'l Lifeline (TILL)**: 028-621-7622 Tues.–Fri. 10:30 A.M.–3:30 P.M.; **Chiba Pref. Foreigners' Telephone Counseling Service**: 043-222-6652 Mon.–Fri. 9:00 A.M.–12:00 noon and 1:00–4:00 P.M.; **Kanagawa Pref. Counseling Center for Foreign Residents** (comprehensive list of doctors): 045-324-2299 Mon., Tues., Fri. 9:00 A.M.–4:00 P.M.; **Yokohama Community Lounge Information Corner (YOKE)**: 045-671-7209 Mon.–Fri. except 3rd Tues. 10:00 A.M.–4:00 P.M.; **Aoba (Yokohama) Int'l Lounge**: 045-971-2040 Tues. –Sun. 9:00 A.M.–9:00 P.M.; **Hodogaya (Yokohama) Int'l Exchange Center**: 045-337-0012 Tues.–Sun. 10:00 A.M.–8:00 P.M.; **Volunteer Ms. Takamatsu**: 045-413-3628 (will accompany to doctor; leave message); **Kawasaki Int'l Center Foreign Residents' Counseling Service**: 044-435-7000 Tues.–Sun. 9:00 A.M.–9:00 P.M.; **Tokyo Metropolitan Health and Medical**

Information Center (Himawari): see endpapers; **AMDA Int'l Med. Information Center (Tokyo)**, see endpapers; **Tokyo Family Network**, see page 236; **Tokyo Foreign Residents' Advisory Center:** 03-5320-7744 Mon.–Fri. 9:30 A.M.–noon and 1:00–4:00 P.M.

B. *Ibaraki Pref. Medical Handbook; Ibaraki Pref. Gaikokujin Iryo Kyoryokusha List* (List of doctors); *Urawa City Guide Book for Foreign Residents; Guide to Living in Yokohama; Hello Kanagawa* (3x a year); *Tamatebako and Seikatsu Mini Joho* (monthly, for Yokohama); *Guidebook for Friendly Exchanges* (Kawasaki); *A Guide to Emergency Medical Treatment in Tokyo;* Tokyo city and ward publications.

C. Ibaraki Pref. Emergency Medical Care Information Control Center: 029-241-4199 (J. only); **Saitama Emergency Medical Information Center** (no dentists): 048-824-4199 (J. only) 24 hrs.; **Chiba Pref. Emergency Hospital Information Service**: 043-279-2211 (J. only) 24 hrs.; **Tokyo Fire Department Disaster and Emergency Information**: 03-3212-2323 (within 23 wards) and 042-521-2323 (outside 23 wards), (in both J. and Eng.) 24 hrs.; **Yokohama Emergency Medical Information Center**: 045-201-1199 (J. only) 24 hrs.

D. Yokohama City web site:
[http://www.city.yokohama.jp/]

■ IBARAKI-KEN
Hitachi Seisakusho Hitachi Sogo Byoin
日立製作所日立総合病院
2-1-1 Jyonan-cho, Hitachi-shi
0294-23-1111

Kokuritsu Mito Byoin (T)
国立水戸病院
3-2-1 Higashihara, Mito-shi 0292-31-5211

Tsuchiura Kyodo Byoin (T)
土浦協同病院
11-7 Shinmachi, Manabe, Tsuchiura-shi
0298-23-3111

Tsukuba Daigaku Byoin
筑波大学附属病院
2-1-1 Amakubo, Tsukuba-shi
0298-53-3900 http://www.sec.tsukuba.ac.jp

■ TOCHIGI-KEN
Dokkyo Ika Daigaku Byoin
獨協医科大学病院
880 Oaza Kita Kobayashi, Mibu-machi
Shimotsuga-gun
0282-86-1111

Kokuritsu Tochigi Byoin
国立栃木病院
1-10-37 Nakatomatsuri, Utsunomiya-shi
0286-22-5241

Oyama Shimin Byoin
小山市民病院
1-1-5 Wakaki-cho, Oyama-shi
0285-21-3800

Saisei-kai Utsunomiya Byoin (T)
済生会宇都宮病院
911-1 Takebayashi, Utsunomiya-shi
028-626-5500

■ GUNMA-KEN
Fuji Jukogyo Kenko Hoken Kumiai Sogo Ota Byoin
富士重工業健康保険組合総合太田病院
29-5 Hachiman-cho, Ota-shi 0276-22-6631

Gunma Daigaku Igakubu Fuzoku Byoin
(Gundai Byoin) 群馬大学医学部附属病院
3-39-15 Showa-machi, Maebashi-shi
027-220-7111
http://www.gunma-u.ac.jp/index-j.html

Kokuritsu Takasaki Byoin (T)
国立高崎病院
36 Takamatsu-cho, Takasaki-shi
0273-22-5901

■ SAITAMA-KEN
Boei Medical University Hospital
Boei Ika Daigakko Byoin
(Boei Idai Byoin) 防衛医科大学校病院
3-2 Namiki, Tokorozawa-shi
0429-95-1511

Dokkyo Ika Daigaku Koshigaya Byoin
獨協医科大学越谷病院
2-1-50 Minami Koshigaya, Koshigaya-shi
0489-65-1111

National Saitama Hospital
Kokuritsu Saitama Byoin

国立埼玉 病院
2-1 Suwa, Wako-shi 048-462-1101

Omiya Sekijuji Byoin (T)
大宮赤十字病院
8-3-33 Kami-Ochiai, Yono-shi
048-852-1111

Saitama Ika Daigaku Fuzoku Byoin
(Saitama Idai Fuzoku Byoin)
埼玉 医科大学附属病院
38 Moro Hongo, Moroyama-machi, Iruma-gun
0492-76-1127 http://www.saitama-med.ac.jp/

Saitama Ika Daigaku Sogo Iryo Center (T)
埼玉 医科大学総合医療センター
1981 Kamoda, Kawagoe-shi 0492-25-7811

■ **CHIBA-KEN**
Chiba Daigaku Igakubu Fuzoku Byoin
(Chiba Dai Byoin) 千葉大学医学部附属病院
1-8-1 Inohana, Chuo-ku, Chiba-shi
043-222-7171

Kameda General Hospital (T)
(Kameda Sogo Byoin)
医療法人鉄薫会亀田総合病院
929 Higashi-cho, Kamogawa-shi
0470-92-2211

Juntendo Daigaku Igakubu Fuzoku Juntendo Urayasu Byoin
(Juntendo Daigaku Urayasu Byoin)
順天堂大学医学部附属順天堂浦安病院
2-1-1 Tomioka, Urayasu-shi 0473-53-3111

Narita Sekijuji Byoin (T)
(Nisseki Byoin) 成田赤十字病院
90-1 Iida-cho, Narita-shi 0476-22-2311

Tokyo Dental University Ichikawa General Hospital
Tokyo Shika Daigaku Ichikawa Sogo Byoin
東京歯科大学市川総合病院
5-11-13 Sugano, Ichikawa-shi
0473-22-0151

■ **TOKYO**
International Medical Center Japan
Kokuritsu Kokusai Iryo Center
国立国際医療センター
1-21-1 Toyama, Shinjuku-ku
03-3202-7181 http://www.imcj.go.jp

Japanese Red Cross Medical Center
Nihon Sekijuji Iryo Center (Nisseki Iryo Center)
日本赤十字社医療センター
4-1-22 Hiroo, Shibuya-ku
03-3400-1311

Jikei Medical University Hospital
Tokyo Jikei Ika Daigaku Fuzoku Byoin
(Jikei Idai Byoin)
東京慈恵会医科大学附属病院
3-19-18 Nishi-Shimbashi, Minato-ku
03-3433-1111

Juntendo University Hospital
Juntendo Daigaku Igakubu Fuzoku Juntendo Iin
順天堂大学医学部附属順天堂医院
3-1-3 Hongo, Bunkyo-ku
03-3813-3111

Keio University Hospital
Keiogijuku Daigaku Byoin (Keio Byoin)
慶應義塾大学病院
35 Shinano-machi, Shinjuku-ku
03-3353-1211

Kokuritsu Byoin Tokyo Iryo Center (T)
国立病院東京医療センター
2-5-1 Higashigaoka, Meguro-ku
03-3411-0111

Kokuritsu Byoin Tokyo Saigai Iryo Center
国立病院東京災害医療センター
3256 Midori-cho, Tachikawa-shi
042-526-5511

Mitsui Memorial Hospital
Mitsui Kinen Byoin 三井記念病院
1 Kanda Izumi-cho, Chiyoda-ku
03-3862-9111

Seibo International Catholic Hospital
Seibo-kai Seibo Byoin 聖母会聖母病院
2-5-1 Naka-Ochiai, Shinjuku-ku
03-3951-1111

Shisei-Kai Second Hospital
Shisei-Kai Daini Byoin 至誠会第二病院
5-19-1 Kami-Soshigaya, Setagaya-ku
03-3300-0366

Showa University Hospital
Showa Daigaku Byoin 昭和大学病院
1-5-8 Hatanodai, Shinagawa-ku
03-3784-8000

St. Luke's International Hospital
Seiroka Kokusai Byoin 聖路加国際病院
9-1 Akashi-cho, Chuo-ku 03-3541-5151

Teikyo University Hospital (T)
Teikyo Daigaku Igakubu Fuzoku Byoin
帝京大学医学部付属病院
2-11-1 Kaga, Itabashi-ku
03-3964-1211
http://www-admin@teikyo-u.ac.jp

Toho University Omori Hospital (T)
Toho Daigaku Igakubu Fuzoku Omori Byoin
東邦大学医学部附属大森病院
6-11-1 Omori-Nishi, Ota-ku
03-3762-4151

Tokai University Hospital
Tokai Daigaku Igakubu Fuzoku Tokyo Byoin
東海大学医学部付属東京病院
1-2-5 Yoyogi, Shibuya-ku 03-3370-2321

Tokyo Adventist Hospital
Tokyo Eisei Byoin 東京衛生病院
3-17-3 Amanuma, Suginami-ku
03-3392-6151

Tokyo University Hospital
Tokyo Daigaku Igakubu Fuzoku Byoin
(Todai Byoin) 東京大学医学部附属病院
7-3-1 Hongo, Bunkyo-ku
03-3815-5411 http://www.cc.h.u-tokyo.ac.jp/

Tokyo Metropolitan Otsuka Hospital
Tokyo Toritsu Otsuka Byoin
東京都立大塚病院
2-8-1 Minami-Otsuka , Toshima-ku
03-3941-3211

Tokyo Metropolitan Fuchu Hospital (T)
Tokyo Toritsu Fuchu Byoin
東京都立府中病院
2-9-2 Musashidai, Fuchu-shi
0423-23-5111

Tokyo Toritsu Hiroo Byoin (T)
東京都立広尾病院
2-34-10 Ebisu, Shibuya-ku 03-3444-1181

Tokyo Metropolitan Komagome Hospital
Tokyo Toritsu Komagome Byoin
東京都立駒込病院
3-18-22 Hon-Komagome, Bunkyo-ku
03-3823-2101

Tokyo Women's Medical University Hospital (T)
Tokyo Joshi Ika Daigaku Byoin (Joshi Idai)
東京女子医科大学病院
8-1 Kawada-cho, Shinjuku-ku
03-3353-8111

Tokyo Women's Medical University Second Hospital
Tokyo Joshi Ika Daigaku Fuzoku Daini Byoin
(Tokyo Joshi Idai Daini Byoin)
東京女子医科大学附属第二病院
2-1-10 Nishi-Ogu, Arakawa-ku
03-3810-1111

Toranomon Hospital
Kokka Komuin Kyosai Kumiai Rengo-kai Toranomon Byoin
国家公務員共済組合連合会虎の門病院
2-2-2 Toranomon, Minato-ku
03-3588-1111

■**KANAGAWA-KEN**
Kitazato University Hospital (T)
Kitazato Daigaku Byoin 北里大学病院
1-15-1 Kitazato, Sagamihara-shi
0427-78-8111

Kokuritsu Sagamihara Byoin
国立相模原病院
18-1 Sakuradai, Sagamihara-shi
0427-42-8311

Kokuritsu Yokohama Byoin (T)
国立横浜病院
252 Harajuku-cho, Totsuka-ku, Yokohama-shi
045-851-2621

Kokuritsu Yokosuka Byoin
国立横須賀病院
2-36 Uwa-machi, Yokosuka-shi
0468-22-2630

Nihon Ika Daigaku Fuzoku Daini Byoin
日本医科大学付属第二病院
1-396 Kosugi-cho, Nakahara-ku, Kawasaki-shi
044-733-5181

Sei Marianna Ika Daigaku Toyoko Byoin
聖マリアンナ医科大学東横病院
3-435 Kosugi-cho, Nakahara-ku, Kawasaki-shi
044-722-2121

Sei Marianna Ika Daigaku Yokohama-shi Seibu Byoin (T)
聖マリアンナ医科大学横浜市西部病院
1197-1 Yazashi-cho, Asahi-ku, Yokohama-shi
045-366-1111

Sei Marianna Medical University Hospital (T)
Sei Marianna Ika Daigaku Byoin
聖マリアンナ医科大学病院
2-16-1 Sugao, Miyamae-ku, Kawasaki-shi
044-977-8111

Shonan Kamakura General Hospital
Shonan Kamakura Sogo Byoin
湘南鎌倉総合病院
1202-1 Yamazaki, Kamakura-shi
0467-46-1717

Tokai Daigaku Igakubu Fuzoku Byoin (T)
(Tokai Dai Fuzoku Byoin)
東海大学医学部附属病院
143 Shimo-Kasuya, Isehara-shi
0463-93-1121

Chubu Region: Niigata, Toyama, Ishikawa, Fukui, Yamanashi, Nagano, Gifu, Shizuoka, Aichi. A largely mountainous region including Mt. Fuji, great for hiking and outdoor vacations. But the industrial zones along the Pacific side produce smog and pollute the ocean water. Hospital patients in Nagano Prefecture are discharged more quickly than in other parts of Japan. Fukui was named the best place to live in Japan from 1991–96. Ishikawa was second and Nagano third. Medical care in Fukui had the highest rating because of the availability of facilities for the disabled and the elderly.

A. Niigata Int'l Exchange Division (Pref.): 025-283-3372 Mon.–Fri. 8:30 A.M.–5:15 P.M.; **Toyama Int'l Center**: 0764-44-2500 Mon.–Fri. 9:00 A.M.–6:00 P.M.; **Ishikawa Foundation for Int'l Exchange**: 0762-62-5931 Mon.–Fri. 9:00 A.M.–5:00 P.M.; **Fukui Int'l Assoc.**: 0776-28-8818 Tues.–Sun. 9:00 A.M.–5:00 P.M.; **Yamanashi Int'l Exchange Center**: 0552-28-5419 Tues.–Sun. 9:00 A.M.–5:00 P.M; **Gifu Int'l Center**: 058-277-1013 Mon.–Fri. 10:00 A.M.–4:00 P.M.; **Aichi-ken Int'l Exchange Assoc.**: 052-961-7902 Mon.–Thurs. 10:00 A.M.–6:00 P.M., Fri. until 8:00 P.M.; **Nagoya Int'l Center Information Counter**:

052-581-0100 Tues.–Sat. 9:00 A.M.–8:30 P.M., Sun. and hols. until 5:00 P.M.

B. *Niigata: A Prefectural Living Guide; Toyama Life Handbook* (Pref.); *Ishikawa Medical Handbook* (Pref.); *Fukui Pref. List of Hospitals and Doctors; Yamanashi Dental Clinics; A Living Guide for Foreign Residents in Yamanashi* (Pref.); *A Guide to Living in Gifu* (City); *Gifu Prefectural Guidebook; Nagoya Living Guide.*

C. Nagoya Emergency Treatment Information Center: 052-263-1133 (J.only) 24 hrs.

■ **NIIGATA-KEN**
Nagaoka Sekijuji Byoin (T)
長岡赤十字病院
297-1 Terashima-machi, Nagaoka-shi
0258-28-3600

Niigata Daigaku Igakubu Fuzoku Byoin
新潟大学医学部附属病院
1-754 Asahi-machi Dori , Niigata-shi
025-223-6161

Niigata Shimin Byoin (T)
新潟市民病院
2-6-1 Shichikuyama, Niigata-shi
025-241-5151

■ **TOYAMA-KEN**
Takaoka Shimin Byoin
高岡市民病院
4-1 Takara-machi, Takaoka-shi
0766-23-0204

Toyama Kenritsu Chuo Byoin (T)
富山県立中央病院
2-2-78 Nishi-Nagae, Toyama-shi
0764-24-1531

Toyama Sekijuji Byoin
富山赤十字病院
2-1-58 Ushijima-honmachi, Toyama-shi
0764-33-2222

■ **ISHIKAWA-KEN**
Ishikawa Kenritsu Chuo Byoin (T)
石川県立中央病院
153 Nu Minami Shinbo-machi, Kanazawa-shi
0762-37-8211

Kanazawa Daigaku Igakubu Fuzoku Byoin
金沢大学医学部附属病院
13-1 Takara-machi, Kanazawa-shi
076-265-2000

Kanazawa Ika Daigaku Byoin
金沢医科大学病院
1-1 Daigaku, Uchinada-machi, Kahoku-gun
0762-86-2211 http://www.kanazawa-med.ac.jp

Komatsu Shimin Byoin
小松市民病院
60 Ho, Mukaimotoori-machi, Komatsu-shi
0761-22-7111

■**FUKUI-KEN**
Fukui Ika Daigaku Byoin
福井医科大学医学部附属病院
23-3 Shimoaizuki, Matsuoka-cho, Yoshida-gun
0776-61-3111

Fukui Kenritsu Byoin (T)
福井県立病院
2-8-1 Yotsui, Fukui-shi 0776-54-5151

Fukui Sekijuji Byoin
福井赤十字病院
2-4-1 Tsukimi, Fukui-shi 0776-36-3630

■**YAMANASHI-KEN**
Fujiyoshida Shiritsu Byoin
富士吉田市立病院
2-8-1 Midorigaoka, Fujiyoshida-shi
0555-22-4111

Kofu Kyoritsu Byoin
甲府共立病院
1-9-1 Takara, Kofu-shi 0552-26-3131

Yamanashi Kenritsu Chuo Byoin (T)
山梨県立中央病院
1-1-1 Fujimi, Kofu-shi 0552-53-7111

■**NAGANO-KEN**
Nagano Sekijuji Byoin (T)
長野赤十字病院
1512-1 Wakasato, Nagano-shi
0262-26-4131

Saku Sogo Byoin (T)
佐久総合病院
197 Oaza Usuda, Usuda-machi, Minamisaku-gun
0267-82-3131

Shinshu Daigaku Igakubu Fuzoku Byoin
(Shin Dai Byoin) 信州大学医学部附属病院
3-1-1 Asahi, Matsumoto-shi 0263-35-4600

Showa Inan Sogo Byoin (T)
昭和伊南総合病院
3230 Akaho, Komagane-shi 0265-82-2121

■**GIFU-KEN**
Gifu Kenritsu Gifu Byoin (T)
岐阜県立岐阜病院
4-6-1 Noisshiki, Gifu-shi 0582-46-1111

Gifu Kenritsu Tajimi Byoin (T)
岐阜県立多治見病院
5-161 Maebata-cho, Tajimi-shi
0572-22-5311

Takayama Sekijuji Byoin
高山赤十字病院
3-11 Tenman-machi, Takayama-shi
0577-32-1111

Tokai Chuo Byoin
東海中央病院
4-6-2 Sohara-Higashijima-cho, Kagamigahara-shi
0583-82-3101

■**SHIZUOKA-KEN**
Fuji Shiritsu Chuo Byoin
富士市立中央病院
50 Takashima-cho, Fuji-shi 0545-52-1131

Hamamatsu Ika Daigaku Igakubu Fuzoku Byoin
浜松医科大学医学部附属病院
3600 Handa-cho, Hamamatsu-shi
053-435-2111 http://www.hama-med.ac.jp.

Shimizu Kosei Byoin
清水厚生病院
578-1 Ihara-cho, Shimizu-shi 0543-66-3333

Shizuoka Kenritsu Sogo Byoin
静岡県立総合病院
4-27-1 Kita-Ando, Shizuoka-shi
0542-47-6111

■**AICHI-KEN**
Aichi Ika Daigaku Fuzoku Byoin (T)
愛知医科大学附属病院
21 Aza Karimata, Oaza Yazako, Nagakute-cho
Aichi-gun 0561-62-3311

Kokuritsu Toyohashi Byoin
国立豊橋病院
100 Aza Nakahara, Nakano-cho, Toyohashi-shi
0532-45-6121

Nagoya Daigaku Igakubu Fuzoku Byoin
名古屋大学医学部附属病院
65 Tsurumai-cho, Showa-ku, Nagoya-shi
052-741-2111

Toyota Kinen Byoin
トヨタ記念病院
1-1 Heiwa-cho, Toyoda-shi 0565-28-0100

Kinki Region: Mie, Shiga, Kyoto, Osaka, Hyogo, Nara, Wakayama. Osaka is the second smallest prefecture (fu) in land area, but is second only to Tokyo in population; crowded!

A. Mie Int'l Exchange Foundation (Pref.): 059-223-5006 Mon.–Thurs. 8:30 A.M.–5:15 P.M.; **Nagoya Int'l Center**: 052-581-0100 Tues.–Sat. 9:00 A.M.–8:30 P.M., Sun. and hol. until 5:00 P.M.; **Shiga Int'l Friendship Assoc.** (Pref.): 0775-26-0931 Mon.–Fri. 8:15 A.M.–5:00 P.M.; **Kyoto City Int'l Community House**: 075-752-3010 Tues.–Sun. 9:00 A.M.– 9:00 P.M.; **Osaka Information Services for Foreign Residents** (Pref.): 06-941-2297 Mon.–Fri. 9:00 A.M.–5:00 P.M.; **INTERMEDIX** (Japan Educational Clinical Cardiology Society): 06-309-7535 Mon., Tues., Wed., Fri. 9:00 A.M.–5:00 P.M.; **AMDA Int'l Med. Information Center (Kansai)**, see endpapers; **Community House and Information Center-Kobe (CHIC)** 078-857-6540 Mon.–Fri. 9:30 A.M.–4:30 P.M. Sept.–June; **Nara Int'l Foundation Commemorating the Silk Road Exposition**: 0742-27-2436 Tues.–Sat. 10:00 A.M.–6:00 P.M.; **Wakayama Pref. Int'l Exchange Division** (Int'l Center open from Dec. '98) 0734-31-4344 Mon.–Thurs. 9:00 A.M.–5:45 P.M., Fri. until noon.

B. *Easy Living in Kyoto* (City); *Medical Passport* (Osaka Pref.); *Medical Access: A Foreigner's Guide to Health Care in Kobe* (order from CHIC); *Wakayama Pref. Medical Guide.*

■ MIE-KEN
Keio Gijuku Daigaku Ise Keio Byoin
(Keio Byoin) 慶應義塾大学伊勢慶應病院
2-7-28 Tokiwa, Ise-shi 0596-22-1155

Mie University Hospital
Mie Daigaku Igakubu Fuzoku Byoin
三重大学医学部附属病院
2-174 Edobashi, Tsu-shi
0592-32-1111

Mie Kenritsu Sogo Iryo Center
三重県立総合医療センター
5450-132 Oazahin, Yokkaichi-shi
0593-45-2321

Yamada Sekijuji Byoin (T)
山田赤十字病院
810 Takabuku, Misonomura, Watarai-gun
0596-28-2171

■ SHIGA-KEN
Hikone Shiritsu Byoin
彦根市立病院
2-1-45 Hon-machi, Hikone-shi
0749-22-6050

Otsu Sekijuji Byoin (T)
大津赤十字病院
1-1-35 Nagara, Otsu-shi 0775-22-4131

Seiko-kai Kusatsu Sogo Byoin
誠光会草津総合病院
4-2-31 Kamigasa, Kusatsu-shi
0775-63-8866

Shiga Ika Daigaku Igakubu Fuzoku Byoin
滋賀医科大学医学部附属病院
Seta Tsukinowa-cho, Otsu-shi
0775-48-2111

■ KYOTO-FU
Japan Baptist Hospital
Nihon Baputisuto Byoin 日本バプテスト病院
47 Kita-Shirakawa Yamanomoto-cho, Sakyo-ku
Kyoto-shi 075-781-5191

Kyoto Daigaku Igakubu Fuzoku Byoin
(Kyoto Daigaku Byoin)
京都大学医学部附属病院
54 Shogoin Kawahara-cho, Sakyo-ku, Kyoto-shi
075-751-3111 http://www.kuhp.kyoto-u.ac.jp/

Kyoto Daini Sekijuji Byoin (T)
(Daini Sekijuji Byoin) 京都第二赤十字病院
355-5 Haruobi-cho, Marutamachi-agaru, Kamanza-dori, Kamigyo-ku, Kyoto-shi
075-231-5171

Kyoto Furitsu Medical University Hospital
Kyoto Furitsu Ika Daigaku Fuzoku Byoin
京都府立医科大学附属病院
465 Kajii-cho, Hirokoji Agaru, Kawaramachi-dori
Kamigyo-ku, Kyoto-shi 075-251-5111

■ **OSAKA-FU**
Kokuritsu Osaka Byoin (T)
国立大阪病院
2-1-14 Hoenzaka, Chuo-ku, Osaka-shi
06-942-1331 http://www.onh.go.jp/onh-e.html

Osaka Daigaku Igakubu Fuzoku Byoin
大阪大学医学部付属病院
1-1-50 Fukushima, Fukushima-ku, Osaka-shi
06-879-5111

Osaka Ika Daigaku Fuzoku Byoin
大阪医科大学附属病院
2-7 Daigaku-cho, Takatsuki-shi 0726-83-1221

Osaka Shiritsu Daigaku Igakubu Fuzoku Byoin
(Shiritsu Dai Byoin)
大阪市立大学医学部附属病院
1-5-7 Asahi-machi, Abeno-ku, Osaka-shi
06-645-2121
http://www.med.osaka-cu.ac.jp/hosp/

Yodogawa Christian Hospital
Yodogawa Kirisutokyo Byoin
淀川キリスト教病院
2-9-26 Awaji, Higashi-Yodogawa-ku, Osaka-shi
06-322-2250

■ **HYOGO-KEN**
Hyogo Ika Daigaku Byoin (T)
兵庫医科大学病院
1-1 Mukogawa-cho, Nishinomiya-shi
0798-45-6111

Kobe Adventist Hospital
Kobe Adobentisuto Byoin
神戸アドベンティスト病院
8-4-1 Arino-dai, Kita-ku, Kobe-shi
078-981-0161

Kobe Kaisei Hospital
Iryo Hojin Kobe Kaisei Byoin
医療法人神戸海星病院
3-11-15 Shinoharakita-machi, Nada-ku, Kobe-shi
078-871-5201

Kobe Shiritsu Chuo Shimin Byoin
(Shimin Byoin) 神戸市立中央市民病院
4-6 Naka-machi, Minatojima, Chuo-ku, Kobe-shi
078-302-4321

Kobe University Hospital
Kobe Daigaku Igakubu Fuzoku Byoin
神戸大学医学部附属病院
7-5-1 Kusunoki-cho, Chuo-ku, Kobe-shi
078-341-7451

Konan Hospital
Konan Byoin 甲南病院
1-5-16 Kamokogahara, Higashi-Nada-ku, Kobe-shi
078-851-2161

Koritsu Toyooka Byoin (T)
公立豊岡病院
6-35 Tachino-cho, Toyooka-shi
0796-22-6111

Rokko Island Hospital
Zaidanhojin, Konan Byoin, Rokko Airando Byoin
財団法人甲南病院六甲アイランド病院
2-11 Koyo-cho Naka, Higashi-Nada-ku, Kobe-shi
078-858-1111

■ **NARA-KEN**
Kokuritsu Nara Byoin
国立奈良病院
1-50-1 Higashi-Kidera-cho, Nara-shi
0742-24-1251

Nara Kenritsu Nara Byoin (T)
(Kenritsu Byoin) 奈良県立奈良病院
1-30-1 Hiramatsu-cho, Nara-shi
0742-46-6001

Tenri Yorozu Sodan-sho Byoin
天理よろづ相談所病院
200 Mishima-cho, Tenri-shi
07436-3-5611

■ **WAKAYAMA-KEN**
Kokuritsu Minami Wakayama Byoin
国立南和歌山病院
27-1 Takinai-cho, Tanabe-shi 0739-26-7050

Nippon Sekijujisha Wakayama Iryo Center (T)
日本赤十字社和歌山医療センター
4-20 Komatsubara-dori, Wakayama-shi
0734-22-4171

Shingu Shiritsu Shimin Byoin
新宮市立市民病院
451 Shingu, Shingu-shi 0735-22-6265

Wakayama Kenritsu Ika Daigaku Fuzoku Byoin
(Kenritsu Fuzoku Byoin)
和歌山県立医科大学附属病院
7-27 Wakayama-shi 0734-31-2151

Chugoku Region: Tottori, Shimane, Okayama, Hiroshima, Yamaguchi. Shimane has the fewest pharmacies (186) of any prefecture and the highest number of elderly householders, followed by Yamaguchi. Yamaguchi has the longest hospital stays.

A. Shimane (Pref.) Int'l Center 0852-31-5056 Mon.–Fri. 8:30 A.M.–7:00 P.M., Sat.–Sun. until 5:00 P.M.; **Okayama Pref. Int'l Exchange Foundation's Information Services**: 086-256-2914/5 Tues.–Sun. 9:00 A.M.–5:00 P.M.; **Hiroshima Int'l Center**: 082-541-3777 Tues.–Sat. 9:00 A.M.–8:30 P.M., Sun. 9:30 A.M.–6:00 P.M.; **Yamaguchi Int'l Exchange Assoc.** (Pref.): 0839-28-8000 Mon.–Fri. 8:30 A.M.–5:15 P.M.

B. *Shimane Handbook* (Pref.); *Yamaguchi Living Guidebook* (Pref.).

C. Emergency Medical Facilities, Hiroshima 0120-169-912 (toll-free from within pref.) Mon.–Sat. 6:00–9:00 P.M., Sun. and hols. 24 hours; **Hiroshima Hint for Health** 0120-169-913 (toll-free from within pref.).

D. **Hiroshima Pref. web site**:
http://www.qq.pref.hiroshima.jp

■ **TOTTORI-KEN**
Kokuritsu Yonago Byoin
(Kokuritsu Byoin) 国立米子病院
1293-1 Kuzumo, Yonago-shi 0859-33-7111

Tottori Daigaku Igakubu Fuzoku Byoin
鳥取大学医学部附属病院
36-1 Nishi-machi, Yonago-shi
0859-33-1111

Tottori Kenritsu Chuo Byoin (T)
鳥取県立中央病院
730 Ezu, Tottori-shi 0857-26-2271

Tottori Sekijuji Byoin
鳥取赤十字病院
117 Shotoku-cho, Tottori-shi
0857-24-8111

■ **SHIMANE-KEN**
Matsue Shiritsu Byoin
(Shiritsu Byoin) 松江市立病院
101 Nada-machi, Matsue-shi
0852-23-1000

Shimane Ika Daigaku Igakubu Fuzoku Byoin
島根医科大学医学部附属病院
89-1 Enya-cho, Izumo-shi
0853-23-2111 http://www.shimane-med.ac.jp

Shimane Kenritsu Chuo Byoin (T)
(Chuo Byoin) 島根県立中央病院
116 Imaichi-cho, Izumo-shi 0853-22-5111

■ **OKAYAMA-KEN**
Kawasaki Ika Daigaku Fuzoku Byoin (T)
川崎医科大学附属病院
577 Matsushima, Kurashiki-shi 0864-62-1111

Okayama Daigaku Igakubu Fuzoku Byoin
岡山大学医学部附属病院
2-5-1 Shikata-cho, Okayama-shi
0862-23-7151

Sogo Byoin Okayama Sekijuji Byoin (T)
総合病院岡山赤十字病院
65-1 Aoe, Okayama-shi
0862-22-8811

Tsuyama Jihukai Tsuyama Chuo Byoin
(Chuo Byoin)
財団法人津山滋風会津山中央病院
67 Nikai-machi, Tsuyama-shi 0868-22-6111

■ **HIROSHIMA-KEN**
Hiroshima Tetsudo Byoin
広島鉄道病院
3-1-36 Futabanosato, Higashi-ku, Hiroshima-shi
082-262-1170

Hiroshima University Hospital
Hiroshima Daigaku Igakubu Fuzoku Byoin
(Daigaku Byoin)
広島大学医学部附属病院
1-2-3 Kasumi, Minami-ku, Hiroshima-shi
082-257-5555

Kokuritsu Kure Byoin (T)
国立呉病院
3-1 Aoyama-cho, Kure-shi 0823-22-3111

Shakai Hoken Hiroshima Shimin Byoin (T)
(Shimin Byoin) 社会保険広島市民病院
7-33 Moto-machi, Naka-ku, Hiroshima-shi
082-221-2291

■ **YAMAGUCHI-KEN**
Kokuritsu Iwakuni Byoin (T)
国立岩国病院
2-5-1 Kuroiso-machi, Iwakuni-shi
0827-31-7121

Saisei-kai Yamaguchi Sogo Byoin
済生会山口総合病院
2-11 Midori-machi, Yamaguchi-shi
0839-22-2430

Shimonoseki Shiritsu Chuo Byoin
(Chuo Byoin) 下関市立中央病院
1-13-1 Koyo-cho, Shimonoseki-shi
0832-31-4111

Yamaguchi Daigaku Igakubu Fuzoku Byoin
山口大学医学部附属病院
1144 Owada Kogushi, Ube-shi
0836-22-2111

Shikoku Region: Tokushima, Kagawa, Ehime, Kochi. Kochi has the largest number of hospital beds per 100,000 population and the longest average hospital stays, as well as a large number of elderly householders.

A. Tokushima Pref. Int'l Assoc. 0886-56-3303 daily 10:00 A.M.–6:00 P.M.; **Kagawa Int'l Exchange Center**: 0878-37-5901 Tues.–Sun. 9:00 A.M.–6:00 P.M.

B. *Welcome to Tokushima* (Pref.)

■ **TOKUSHIMA-KEN**
Kenko Hoken Naruto Byoin
健康保険鳴門病院
32-1 Aza Kotani Kurosaki, Muya-cho, Naruto-shi
0886-85-2191

Tokushima Daigaku Igakubu Fuzoku Byoin
徳島大学医学部附属病院
2-50-1 Kuramoto-cho, Tokushima-shi
0886-31-3111 http://www.tokushima-u.ac.jp

Tokushima Kenritsu Chuo Byoin (T)
(Chuo Byoin) 徳島県立中央病院
1-10-3 Kuramoto-cho, Tokushima-shi
0886-31-7151

■ **KAGAWA-KEN**
Kagawa Ika Daigaku Igakubu Fuzoku Byoin
(Kagawa Idai) 香川医科大学医学部附属病院
1750-1 Oaza Ikenobe, Miki-cho, Kita-gun
087-898-5111

Kagawa Kenritsu Chuo Byoin (T)
(Chuo Byoin) 香川県立中央病院
5-4-16 Ban-cho, Takamatsu-shi 0878-35-2222

Takamatsu Sekijuji Byoin
(Nisseki) 高松赤十字病院
4-1-3 Ban-cho, Takamatsu-shi 0878-31-7101

■ **EHIME-KEN**
Ehime Daigaku Igakubu Fuzoku Byoin
愛媛大学医学部附属病院
Shitsukawa, Shigenobu-cho, Onsen-gun
0899-64-5111

Ehime Kenritsu Chuo Byoin (T)
愛媛県立中央病院
83 Kasuga-machi, Matsuyama-shi
0899-47-1111

Sogo Byoin Matsuyama Sekijuji Byoin
(Nisseki Byoin) 総合病院松山赤十字病院
1 Bunkyo-cho, Matsuyama-shi 0899-24-1111

Juzen Sogo Byoin
積善会附属十全総合病院
1-5 Kita-Shin-machi, Niihama-shi
0897-33-1818

■ **KOCHI-KEN**
Kochi Ika Daigaku Igakubu Fuzoku Byoin
高知医科大学医学部附属病院
Konasu, Oko-cho, Nankoku-shi 0888-66-5811

Kochi Sekijuji Byoin
高知赤十字病院
2-13-51 Shinhon-machi, Kochi-shi
0888-22-1201

Kochi Shiritsu Shimin Byoin
(Shimin Byoin) 高知市立市民病院
1-7-45 Marunouchi, Kochi-shi
0888-22-6111

Tosa Shiritsu Tosa Shimin Byoin
土佐市立土佐市民病院
1867 Ko, Takaoka-cho, Tosa-shi 0888-52-2151

Kyushu Region: Fukuoka, Saga, Nagasaki, Kumamoto, Oita, Miyazaki, Kagoshima, Okinawa. Okinawa is a pretty healthy place to live. It has the lowest incidence in Japan of death from cancer, heart disease, cardiovascular disease, or kidney failure. It has the most residents aged 100 years or above. It also has the highest birthrate, 1.87, vs. 1.1 for women in Tokyo (1995 census).

A. Kitakyushu Int'l Assoc.: 093-662-0055 Tues.–Sun. 9:00 A.M.–5:30 P.M.; **Saga Pref. Int'l Exchange**: 095-225-7004 Mon.–Fri. 9:00 A.M.–5:00 P.M.; **Nagasaki Int'l Assoc.** (Pref.): 0958-23-3931 Mon.–Fri. 9:00 A.M.–5:30 P.M.; **Kumamoto Pref. Int'l Affairs Division** 096-383-1502 Mon.–Fri. 9:15 A.M.–5:15 P.M.; **Oita Pref. Int'l Center**: 0975-38-5161 Mon.–Fri. 9:00 A.M.–5:00 P.M., 1st and 3rd Sat. until 12:30; **Miyazaki Int'l Center**: 0985-32-8457 Mon.–Fri. 8:30 A.M.–5:15 P.M.; **Int'l Exchange Plaza** (Kagoshima Pref.) 099-225-3279 Mon.–Sat. 9:00 A.M.–5:30 P.M.

B. *1997 Hospital Guide in Fukuoka* (City); *Heart-full Communication in Kitakyushu*; *Kitakyushu A Healthy City*; *Saga Health Care Guide* (Pref.); *Nagasaki Hospital Guide* (Pref.); *Kumamoto Emergency Handbook* (Pref.); *Oita City Guide*; *Oita Pref. Int'l Center's Living Guide*; *Miyazaki Pref. Hospital Guide*.

C. Fukuoka Pref. Emergency Hospital Information Center: 092-471-0099 (J. only) Daily 24 hrs.; **Kitakyushu Emergency Treatment Information Center**: 093-582-9999 (J.only) Mon.–Sat.7:30 P.M.–7:00 A.M., Sun. and hols. 9:00 P.M.–7:00 A.M.

■ FUKUOKA-KEN
Fukuoka Daigaku Byoin
(Fukudai Byoin) 福岡大学病院
7-45-1 Nanakuma, Jonan-ku, Fukuoka-shi
092-801-1011

St. Mary's Hospital
Sei Maria Byoin

聖マリア病院
422 Tsubuku-honmachi, Kurume-shi
0942-35-3322

Kurume Daigaku Byoin (T)
久留米大学病院
67 Asahi-machi, Kurume-shi 0942-35-3311

Kyushu University Hospital
Kyushu Daigaku Byoin
九州大学医学部附属病院
3-1-1 Maidashi, Higashi-ku, Fukuoka-shi
092-641-1151

Nippon Sekijujisha Karatsu Sekijuji Byoin
(Nisseki Byoin) 日本赤十字社唐津赤十字病院
1-5-1 Futago, Karatsu-shi 0955-72-5111

■ SAGA-KEN
Saga Ika Daigaku Igakubu Fuzoku Byoin
佐賀医科大学医学部附属病院
5-1-1 Nabeshima, Saga-shi 0952-31-6511

Saga Kenritsu Byoin Kosei-kan (T)
(Saga Kenritsu Byoin) 佐賀県立病院好生館
1-12-9 Mizugae, Saga-shi 0952-24-2171

■ NAGASAKI-KEN
Kokuritsu Nagasaki Chuo Byoin (T)
国立長崎中央病院
2-1001-1 Kubara, Omura-shi 0957-52-3121
http://www.usl.nagasaki-noc.or.jp/~nagachuo/EN/

Nagasaki Daigaku Igakubu Fuzoku Byoin
長崎大学医学部附属病院
1-7-1 Sakamoto-machi, Nagasaki-shi
0958-47-2111

Sasebo Shiritsu Sogo Byoin
(Sogo Byoin) 佐世保市立総合病院
9-3 Hirase-machi, Sasebo-shi
0956-24-1515

■ KUMAMOTO-KEN
Kokuritsu Kumamoto Byoin
国立熊本病院
1-5 Ninomaru, Kumamoto-shi 096-353-6501

Kumamoto Daigaku Igakubu Fuzoku Byoin
熊本大学医学部附属病院
1-1-1 Honjo, Kumamoto-shi 096-344-2111

Kumamoto Sekijuji Byoin (T)
熊本赤十字病院
2-1-1, Nanamine-Minami, Kumamoto-shi
096-384-2111

■ **OITA-KEN**
Kokuritsu Beppu Byoin
国立別府病院
1473 Uchikamado Oaza, Beppu-shi
0977-67-1111

Oita Ika Daigaku Igakubu Fuzoku Byoin
大分医科大学医学部附属病院
1-1 Idaigaoka, Hazama-machi, Oita-gun
0975-49-4411 http://www.oita-med.ac.jp.

Oita Kenritsu Byoin
(Kenritsu Byoin) 大分県立病院
476 Bunyo, Oita-shi 0975-46-7111

Oitashi Ishikairitsu Arumeida Byoin (T)
大分市医師会立アルメイダ病院
1315 Miyazaki Oaza, Oita-shi
0975-69-3121

■ **MIYAZAKI-KEN**
Miyazaki Ika Daigaku Igakubu Fuzoku Byoin
宮崎医科大学医学部附属病院
5200 Kihara, Oaza, Kiyotake-cho, Miyazaki-gun
0985-85-1510

Miyazaki Kenritsu Miyazaki Byoin (T)
(Kenritsu Byoin) 宮崎県立宮崎病院
5-35 Kitatakamatsu-cho, Miyazaki-shi
0985-24-4181

Miyazaki Kenritsu Nobeoka Byoin
宮崎県立延岡病院
2-1-10 Shinkoji, Nobeoka-shi 0982-32-6181

■ **KAGOSHIMA-KEN**
Kagoshima Daigaku Byoin
鹿児島大学医学部附属病院
8-35-1 Sakuragaoka, Kagoshima-shi
099-275-5111

Kagoshima Kenritsu Oshima Byoin
鹿児島県立大島病院
18-1 Manabu-cho, Naze-shi 0997-52-3611

Kagoshima Shiritsu Byoin (T)
(Shiritsu Byoin) 鹿児島市立病院
20-17 Kajiya-cho, Kagoshima-shi
099-224-2101

■ **OKINAWA-KEN**
Adventist Hospital
Adobentisuto Eisei Byoin
アドベンティスト衛生病院
868 Aza Kouchi, Nishihara-cho, Nakagami-gun
098-946-2833

Okinawa Kenritsu Chubu Byoin (T)
(Chubu Byoin) 沖縄県立中部病院
208-3 Aza-Miyazato, Gushikawa-shi
098-973-4111

Okinawa Sekijuji Byoin
沖縄赤十字病院
4-11-1 Kohagura, Naha-shi 098-853-3134

Ryukyu Daigaku Igakubu Fuzoku Byoin
琉球大学医学部附属病院
207 Kami-Uehara, Nishihara-cho, Nakagami-gun
098-895-3331

All books with Japanese titles are in Japanese unless stated otherwise.

■ USING THE SYSTEM

Byōin Erabi「病院えらび事典」(Choosing a Hospital), by Shinpei Miyata. Tokyo: Bungei Shunju, 1997.

Medical Access: A Foreigner's Guide to Health Care in Kobe. Medical Access Project Team, 1997. (Comprehensive resource for the Kansai area. Order from CHIC: 078-857-6540, fax 078-857-6541.)

Nihon Zenkoku Byōin Rankingu「日本全国病院ランキング」(Japan Hospital Rankings), edited and published by Takarashimasha, Tokyo, 1994. (Lists the top 30 hospitals nationwide in many different specialties.)

Tokyo Whole Life Pages '98. (Alternative healing resources. Order from: Book Club Kai: 2-7-30-B1 Minami-Aoyama, Minato-ku, Tokyo. 03-3403-1926, fax 03-3403-9849.)

Zenkoku Byōin Gaido「全国病院ガイド」(Nationwide Hospital Guide), edited by Yuichiro Gotoh and Fumimaro Takahisa. Tokyo: Shogakukan, 1996.

■ PREGNANCY, BIRTH, BREAST-FEEDING

Active Birth, by Janet Balaskas, rev. ed. Boston: Harvard Common Press, 1992. Also available in Japanese translation: *Nyū Akutibu Bāsu*「ニュー・アクティブ・バース」rev. ed. Tokyo: Gendai Shokan, 1998.

Atarashii Seimei no Tame ni「新しい生命のために」(For the Sake of New Life), edited and published by Tokyo Health Bureau, 1994. (Text used at public health center childbirth preparation classes.)

The Baby Book: Everything You Need to Know about Your Baby from Birth to Age Two, by William Sears, M.D. and Martha Sears, R.N. Boston: Little, Brown and Co., 1993.

Complete Book of Pregnancy and Childbirth, by Sheila Kitzinger. New York: Alfred Knopf, 1997. Also in Japanese translation: *Shīra Obasan no Ninshin to Shussan no Hon*「シーラおばさんの妊娠と出産の本」Tokyo: Nobunkyo, 1994.

A Good Birth, A Safe Birth, by Diana Korte and Roberta Scaer, 3rd ed. Boston: The Harvard Common Press, 1992.

Having Your Baby with a Nurse-Midwife: Everything you Need to Know to Make an Informed Decision, by The American College of Nurse-Midwives and Sandra Jacobs. New York: Hyperion, 1993.

Koko de Umitai「ここで産みたい!」(I Want to Give Birth Here!), edited by Natural Birth Club. Tokyo: Shoppan, 1997. (Experiences of 400 mothers at 364 birthing facilities in Tokyo.)

Boshi Hoken no Omonaru Tōkei「母子保健の主たる統計」(Maternal and Child Health Statistics of Japan), by the Maternal and Child Health Division; Children and Families Bureau, and the Statistics and Information Department, Minister's Secretariat of the Ministry of Health and Welfare, Japan. (Bilingual publication in English and Japanese. Order from Boshi Hoken Jigyodan: 03-3499-3111.)

Mothering Multiples—Breast-feeding and Caring for Twins, by Karen Kerkhoff Gromada. Schaumburg, IL: La Leche League International, 1991.

Preconception: A Woman's Guide to Preparing for Pregnancy and Parenthood, by Brenda Aikey-Keller. Santa Fe, NM: John Muir Publications, 1990.

Preventing Miscarriage: The Good News, by Jonathan Scher and Carol Dix. New York: Harper Collins, 1990.

Sanka/San'in Dēta Bukku「産科・産院データブック」(Databook of Obstetric Departments and Birth Clinics), edited and published by Kodansha, Tokyo, 1996. (Information on selected birthing facilities from Hokkaido to Kyushu.)

What to Expect When You're Expecting, by Eisenberg, Murkoff, and Hathaway. New York: Workman Publishing, 1991.

The Womanly Art of Breastfeeding, by La Leche League International, 6th ed., 1998. (Order in English or Japanese from La Leche League: see page 119.)

Zenkoku Josan'in Mappu「全国助産院マップ」

(Nationwide Map of Midwife Clinics). Tokyo: Japanese Midwives' Association, 1997. (To order: 03-3262-9910 or fax 03-3262-8933.)

■ CHILDREN'S HEALTH

Baby and Child, by Penelope Leach. Penguin, 1989.

Educating Andy, by Anne Conduit. Tokyo: Kodansha International, 1996. (The experiences of a foreign family in the Japanese public school system.)

Gakushū Shōgai-ji no Kyōiku「学習障害児の教育」(Education For the Learning Disabled Child). Kazuhiko Ueno and Etsuko Muta. Tokyo: Nihon Bunka Kagakusha, 1993. (Lists centers and hospitals nationwide for testing and therapy in Japanese.)

Japanese Lessons: A Year in a Japanese School Through the Eyes of an American Anthropologist and Her Children, by Gail Benjamin. New York: New York University Press, 1997.

The Portable Pediatrician for Parents: Birth to Five, by Laura Nathanson. New York: Harper Perennials, 1994.

Smart Kids with School Problems, by Priscilla L. Vail. New York: Plume, 1987. (General introduction to learning disabilities, with strategies for overcoming problems; detailed section on the WISC-R test.)

Teenage Health Care, by Gail B. Slap and Martha Jablow. New York: Pocket Books, 1994.

Your Child's Health: A Pediatric Guide for Parents, by Barton D. Schmitt. New York: Bantam Books, 1991.

■ THE DISABLED AND THE ELDERLY

Accessible Tokyo. Japanese Red Cross Language Service Volunteers. (For people using wheelchairs. Order a free copy from the Red Cross: 1-1-3 Shiba-Daimon, Minato-ku, Tokyo, or fax 03-3432-5507, and note your reasons for wanting the book.)

How to Care for Aging Parents, by Virginia Morris. New York: Workman Publishing, 1996.

Zenkoku Ryōiku Meibo Shinshin Shōgai-ji Kankei Iryō Kyōiku Shisetsu Dantai tō Ichiran「全国療育名簿・心身障害児者関係医療・福祉・教育・施設団体等一覧」(Nationwide Resources for Handicapped Children). Tokyo: Zenkoku Shinshin Shogai-ji Fukushi Zaidan, 1991. (Lists facilities, treatment centers, hospitals, and dental clinics which treat handicapped children.)

■ MENTAL HEALTH

Adikushon「アディクション」(Addiction), edited by Arukoru Mondai Zenkoku Shimin Kyokai. Tokyo: ASK Human Care, 1995. (Lists 260 facilities nationwide treating addictions and also self-help groups for addicts. Order from ASK Human Care; see page 242.)

Andrew's Home Page: http://www2.gol.com/users/andrew/ (Home page of Andrew Grimes, British clinical psychologist at the Ikebukuro Counseling Center. Provides lists of hospitals with English-speaking psychiatrists and other information.)

Harukanaru Nami no Oto: Gaikokujinzumatachi no Saigetsu「はるかなる波の音: 外国人妻たちの歳月」(The Distant Sound of Waves: Stories of Foreign Wives of Japanese), by International Bridges and International Videoworks. Color, 73 min., 1996. Video tracing the history of the earliest foreign wives in the Meiji period and interviewing women in their eighties and nineties married to Japanese men since before World War II. Order from International Videoworks: 03-3333-5335; ivw@gol.com)

International Marriage Handbook: A Handbook on the Social Security System and Residential Status for People in Cross-cultural Marriages in Japan, by Asian People's Friendship Society. Tokyo: Happy House, 1995. To order, call APFS: 03-3964-8739.

Kokusai Kekkon Handobukku「国際結婚ハンドブック」(International Marriage Handbook). Tokyo: Akashi Shoten, 1998.

■ ALTERNATIVE HEALING

Back to Balance: A Holistic Self-Help Guide to Eastern Remedies, by Dylana Accolla with Peter

Yates. Tokyo: Kodansha International, 1996.

The Complete Book of Shiatsu Therapy , by Toru Namikoshi. Tokyo: Japan Publications, Inc., 1981.

A Guide to Japanese Hot Springs, by Anne Hotta with Yoko Ishiguro. Tokyo: Kodansha International, 1986.

Japan's Hidden Hot Springs, by Robert Neff. Tokyo: Charles E. Tuttle, 1995.

Understanding Chinese Medicine: The Web that Has No Weaver, by Ted Kaptchuk. New York: Congdon E. Weed, 1983.

Zen Imagery Exercises: Meridian Exercises for the Whole Body, by Shizuto Matsunaga. Tokyo: Japan Publications, Inc., 1987.

■ **NUTRITION**

The Book of Soba, by James Udesky. Tokyo: Kodansha International, 1996. (Recipes for various dishes, how to make noodles at home, and where to eat out in Japan.)

A Dictionary of Japanese Food: Ingredients and Culture, by Richard Hosking. Tokyo: Charles E. Tuttle, 1996. (A book for native speakers of English that includes romanized and Japanese terms together with the English translations. Gives background information on food items and tells how they are used in cooking.)

Gaishoku Teikuauto no Karorī Gaidobukku「外食テイクアウトのカロリーガイドブック」(A Calorie Guidebook for Restaurant and Take-out Food). Tokyo: Joshi Eiyo Daigaku Shuppan-bu, 1997. (Illustrated menus of all your favorite fast-food and restaurant chains, with information on the nutritional value of the dishes they serve. Explanation is all in Japanese, but the code is easy to understand: P=protein; F=fat; C=carbohydrate; and 塩 is salt.)

A Guide to Food Buying in Japan, by Carolyn R. Krouse. Tokyo: Charles E. Tuttle, 1986.

Healthy Vegetable Cooking, by Asako Tohata, M.D. Tokyo: Graph-sha, Ltd., 1995. (Guide to medicinal properties of Japanese vegetables. Beautiful photographs and easy-to-follow recipes from a popular diet and nutrition specialist.)

Japanese Cooking for Health and Fitness, by Kiyoko Konishi. Tokyo: Gakken, 1983. (Traditional and innovative recipes.)

The Mount Sinai School of Medicine Complete Book of Nutrition, by Victor Herbert, et. al. New York: St. Martin's Press, 1990. (Covers all aspects of nutrition, including nutrition and disease.)

My Japanese Kitchen: Thoughts on Housekeeping, Working Women and Japanese Life, by Sadako Sawamura, translated by Mary Goebel Noguchi. Tokyo: Japan International Cultural Exchange Foundation, 1994. (Essays about food, housekeeping, and combining a career with married life, by a stage actress born in 1908.)

Natural Restaurant Guide「ナチュラルレストランガイド」. Shibata Shoten, 1998. (Order from any Japanese bookstore. Lists over 100 vegetarian, organic, and macrobiotic restaurants in Japanese. Short summaries, names, and addresses in English. Covers both Kanto and Kansai areas.)

Tofu and Soybean Cooking, by Kyoko Honda. Tokyo: Graph-sha, Ltd., 1997. (Easy to follow delicious, healthy recipes from a well-known nutritionist.)

Yontei Shokuhin Seibun-hyō 1998「四訂食品成分表1998」(Standard Tables of Food Composition 1998), edited by Yoshiko Kagawa, 4th ed. Tokyo: Joshi Eiyo Daigaku Shuppan-bu, 1998. (Comprehensive list of all Japanese foods with nutritional content analysis. Foods are listed in English, but the rest is in Japanese.)

Zen Vegetarian Cooking, by Soei Yoneda with Koei Hoshino. Tokyo: Kodansha International, 1998 (first published 1982 as *Good Food from a Japanese Temple*). (Written by the late abbess of the Sanko-in Buddhist nunnery in Tokyo.)

■ **DEATH AND DYING**

Dying in a Japanese Hospital, by Fumio Yamazaki. Tokyo: The Japan Times, 1996.

■ **MEDICAL VOCABULARY AND CONVERSATION AIDS**

Conversation Aid for Obtaining Medication in 9

Languages. AMDA Medical Information Center, Tokyo. (Written for pharmacists to use with foreign patients. Order from AMDA 03-5285-8088.)

Gaikoku de Byōki ni Natta Toki Anata o Sukū Hon「外国で病気になったときあなたを救う本」(Sick in a Foreign Country: A Book to Rescue You), by Kenji Sakurai. Tokyo: The Japan Times, 1995. (Written for speakers of Japanese receiving medical care in English, but full of vocabulary and examples of doctor-patient conversations useful for Japanese learners too.)

Physician/Patient Conversation Aid in 11 Languages. AMDA Medical Information Center, Tokyo. (Written for Japanese physicians to use with foreign patients. Order from AMDA: 03-5285-8088.)

■ HEALTH GUIDES

American Medical Association Family Medical Guide. New York: Random House, 1994.

The Encyclopedia of Family Health, by the Royal Society of Medicine. Surrey, U.K.: Bloomsbury, 1995.

Health Information for International Travel. (Updated annually; gives information on disease prevalence and inoculation requirements for many countries. Order from U.S. Government Printing Office, Superintendent of Documents: Mail Stop, SSOP Washington D.C. 20402-9328 U.S.; 202-783-3238; http://www.cdc.gov/travel/)

Hoken Dōjin Handi Shin Akahon Katei no Igaku「保健同人ハンディ新赤本家庭の医学」(Hoken Dojin Handy New Red Book of Home Medicine). Tokyo: Hoken Dojinsha, 1994.

The New Our Bodies, Ourselves, by Boston Women's Health Collective Staff. New York: Touchstone Books, 1996.

■ IDEAS FOR RAISING BILINGUAL KIDS

The Bilingual Family: A Handbook for Parents, by Edith Harding and Philip Riley. Cambridge, U.K.: Cambridge University Press, 1986.

The Bilingual Family Newsletter, c/o Multilingual Matters, Frankfurt Lodge, Clevedon Hall, Victoria Road, Clevedon, England BS21 7SJ, tel 44-1275-876519, fax 44-1275-343096. (A quarterly informational and support newsletter for parents.)

Japan for Kids, by Diane Wiltshire Kanagawa and Jeanne Erickson. Tokyo: Kodansha International, 1992.

A Parents' and Teachers' Guide to Bilingualism, by Colin Baker. Clevedon, U.K.: Multilingual Matters, 1995.

■ CONSUMER DRUG GUIDES

The Complete Guide to Prescription and Nonprescription Drugs, by W. Griffith and J. J. Rybacki. New York: Putnam, 1994.

Essential Guide to Prescription Drugs, by J. W. Long. New York: Harper Perennial, 1994.

98 Kusuri no Jiten Piru Bukku「'98薬の事典ピルブック」('98 Medication Encyclopedia Pill Book, 9th edition). Tokyo: Yakugyoji Hosha, 1997. (Pictures, descriptions, and identifying numbers of more than 2,000 prescription drugs in Japan.)

'98-'99 Taishūyaku Jiten「'98-'99大衆薬事典」('98–'99 OTC Encyclopedia), by the Propriety Association of Japan, 6th ed. Tokyo: Yakugyoji-hosha, 1998. (Detailed descriptions of more than 2,900 over-the counter (nonprescription) drugs. Also lists all Japanese drug companies and their customer-service phone numbers.)

■ GENERAL BOOKS ON JAPAN

Japanese Etiquette: An Introduction, compiled by the Tokyo Y.W.C.A.. Tokyo: Charles E. Tuttle, 1955. (Includes detailed description of funeral customs in Japan, surprisingly not out of date.)

Japanese Etiquette Today, by James and Michiko Vardaman. Tokyo: Charles E. Tuttle, 1994. (Includes information on funeral customs.)

Kodansha Encyclopedia of Japan, edited and published by Kodansha, Tokyo, 1993.

Living in Japan, by International Videoworks, Spinfish (VIS, Inc.), and Arati Co. Color, 90 min., 1998. (The only detailed video available about daily life in Japan for foreigners. Order from the American Chamber of Commerce in Japan: 03-3433-5381.)

Manual for Migrants: Information for Living in

Japan, by the Catholic Diocese of Yokohama Solidarity Center for Migrants, rev. ed., 1997. (Order from the Center: 044-549-7678, fax 044-511-9495.)

Q & A : A Guide to Your Life in Japan 「Q & A 外国人相談ハンドブック」. Tokyo Foreign Residents Advisory Center, 1998. (Available at the Tokyo Metropolitan Government Office Building Bookstore, Shinjuku.)

Volunteering in the Tokyo Area, by Foreign Executive Women (FEW). (To order, call TELL for the current FEW telephone number.)

■ BACKGROUND ON THE JAPANESE HEALTH CARE SYSTEM

Annual Report on Health and Welfare 1996–1997. Ministry of Health and Welfare, Tokyo, 1997.

Containing Health Care Costs in Japan. Edited by Naoki Ikegami and John Creighton Campbell. Ann Arbor, MI: University of Michigan Press, 1996.

Getting Sick in Japan, by Dr. Satoshi Tanaka and Dr. Tomofumi Sone. Kyoto: Kobunshi Kankokai, 1996.

Nihon no Iryo/Fukushi Seido Gaido 「日本の医療・福祉制度ガイド」 (A Guide to the Japanese Health Care System) by Yoneyuki Kobayashi, M.D. Tokyo: Nakayama Shoten, 1993. (Multilingual volume in Chinese, English, Japanese, Korean, Portuguese, and Spanish.)

Human Rights in Mental Health: Japan, by Larry Gostin. Boston: World Health Organization and Harvard University, 1987.

Illness and Culture in Contemporary Japan: An Anthropological View, by Emiko Ohnuki-Tierney. New York: Cambridge University Press, 1984.

Iryō Seido Kōzō Kaikaku e no Suteppu 「医療制度構造改革へのステップ」 (Steps towards Structural Reform of the Medical System), by Yakugyojihosha. Tokyo: Yakugyojihosha, 1997.

Kaigo Hoken wa kō Kimatta! 「介護保険はこう決まった！」 (So This is the Nursing Insurance Decision!), by Yoshio Sato. Tokyo: Nihon Horei, 1998.

Kokumin Eisei no Dōkō 「国民衛生の動向」 (Trends in National Health). Edited and published by the Health and Welfare Statistics Association, Tokyo, 1997.

Maternal and Child Health Statistics of Japan, compiled under the supervision of the Ministry of Health and Welfare. Tokyo: Mothers' and Children's Health Organization, 1997.

1997 Health and Welfare Statistics in Japan, compiled by the Ministry of Health and Welfare. Tokyo: Health and Welfare Statistics Association, 1997.

Outline of Health Insurance, National Health Insurance, National Pension and Employees' Pension Insurance Systems, (Kenko Hoken, Kokumin Kenko Hoken, Kokumin Nenkin, Eisei Nenkin, Hoken no Aramashi) 「健康保健・国民健康保健・国民年金・厚生年金保健のあらまし」 1997. (Multilingual volume in English, Korean, Chinese, and Japanese. Compiled by and available from the Tokyo Metropolitan Government Social Insurance Management Division, Bureau of Social Welfare, 03-5320-4191.)

Prefectural, city, and ward handbooks (See "Regional Resources."

Shakai Hoken Techō '94 「社会保険手帳'94」 (Social Insurance Handbook), edited and published by Shakai Hokencho Kosei Shuppansha, Tokyo, 1993.

Zenkoku Kango, Iryō, Fukushi, Senshū, Kakushu Gakko Gaido 「全国看護医療福祉専修各種学校ガイド」 (Nationwide Technical Schools for Nursing, Health, and Social Service Specialties). Tokyo: Shobunsha Shuppan, 1994.

■ PROFESSIONAL MEDICAL REFERENCES

Harrison's Principles of Internal Medicine, by Anthony Fauci et. al. New York: McGraw Hill, 1991.

Konnichi no Iryo Shishin 1998 「今日の医療指針 1998」 (Today's Therapy 1998), edited by Shigeaki Hinohara, M.D., and Masakazu Abe, M.D. Tokyo: Igaku Shoin, 1998.

Martindale:The Extra Pharmacopoeia, 30th ed. London: The Pharmaceutical Press, 1993.

National Library of Medicine (U.S.) web site: http://www4.ncbi.nlm.nih.gov/PUB/MED/ (Information on new medical reports.)

1997 Red Book Report of the Committee on Infectious Diseases. Elk Grove Village, IL: American Academy of Pediatrics, 1997.

NOTE: Vocabulary words are listed separately, within the individual chapters of the book, for the following categories:
breast-feeding: page 148
first-aid kit supplies: page 51
drugstore supplies: page 261
laboratory tests: page 90
medications: page 252
prenatal and childbirth: page 146

A

abdomen; tummy *hara; o-naka* 腹; おなか

abnormal *ijō na* 異常な

abortion, elective *ninshin chūzetsu, jinkō chūzetsu* 妊娠中絶, 人工中絶

abscess *nōyō* 膿瘍

accident *jiko* 事故

acne *nikibi* にきび

acute *kyū-sei* 急性

adenoids *adenoido* アデノイド

adolescent outpatient clinic *shishunki-ka* 思春期科

alcohol dependency *arukōru izonshō* アルコール依存症

allergic rhinitis *arerugī-sei bien* アレルギー性鼻炎

allergy *arerugī* アレルギー

alopecia; hair loss *datsumōshō* 脱毛症

Alzheimer's dementia *arutsuhaimā-gata chihōshō* アルツハイマー型痴呆症

amputation *setsudan* 切断

anemia *hinketsu* 貧血

iron deficiency ~ *tetsuketsubō-sei hinketsu* 鉄欠乏性貧血

anesthesia *masui* 麻酔

epidural ~ *kōmakugai masui* 硬膜外麻酔

general ~ *zenshin masui* 全身麻酔

local ~ *kyokubu masui* 局部麻酔

spinal ~ *sekizui masui* 脊髄麻酔

aneurysm *dōmyaku-ryū* 動脈瘤

aortic ~ *daidōmyaku-ryū* 大動脈瘤

angina pectoris *kyōshinshō* 狭心症

angiography *kekkan zōei* 血管造影

ankle *ashi kubi* 足首

anorexia nervosa *shinkei-sei shokushi-fushinshō* 神経性食思不振症

antibody *kōtai* 抗体

anus *kōmon* 肛門

anxiety *fuan-kan* 不安感

anxiety neurosis *fuan shinkeishō* 不安神経症

aphasia *shitsugoshō* 失語症

appendectomy *chūsui setsujo-jutsu* 虫垂切除術

appendicitis *mōchōen; chūsuien* 盲腸炎; 虫垂炎

appendix *mōchō; chūsui* 盲腸; 虫垂

appetite *shokuyoku* 食欲

~ loss *shokuyoku fushin* 食欲不振

appointment *yoyaku* 予約

arm *ude* 腕

armpit *waki* わき

arrhythmia *fusei-myaku* 不整脈

arteriosclerosis *heisoku-sei dōmyaku kōkashō* 閉塞性動脈硬化症

artery *dōmyaku* 動脈

arthritis *kansetsuen* 関節炎

rheumatoid ~ *kansetsu riumachi* 関節リウマチ

arthroplasty *kansetsu keisei-jutsu* 関節形成術

asthma *zensoku* 喘息

astigmatism *ranshi* 乱視

athlete's foot *mizumushi* 水虫

atopic dermatitis *atopī-sei hifuen* アトピー性皮膚炎

attention deficit disorder *tadōshō* 多動症

autism *jiheishō* 自閉症

B

back *senaka* 背中

lower ~ pain *yōtsū(shō)* 腰痛（症）

sprain lower ~ *gikkuri-goshi* ぎっくり腰

bacteria *baikin* ばい菌

bacterial *saikin-sei* 細菌性

barium enema *bariumu chūchō kensa* バリウム注腸検査

basin *senmenki* 洗面器

bed *beddo* ベッド

bedpan *benki* 便器

bedrest *ansei* 安静

bedridden *netakiri* 寝たきり

bedside commode *shitsunai benki* 室内便器

bedsore *tokozure* 床ずれ

belch; burp *geppu* げっぷ

Bell's palsy; partial facial paralysis *ganmen shinkei mahi* 顔面神経麻痺

benign *ryō-sei* 良性

biopsy *seiken* 生検

   needle ~ *shin-seiken* 針生検

birthmark *aza; bohan* あざ; 母斑

bladder *bōkō* 膀胱

   ~ inflammation; cystitis *bōkōen* 膀胱炎

bleed *chi ga deru* 血が出る

blister *mizubukure* みずぶくれ

blood *chi; ketsueki* 血; 血液

   fasting ~ sugar *kūfukuji kettōchi* 空腹時血糖値

   ~ gas *ketsueki gasu* 血液ガス

   ~ pressure *ketsuatsu* 血圧

   ~ pressure instrument *ketsuatsukei* 血圧計

   take (withdraw) ~ *saiketsu suru* 採血する

   ~ test *ketsueki kensa* 血液検査

   ~ transfusion *yuketsu* 輸血

   ~ type *ketsueki-gata* 血液型

   ~ vessel *kekkan* 血管

boil; furuncle *dekimono; setsu* できもの; せつ

bone *hone* 骨

   ~ marrow aspiration *kotsuzui senshi* 骨髄穿刺

   ~ marrow transplant *kotsuzui ishoku* 骨髄移植

   ~ mineral density test *kotsusoshōshō ken-shin* 骨粗鬆症検診

bowel movement; evacuation *o-tsūji; haiben* お通じ; 排便

bowleg *O kyaku* O脚

braces (orthodontic) *(ha no) kyōseiki* （歯の）矯正器

brain *nō* 脳

   ~ concussion *nōshintō* 脳震盪

   ~ tumor *nōshuyō* 脳腫瘍

breast *mune; chichi* 胸; ちち

   ~ cancer *nyūgan* 乳癌

breath, to be short of *ikigire ga suru* 息切れがする

breathe, to *kokyū suru* 呼吸する

bridge (dental) *buridji* ブリッジ

bronchitis *kikanshien* 気管支炎

bronchoscopy (fiberscope) *kikanshikyō kensa* 気管支鏡検査

bruise; contusion *uchimi; daboku* うちみ, 打撲

bulimia *burimia* ブリミア

bunions; hallux vulgus *gaihan boshi* 外反母趾

burns *yakedo; nesshō* やけど; 熱傷

buttocks *o-shiri* お尻

C

cancer *gan* 癌; がん

canker sore; aphthous ulcer *afuta-sei kaiyō* アフタ性潰瘍

cap (dental) *jaketto* ジャケット

cardiopulmonary resuscitation (CPR) *shinpai sosei; CPR* 心肺蘇生; CPR

cardiovascular medicine *junkanki-ka* 循環器科

cardiovascular surgery (dept. of) *shinzōkekkan geka* 心臓血管外科

carpal tunnel syndrome *shukonkan-shōkō-gun* 手根管症候群

cartilage *nankotsu* 軟骨

cast, plaster *gibusu* ギブス

cataract *hakunaishō* 白内障

cavity; dental caries *mushiba* むし歯

cerebral palsy *nō-sei mahi* 脳性麻痺

cerebrovascular accident; stroke *nōkekkan shōgai; nōsotchū* 脳血管障害; 脳卒中

certificate of health *kenkō shindansho* 健康診断書

cervical erosion *shikyū chitsubu biran* 子宮膣部ビラン

cervix *shikyūkei* 子宮頸

chart (hospital) *karute* カルテ

cheek *hoho; hō* ほほ; ほお

chest *mune* 胸

chickenpox; varicella zoster *mizu bōsō; suitō* みずぼうそう; 水痘

chilblain *shimoyake* しもやけ

child abuse *shōni gyakutai* 小児虐待

chills *samuke* 寒気

chin *ago* あご

chlamydia *kuramijia* クラミジア

cholecystitis *tannōen* 胆嚢炎

cholera *korera* コレラ

chronic *mansei* 慢性

cleaning (dental) *sukēringu* スケーリング

clitoris *kuritorisu* クリトリス

cold, common *kaze* 風邪

colon. *See* intestines

colon cancer *ketchō gan* 結腸癌

color blindness *shikikaku ijō; shikimō* 色覚異常; 色盲

colostomy surgery *jinkō kōmon keisei-jutsu* 人工肛門形成術

congenital *senten-sei* 先天性

  ~ dislocation of hip *senten-sei kokansetsu dakkyū* 先天性股関節脱臼

  ~ heart disease *senten-sei no shinzō-byō* 先天性の心臓病

congestive heart failure *ukketsu-sei shinfuzen* うっ血性心不全

conjunctiva *ketsumaku* 結膜

conjunctivitis *ketsumakuen* 結膜炎

  acute hemorrhagic ~ *kyū-sei shukketsusei ketsumakuen* 急性出血性結膜炎

  epidemic kerato ~ *hayarime; ryūkō-sei kakuketsumakuen* はやり目; 流行性角結膜炎

constipation *benpi* 便秘

consultation room *shinsatsu shitsu* 診察室

convulsion *keiren; hikitsuke* けいれん; ひきつけ

  febrile ~ *nes-sei keiren* 熱性痙攣

corn *uo no me; tako* うおの目; たこ

cornea *kakumaku* 角膜

corneal ulcer *kakumaku kaiyō* 角膜潰瘍

coronary artery *kandōmyaku* 冠動脈

  ~ bypass surgery *kandōmyaku baipasu shu-jutsu* 冠動脈バイパス手術

  ~ disease *kandōmyaku shikkan* 冠動脈疾患

cosmetic surgery *biyō geka* 美容外科

cough *seki* 咳

counseling *kaunseringu* カウンセリング

cradle cap *shirō-sei shisshin* 脂漏性湿疹

Crohn's disease *kurōn-byō* クローン病

crown (dental) *shikan* 歯冠

crutches *matsubazue* 松葉杖

CT scan; computerized axial tomography *CT sukyan; dansō satsuei* CTスキャン; 断層撮影

culture shock *karuchā shokku* カルチャーショック

cure, to *naosu* 治す

cyst *nōshu* 嚢腫

D

dandruff *fuke* ふけ

defecate, to *haiben suru* 排便する

  have urge to ~ *ben'i ga aru* 便意がある

dehydration *dassuishō* 脱水症

dental hygienist *shika eiseishi* 歯科衛生士

dentist *haisha; shika'i* 歯医者; 歯科医

dentistry *shika* 歯科

dentures; false teeth *gishi; ireba* 義歯; 入れ歯

  partial ~ *kyokubu gishi* 局部義歯

depression *utsu-byō* うつ病

dermatology *hifu-ka* 皮膚科

deviated septum *bichūkaku wankyokushō* 鼻中隔湾曲症

diabetes *tōnyō-byō* 糖尿病

diagnosis *shindan* 診断

dialysis *tōseki* 透析

  peritoneal ~ *fukumaku tōseki* 腹膜透析

diaper rash *omutsukabure* おむつかぶれ

diaphragm (anat.) *ōkakumaku* 横隔膜

diarrhea *geri* 下痢

dilatation and curettage (D&C) *sōha-jutsu* 掻爬術

diphtheria *jifuteria* ジフテリア

disability *shōgai* 障害

  learning ~ *gakushū shōgai* 学習障害

  mental ~ *seishin shōgai* 精神障害

  physical ~ *shintai shōgai* 身体障害

disease *byōki* 病気

dislocation *dakkyū* 脱臼

diverticular disease *keishitsuen* 憩室炎

dizziness; vertigo *memai* めまい

  ~ on standing *tachikurami* 立ちくらみ

doctor. *See* physician

Down syndrome *daunshō* ダウン症

drug; medication *kusuri; yakuzai* 薬; 薬剤

  ~ prescription *shohōsen* 処方せん

  nonprescription ~ *shihanyaku* 市販薬

  prescription ~ *shohōsen chōzai* 処方せん調剤

drug reaction (rash) *yakushin* 薬疹

E

ear *mimi* 耳

  ~ discharge *mimidare* 耳だれ

  ~ infection. *See* otitis media

ringing in ~ *miminari* 耳鳴り

eardrum; tympanic membrane *komaku* 鼓膜

 ruptured ~ *komaku haretsu* 鼓膜破裂

ear, nose and throat (ENT) clinic *jibi-ka; jibi-inkō-ka* 耳鼻科；耳鼻咽喉科

early detection *sōkihakken* 早期発見

eczema *shisshin* 湿疹

edema *mukumi; fushu* むくみ；浮腫

egg; ovum *ranshi* 卵子

electrocardiogram (EKG/ECG) *shindenzu* 心電図

elbow *hiji* 肘

 ~ joint *chūkansetsu* 肘関節

electroencephalogram *nōha-zu* 脳波図

electroshock therapy *denki shokku ryōhō* 電気ショック療法

embolism *kansen-shō* 塞栓症

 cerebral ~ *nō sokusenshō* 脳塞栓症

 pulmonary ~ *hai sokusenshō* 肺塞栓症

emergency room *kyūkyū gairai* 救急外来

electromyogram (EMG) *kindenzu* 筋電図

emphysema *haikishu* 肺気腫

encephalitis *nōen* 脳炎

endocarditis *shinnai makuen* 心内膜炎

endocrinology and metabolism clinic *naibunpitsu taisha-ka* 内分泌代謝科

endometriosis *shikyū naimakushō* 子宮内膜症

endoscopy *naishikyō kensa* 内視鏡検査

enema *kanchō* 浣腸

epidemic (adj.; n.) *ryūkō-sei no; ryūkōbyō* 流行性の；流行病

epilepsy *tenkan* てんかん

epileptic seizure *tenkan hossa* てんかん発作

esophagus *shokudō* 食道

exercise tolerance test *undō fuka shiken* 運動負荷試験

eye *me* 目

 ~ discharge *meyani* 目やに

eyeball *gankyū* 眼球

eyedrops *tenganyaku* 点眼薬

eyeglasses *megane* 眼鏡

eyelash *matsuge* まつげ

eyestrain *gansei hiro* 眼精疲労

F

face *kao* 顔

faint (v.) *shisshin suru* 失神する

fallopian tube *rankan* 卵管

false teeth. *See* denture

farsightedness; hyperopia *enshi* 遠視

 ~ due to old age *rōgan* 老眼

fecal (stool) test (for blood) *kenben (ketsuben kensa)* 検便（血便検査）

feces; stool *(dai) ben; unchi (child's)* （大）便；うんち

 blood in ~ *ketsuben* 血便

fever *netsu* 熱

 high ~ *kōnetsu* 高熱

 slight ~ *binetsu* 微熱

fibroma. *See* uterine tumor

fibromyalgia *kinmakuen* 筋膜炎

Fifth disease *ringo-byō* リンゴ病

filling (dental) *tsumemono* 詰め物

finger *yubi* 指

 sprained (jammed) ~ *tsuki yubi* つき指

food refusal *kyoshoku* 拒食

foot *ashi* 足

 flat ~ *henpeisoku* 扁平足

forehead *hitai; o-deko* 額；おでこ

foreskin of penis *penisu no hōhi* ペニスの包皮

fracture *kossetsu* 骨折

 stress ~ *hirō kossetsu* 疲労骨折

freckles *sobakasu* そばかす

frigidity *fukanshō* 不感症

fungus; mycosis; mold *kabi; shinkin* カビ；真菌

G

gallbladder *tannō* 胆嚢

 inflammation of the ~. *See* cholecystitis

gallstone; cholelithiasis *tanseki(shō)* 胆石（症）

gastrectomy *i-setsujo-jutsu* 胃切除術

gastric ulcer *ikaiyō* 胃潰瘍

gastroenteritis *ichōen* 胃腸炎

 infantile ~ *nyūji ōto gerishō* 乳児嘔吐下痢症

gastroenterology *shōkaki-ka; ichō-ka* 消化器科；胃腸科

gastrointestinal (GI) *ichō no* 胃腸の

 lower ~ endoscopy; colon endoscopy *daichō faibāsukōpu* 大腸ファイバースコープ

 upper ~ endoscopy *i kamera* 胃カメラ

 upper ~ series; barium swallow *itōshi; jōbushōkakan zōeikensa* 胃透視；上部消化管造影検査

gene *idenshi* 遺伝子

gingivitis *shinikuen* 歯肉炎

glaucoma *ryokunaishō* 緑内症

glucose tolerance test *budōtō fukashiken* ブドウ糖負荷試験

gonorrhea *rinbyō* 淋病

gonorrheal urethritis *rinkin-sei nyōdōen* 淋菌性尿道炎

gout *tsūfū* 痛風

gum; gingiva *haguki* 歯茎

gynecology *fujinka* 婦人科

H

hair *ke* 毛

  (on head) *kami no ke* 髪の毛

  pubic ~ *inmō* 陰毛

hand *te* 手

hand-foot-and-mouth disease *te ashi kuchi byō* 手足口病

hangover *futsukayoi* 二日酔い

hay fever; pollinosis *kafunshō* 花粉症

head *atama* 頭

health insurance *kenkō hoken* 健康保険

  ~ certificate *hoken-shō* 保険証

hearing acuity *chōryoku* 聴力

hearing aid *hochō ki* 補聴器

hearing loss *nanchō* 難聴

heart *shinzō* 心臓

  ~ attack; myocardial infarction (MI) *shinzō hossa; shinkin kōsoku* 心臓発作; 心筋梗塞

  ~ failure *shinfuzen* 心不全

  ~ murmur *shinzatsuon* 心雑音

heartburn *muneyake* 胸やけ

heat rash *asemo* 汗疹

heel *kakato* かかと

height (of body) *shinchō* 身長

hemodialysis *ketsueki tōseki* 血液透析

hemophilia *ketsuyū-byō* 血友病

hemorrhage *shukketsu* 出血

  subarachnoid ~ *kumomakuka shukketsu* くも膜下出血

  subconjunctival ~ *ketsumakuka shukketsu* 結膜下出血

hemorrhoid *jikaku; ji* 痔核; 痔

hepatitis, viral *uirususei kan'en* ウイルス性肝炎

hernia *herunia* ヘルニア

  hiatal ~ *ōkakumaku herunia* 横隔膜ヘルニア

  inguinal ~ *sokei herunia* 鼠蹊ヘルニア

  intestinal ~ *datchō* 脱腸

  strangulated ~ *kanton herunia* 嵌頓ヘルニア

  umbilical ~ *sai herunia* 臍ヘルニア

herniated disk *tsuikanban herunia* 椎間板ヘルニア

herpangina *herupangīna* ヘルパンギーナ

herpes *herupes* ヘルペス

  ~ genitalis *inbu herupes* 陰部ヘルペス

  ~ gingivostomatis *herupesu-sei shiniku kōnaien* ヘルペス性歯肉口内炎

  ~ labialis *kōshin herupesu* 口唇ヘルペス

  ~ zoster; shingles *taijō hōshin* 帯状疱疹

hiccup *shakkuri* しゃっくり

hip joint *kokansetsu* 股関節

hip replacement surgery *jinkō kottō chikan-jutsu* 人工骨頭置換術

hives; urticaria *jinmashin* じんましん

hoarse (of voice) *(koe ga) kareta* （声が）かれた

hospital *byōin* 病院

  admission to ~ *nyūin* 入院

  ~ chart *karute* カルテ

  discharge from ~ *taiin suru* 退院する

hot water bottle *yutanpo* 湯たんぽ

hydrocele *innōsuishu* 陰嚢水腫

hydrocephalus *suitōshō* 水頭症

hypertension (disorder) *kōketsuatsu(shō)* 高血圧 (症)

hyperthyroidism (disorder) *kōjōsen kinō kōshin(shō)* 甲状腺機能抗進症

hyperventilate *kakokyū suru* 過呼吸する

hyperventilation syndrome *kakokyū shōkōgun* 過呼吸症候群

hypotension *teiketsuatsu(shō)* 低血圧 (症)

  orthostatic ~ *kiritsu-sei teiketsuatsu* 起立性低血圧

hysterectomy *shikyū tekishutsu-jutsu* 子宮摘出術

hysterosalpingography *shikyūrankan zōei* 子宮卵管造影

I

immunity *men'eki* 免疫

impetigo *tobihi* とびひ

implant (dental) *inpuranto* インプラント

incubation period *senpuku kikan* 潜伏期間

incurable *fuji no* 不治の

indigestion *shōka furyō* 消化不良

infarction *kōsoku* 梗塞

  cerebral ~ *nō kōsoku* 脳梗塞

infected *unde iru* 膿んでいる

infectious disease (dept. of) *kansenshō-ka* 感染症科

inflammation *enshō* 炎症

influenza *infuruenza* インフルエンザ

informed consent *infōmudo konsento* インフォームド・コンセント

injection *chūsha* 注射

injury *kega* けが

  mild ~ *keishō* 軽傷

  severe ~ *jūshō* 重傷

inlay (dental) *inrei* インレイ

insomnia *fumin(shō)* 不眠 (症)

intensive care unit; ICU *ICU; shūchūchiryō shitsu;* 集中治療室

  neonatal ~ care unit; NICU *NICU; shinseiji shūchū chiryō shitsu* NICU; 新生児集中治療室

internal medicine *naika* 内科

internal organs *zōki* 臓器

intestines *chō* 腸

  large ~; colon *daichō; ketchō* 大腸; 結腸

  small ~ *shōchō* 小腸

intraocular pressure *gan atsu* 眼圧

intravenous (IV) drip *tenteki* 点滴

iris *kurome; kōsai* 黒目; 虹彩

irritable, be *ira-ira suru* イライラする

irritable bowel syndrome *kabin-sei chōshōkōgun* 過敏性腸症候群

itchy *kayui* かゆい

J

Japanese encephalitis *nihon nōen* 日本脳炎

jaundice *ōdan* 黄疸

joint *kansetsu* 関節

K

kanpōyaku. See oriental medicine

Kawasaki Syndrome *kawasaki-byō* 川崎病

keloid *keroido* ケロイド

kidney *jinzō* 腎臓

knee *hiza* 膝

  (~) cartilage (meniscus) injury *hangetsuban sonshō* 半月板損傷

  (~) collateral ligaments injury *sokufukujintai sonshō* 側副靭帯損傷

  (~) cruciate ligament rupture *jūjijintai dan-retsu* 十字靭帯断裂

  ~ joint *shitsukansetsu* 膝関節

knock-knee *X kyaku* X脚

kyphosis; humpback *kōwanshō* 後湾症

L

laboratory *kensa shitsu* 検査室

  ~ technician *rinshōkensa gishi* 臨床検査技師

laminectomy *tsuikyū setsujo-jutsu* 椎弓切除術

laparotomy *kaifuku-jutsu* 開腹術

laryngitis *kōtōen* 喉頭炎

larynx *kōtō* 喉頭

lead apron, use a *purotekutā o tsukau* プロテクターを使う

leg *ashi* 脚

lens (of eye) *suishōtai* 水晶体

letter of introduction *shōkaijō* 紹介状

leukemia *hakketsu-byō* 白血病

lice *shirami* 虱

ligament *jintai* 靭帯

  stretch a ~ *jintai o nobasu* 靭帯を伸ばす

limp (v.) *ashi o hikizuru* 足を引きずる

lip *kuchibiru* 唇

listless *darui* だるい

liver *kanzō* 肝臓

  ~ cirrhosis *kankōhen* 肝硬変

lordosis; swayback *zenwanshō* 前湾症

lumbar puncture *yōtsui senshi* 腰椎穿刺

lump *shikori* しこり

lumpectomy, breast *nyūbō onzonhō* 乳房温存法

lung *hai* 肺

  ~ cancer *haigan* 肺癌

lymph node *rimpasetsu* リンパ節

  regional ~ *shozoku rimpasetsu* 所属リンパ節

lymphoma, malignant *aku-sei rinpashu* 悪性リンパ腫

M

magnetic resonance imaging (MRI) *MRI; jikikyō meiga zōhō;* 磁気共鳴画像法

malaria *mararia* マラリア

malignant *aku-sei* 悪性

mammography *manmogurafī* マンモグラフィー

manic-depressive psychosis *sō utsu-byō* 躁うつ病

mastectomy *nyubō setsujōjutsu* 乳房切除術

mastitis *nyūsen'en* 乳腺炎

measles *hashika; mashin* はしか; 麻疹

medical (clinical) history *byōreki* 病歴

medications. *See* drugs

melanoma *kokushokushu* 黒色腫

memory loss; amnesia *kioku sōshitsu* 記憶喪失

meningitis *zuimakuen* 髄膜炎

meniscectomy; cartilage removal *hangetsuban setsujo-jutsu* 半月板切除術

mental illness *seishin-byō* 精神病

mental retardation *seishinchitai* 精神遅滞

menopause (termination of menses) *gekkei heisa* 月経閉鎖

　years surrounding ~ *kōnenki* 更年期

　symptoms of ~ *kōnenki shōgai* 更年期障害

menstrual cramp *seiritsū* 生理痛

menstrual period, last *saishū gekkei* 最終月経

menstruation *seiri* 生理

　irregular ~ *seiri fujun* 生理不順

　painful ~; dysmenorrhea *gekkei konnan* 月経困難

metastasis *ten'i* 転移

midwife *josanpu* 助産婦

migraine headache *henzutsū* 偏頭痛

molar *kyūshi* 臼歯

mole; nevus *hokuro* ほくろ

molluscum contagiosum *mizuibo; densen-sei nanzokushu* 水いぼ; 伝染性軟属腫

mongolian spot *mōkohan* 蒙古斑

mononucleosis, infectious ("mono") *densen-sei tankakushō* 伝染性単核症

mouth *kuchi* 口

mucous membrane *nen maku* 粘膜

multiple sclerosis (MS) *tahatsu-sei kōkashō* 多発性硬化症

mumps *otafuku kaze* おたふく風邪

muscle *kinniku* 筋肉

　calf ~ *fukurahagi* ふくらはぎ

　~ pain *kinnikutsū* 筋肉痛

　~ pull *nikubanare* 肉ばなれ

myoma. *See* uterine tumor

N

nail (finger-, toe-) *tsume* 爪

nasal polyps *hanatake* 鼻茸

nasogastric tube; NG tube *keibi ikan* 経鼻胃管

nausea *hakike* 吐き気

navel *o-heso* おへそ

nearsightedness; myopia *kinshi* 近視

neck *kubi* 首

negative reaction *in-sei hannō* 陰性反応

nerve *shinkei* 神経

neurology *shinkei naika* 神経内科

neurosis *shinkeishō* 神経症

neurosurgery (dept. of) *nōshinkei geka* 脳神経外科

nipple *chikubi; nyūtō* 乳首; 乳頭

normal *seijō na* 正常な

nose *hana* 鼻

　runny ~ , have a *hanamizu ga deru* 鼻水が出る

　stuffy ~ *hanazumari* 鼻づまり

nosebleed *hanaji* 鼻血

nostril *bikō* 鼻孔

nothing-by-mouth *zesshoku* 絶食

numbness *shibire* しびれ

nurse *kangofu* 看護婦

　assistant ~ *junkangofu* 准看護婦

　male ~ *kangoshi* 看護士

　professional ~ *seikangofu* 正看護婦

　public health ~ *hokenfu* 保健婦

nursing care *kango* 看護

nutritionist *eiyōshi* 栄養士

O

obese *himan no* 肥満の

obesity *himanshō* 肥満症

obsessive-compulsive neurosis *kyōhaku shinkeishō* 強迫神経症

obstetrics *sanka* 産科

obstetrics-gynecology (Ob-Gyn) *sanfujin-ka* 産婦人科

occupational therapist *sagyō ryōhōshi* 作業療法士

operating room *shujutsu shitsu* 手術室

operation *shujutsu* 手術

ophthalmology *ganka* 眼科

optometrist *kenganshi* 検眼士

oriental medicine *kanpōyaku* 漢方薬

orthodontics *shika kyōsei-jutsu* 歯科矯正術

orthodontist *kyōsei shika'i* 矯正歯科医

orthopedics *seikei geka* 整形外科

osteoarthritis *henkei-sei kansetsuen* 変形性関節炎

osteoporosis *kotsusoshōshō* 骨粗鬆症

osteosarcoma *kotsu nikushu* 骨肉腫

otitis *jien* 耳炎

  ~ externa; swimmer's ear *gaijidōen* 外耳道炎

  ~ media *chūjien* 中耳炎

  serous ~ media *shinshutsu-sei chūjien* 滲出性中耳炎

otolaryngology. *See* ear, nose and throat clinic

outpatient department *gairai* 外来

  receive continued follow-up care in an ~ *tsūin suru* 通院する

ovarian cysts *ransō nōshu* 卵巣嚢腫

ovary *ransō* 卵巣

overeating *kashoku-shō* 過食症

overweight *futorisugi* 太り過ぎ

overwork, death from *karōshi* 過労死

oxygen tent *sanso tento* 酸素テント

P

pain *itami* 痛み

  acute (sudden) ~ *kyū na itami* 急な痛み

  anginal ~ *shinzōtsū; mune no itami* 心臓痛; 胸の痛み

  burning ~ *hiri-hiri suru itami* ひりひりする痛み

  chronic ~ *man-sei no itami* 慢性の痛み

  dull ~ *nibui itami* 鈍い痛み

  intolerable ~ *gaman dekinai itami* 我慢できない痛み

  mild ~ *karui itami* 軽い痛み

  sharp ~ *surudoi itami* 鋭い痛み

palm *te no hira* 手のひら

palpitation *dōki* 動悸

pancreas *suizō* 膵臓

pancreatitis *suien* 膵炎

panic disorder *panikku disuōdā* パニック・ディスオーダー

Pap smear *sumea tesuto; shikyū saibō shin* スメアテスト; 子宮細胞診

Parkinson's disease *pākinson byō* パーキンソン病

patient; sufferer *kanja* 患者

pediatrics *shōni-ka* 小児科

pedometer *manpokei* 万歩計

pelvic exam (internal) *naishin* 内診

pelvic inflammatory disease *kotsubannai kansen(shō)* 骨盤内感染 (症)

pelvis *kotsuban* 骨盤

penis *penisu* ペニス

periodontist *shishū-byō senmon'i* 歯周病専門医

periodontitis; pyorrhea *shishūen; shisōnōrōshō* 歯周炎; 歯槽膿漏症

peritonitis *fukumakuen* 腹膜炎

pertussis; whooping cough *hyakunichi zeki* 百日咳

pharmacist *yakuzaishi* 薬剤師

pharmacy; drugstore *yakkyoku; kusuriya* 薬局; 薬屋

  prescription ~ *chōzai yakkyoku* 調剤薬局

pharyngitis *intōen* 咽頭炎

pharyngoconjunctival fever *intō ketsumaku netsu* 咽頭結膜熱

pharynx *intō* 咽頭

phlebothrombosis *jōmyakukessenshō* 静脈血栓症

phlegm. *See* sputum

phobia *kyōfushō* 恐怖症

physical exam *kenkō shindan* 健康診断

physical therapist *rigaku ryōhōshi* 理学療法士

physician *ishi; isha (sensei)* 医師; 医者 (先生)

  female ~ *joi* 女医

pimple *nikibi* にきび

pinworms *gyōchū* 蟯虫

plastic surgery (dept.of) *keisei geka* 形成外科

pneumonia *haien* 肺炎

polio *shōni mahi; porio* 小児マヒ; ポリオ

polyp, intestinal *daichō porīpu* 大腸ポリープ

positive reaction *yōsei hannō* 陽性反応

predisposition *soshitsu* 素質

pregnancy *ninshin* 妊娠

premenstrual syndrome; PMS *gekkeizen shōkōgun* 月経前症候群

prevention *yobō* 予防

private room *koshitsu* 個室

proctology *kōmon-ka* 肛門科

prostate gland *zenritsusen* 前立腺

enlarged ~ *zenritsusen hidaishō* 前立腺肥大症

psoriasis *kansen* 乾癬

psychiatry *seishin-ka* 精神科

psychosomatic disease *shinshinshō* 心身症

pubic region *inbu* 陰部

pyloric stenosis *yūmonkyōsakushō* 幽門挟窄症

pulse *myaku* 脈

pupil (of eye) *hitomi* 瞳

pus *umi* 膿

pulmonary embolism *haisokusenshō* 肺塞栓症

pyelonephritis *jinujinen* 腎盂腎炎

R

rabies *kyōken-byō* 狂犬病

radiologic technologist/radiology technician *hōshasen gishi* 放射線技師

radiology (dept. of) *hōshasen-ka* 放射線科

raped *gōkan sareta* 強姦された

recovery room *kaifuku shitsu* 回復室

rectum *chokuchō* 直腸

recurrence *saihatsu* 再発

reflux esophagitis *gyakuryū-sei shokudōen* 逆流性食道炎

remission *kankai* 寛解

renal insufficiency *jinfuzen* 腎不全

respiratory *kokyū no* 呼吸の

acute ~ distress syndrome *kyū-sei kokyū shōgai* 急性呼吸障害

~ medicine *kokyūki-ka* 呼吸器科

upper ~ tract infection; URI *jōkidōen* 上気道炎

retina *mōmaku* 網膜

retinal detachment *mōmaku hakuri* 網膜剥離

rheumatic fever *riumachi netsu* リウマチ熱

ringworm fungus *tamushi* たむし

risk factor *kiken inshi* 危険因子

root canal (dental) *shikon no chiryo* 歯根の治療

roseola *toppatsu-sei hosshin* 突発性発疹

rubella; three day measles *fūshin; mikka bashika* 風疹；三日ばしか

S

saliva *daeki* 唾液

salpingitis *rankan'en* 卵管炎

scale (for body weight) *taijūkei* 体重計

scaling, of teeth *sukēringu* スケーリング

scar *kizuato; hankon* 傷跡；瘢痕

scarlet fever *shōkō netsu* 猩紅熱

sciatica *zakotsu shinkeitsū* 坐骨神経痛

schizophrenia *seishin bunretsu-byō* 精神分裂病

scoliosis *sokuwanshō* 側湾症

scrotum *innō* 陰嚢

scrub typhus *tsutsugamushi-byō* つつが虫病

semen *sei eki* 精液

blood in ~; hemospermia *ketsuseiekishō* 血精液症

senile dementia *rōjin-sei chihō* 老人性痴呆

septicemia *haiketsushō* 敗血症

sexual abuse *sei-teki gyakutai* 性的虐待

sexually transmitted disease (STD) *seibyō* 性病

shingles. *See* herpes

shiver *furueru* 震える

shoulder *kata* 肩

stiff ~ *katakori* 肩凝り

~ joint *katakansetsu* 肩関節

side effect; adverse reaction *fuku sayō* 副作用

sinusitis *fukubikōen* 副鼻腔炎

skull; cranium *zugaikotsu* 頭蓋骨

sneeze *kushami* クシャミ

snoring *ibiki* いびき

social worker *sōsharuwākā* ソーシャルワーカー

speech *hanashi kata* 話し方

~ delay *gengo chitai* 言語遅滞

~ therapist *gengo ryōhōshi* 言語療法士

~ therapy *gengo kunren* 言語訓練

sperm *seishi* 精子

spina bifida *nibun sekitsui* 二分脊椎

spinal cord *sekizui* 脊髄

spine; vertebral column *sekitsui* 脊椎

spleen *hizō* 脾臓

spontaneous pneumothroax *shizen kikyō* 自然気胸

sprain *nenza* 捻挫

  ~ an ankle *ashikubi o ~ suru* 足首を~する

sputum; phlegm *tan* 痰

  bloody ~ *kettan* 血痰

  ~ test *tan no kensa* タンの検査

sterility; infertility *funinshō* 不妊症

stitch, one *hitohari* 一針

stitch, remove a *basshi suru* 抜糸する

stomach *i* 胃

strabismus; crossed eye *shashi* 斜視

strep throat *yōrenkin kansenshō* 溶連菌感染症

stress *sutoresu* ストレス

stress incontinence *kyūhakusei nyōshikkin* 急迫性尿失禁

stroke. *See* cerebrovascular accident

stutter, to *domoru* 吃る

sty *bakuryūshu; monomorai* 麦粒腫; ものもらい

suicide *jisatsu* 自殺

surgery (dept. of) *geka* 外科

surgery (operation) *shujutsu* 手術

surgery (removal of whole organ) *zenteki shujutsu* 全摘手術

suture, to *hōgō suru* 縫合する

swallow, be difficult to *nomikomi nikui* 飲み込みにくい

sweat (v.) *ase o kaku* 汗をかく

swollen, be *harete iru* 腫れている

symptom *shōjō* 症状

  withdrawal ~ *kindan shōjō* 禁断症状

syphilis *baidoku* 梅毒

T

tartar *shiseki* 歯石

tears *namida* 涙

  shed ~; cry *naku; namida o nagasu* 泣く; 涙を流す

temperature (of body) *taion* 体温

tendon *ken* 腱

  Achilles ~ *akiresuken* アキレス腱

  ~ rupture *ken danretsu* 腱断裂

  tear a ~ *ken o kiru* 腱を切る

tendonitis *ken'en* 腱炎

tendoplasty; tendon repair *kenkeiseijutsu* 腱形成術

testicles *kōgan* 睾丸

  undescended ~ *teiryūkōgan* 停留睾丸

tetanus *hashōfu* 破傷風

thermometer (for body) *taionkei* 体温計

therapy *ryōhō* 療法

thirsty *nodo ga kawaku* 喉が渇く

throat *nodo* 喉

  sore throat, have a *nodo ga itai* 喉が痛い

thrombosis *kessenshō* 血栓症

  cerebral ~ *nō kessenshō* 脳血栓症

thrush, oral *kōkōkanjida; gakōsō* 口腔カンジダ; 鵞口瘡

tired, be *tsukarete iru* 疲れている

toe *ashi no yubi* 足の指

tongue *shita* 舌

  geographic ~ *chizujōzetsu* 地図状舌

tonsillectomy *hentōsen setsujojutsu* 扁桃腺切除術

tonsillitis *hentōsen* 扁桃腺

tooth *ha* 歯

  ~ abscess *ha no nōyō* 歯の膿瘍

  chipped ~ *kaketa ha* 欠けた歯

  extraction of ~ *basshi* 抜歯

  primary ~; baby ~ *nyūshi* 乳歯

  permanent ~; adult ~ *eikyūshi* 永久歯

  wisdom ~ *oyashirazu; chishi* 親知らず; 智歯

toothache *shitsū* 歯痛

trachea *kikan* 気管

traction (orthopedic) *ken'in* 牽引

transient ischemic attack (TIA) *ikka-sei nōkyoketsu hossa* 一過性脳虚血発作

treat (v.) *chiryō suru* 治療する

treatment *chiryō* 治療

  temporary ~ *ōkyū shochi* 応急処置

  ~ room *chiryō shitsu* 治療室

trunk; torso *dōtai* 胴体

tubal ligation *rankankessatsu* 卵管結紮

tuberculosis *kekkaku* 結核

tumor *shuyō* 腫瘍

  primary ~ *genpatsu-sei shuyō* 原発性腫瘍

typhoid fever *chō chifusu* 腸チフス

U

ulcerative colitis *kaiyō-sei daichōen* 潰瘍性大腸炎

ultrasonography *chōonpa kensahō; ekō* 超音波検査法; エコー

unconscious *ishiki fumei* 意識不明

underweight *yasesugi* やせすぎ

uremia *nyōdokushō* 尿毒症

urethral stricture *nyōdō kyōsaku* 尿道狭窄

urinary *nyō no* 尿の

~ stone *nyōro kesseki* 尿路結石

~ tract infection *nyōro kansenshō* 尿路感染症

~ incontinence *nyō shikkin* 尿失禁

urination *hai'nyō* 排尿

~ difficulty *hai'nyō konnan* 排尿困難

frequency of ~ *hai'nyō no hindo* 排尿の頻度

urine *oshōsui, nyō, oshikko* お小水, 尿, おしっこ

blood in ~ *ketsu'nyō* 血尿

cloudy ~ *nyō kondaku* 尿混濁

~ containing protein *tanpaku nyō* 蛋白尿

~ test *nyō kensa* 尿検査

urology *hi'nyōki-ka* 泌尿器科

uterine cancer *shikyū gan* 子宮がん

uterine tumor; leiomyoma (fibroma/myoma) *shikyū kinshu* 子宮筋腫

uterus *shikyū* 子宮

V

vagina *chitsu* 膣

vaginal discharge *orimono; taige* おりもの; 帯下

vaginal yeast infection , candida *chitsu kanjidashō* 膣カンジダ症

vaginitis *chitsuen* 膣炎

valvular heart disease *shinzō benmakushō* 心臓弁膜症

varicose veins (leg) *jōmyaku ryū (kashi)* 静脈瘤（下肢）

vasectomy *paipukatto* パイプカット

venereal disease *seibyō* 性病

venereal disease (VD) medicine (department of) *seibyō-ka* 性病科

vein *jōmyaku* 静脈

viral; virus *uirusu-sei; uirusu* ウイルス性; ウイルス

vision *shiryoku* 視力

~ test *shiryoku tesuto* 視力検査

~ therapist *shinō kunreshi* 視能訓練士

visual acuity *shiryoku* 視力

visiting hours *menkai jikan* 面会時間

vocal cord polyp *seitai porīpu* 声帯ポリープ

vomit (v.) *haku, modosu, ōto suru* 吐く, 戻す, 嘔吐する

~ blood (V.) *toketsu suru* 吐血する

W

ward *byōtō* 病棟

wart *ibo* いぼ

weight (of body) *taijū* 体重

Weil's Disease *wairu-byō* ワイル病

wheelchair *kurumaisu* 車椅子

wheeze (v.) *zeizei suru* ぜいぜいする

whiplash (injury) *muchiuchi (sonshō)* 鞭打ち（損傷）

wound (n.) *kizu* 傷

wrinkle (n.) *shiwa* しわ

wrist *tekubi* 手首

X

X-ray *rentogen* レントゲン

Delivery (obstetric), 139–40

Dentists 265–67; evaluation of 268–69

Dentistry 265–72; clinics, 271–72; for disabled, 217; emergencies, 265; insurance coverage of, 80, 268–69; oral surgery, 267; orthodontics, 266; scaling, 270; tooth care aids, 271

Dermatology 20; clinics, 33, 184

Designated diseases 60–64, 171

Developmental delays 173–78

Diabetes 186–87; balneotherapy for, 289; meal delivery services, 307–308; nutrition counseling for, 186–87; prevention of, 304; treatment centers, 186–87; urine/blood sugar testing for, 88, 90. See also Pregnancy: government assistance for, prenatal checks

Diagnosis 27–28; oriental medicine, 276–77; understanding of, 197

Diarrhea (acute) 156. See also Infantile gastroenteritis

Diet: counseling on, 310–11; and mental health, 235; foods 302. See also Diabetes; Eating disorders; Macrobiotics; Nutrition

Disabled 213–19; attitudes toward, 21; consultations, 214; evaluation of, 214; financial assistance for, 214–15; health insurance for, 214; help with travel plans, 216; home care, 217; public services for, 217; registration of, 213; specialist care for, 217

Discharge from hospital 43–44

Diseases and disorders: allergies, 181–85; communicable, 122; conditions of middle age, 190–92, 304; congenital, 135, 163; excused absence, 171; designated intractable, 62–63; information center, 197; mental, 175–86; sexually transmitted, 110–12; that are not common in Japan, 163.

Doctors (Physicians): choosing 25–27; communicating with, 27; getting a second opinion, 28; licensing of, 17–18, 58–59. See also Health care professionals

Dogs: guide 216–17; companion: 216–17

Domestic violence. See Battered women; Child abuse

Donation: blood, 209–10; bone marrow, 210; donor card, 208–209; eye bank, 209

Down syndrome 135–36; 176–78

Drugs: to bring from home country, 315; use at birth, 123–24; and drugstores, 249–62; and insurance coverage, 70, 75, 278; and oriental medicine, 277–80; powdered, 252; in treating

pain 253, 258, 330. See also Addictions

Dyslexia 174–75

Dysrhythmias 196–97

E

Ears: infections, 154–55; drugstore products for, 261. See also Hearing

Earthquakes: preparedness, 324; response, 324–25

Eating disorders 243; counseling for, 239–40, 243–44

E. coli-O157 312

Eczema (atopic dermatitis) 183; garlic baths for, 183; pajamas for, 184. See also Allergies

Education. See Schools

Elderly 219–28; assistance to families caring for at home, 222–23; care facilities, 223–25, 227; emergency care for, 227–28; home care, 225–27; insurance for, 72–73

Electricity 320

Embalming 333–34

Emergency care 45–51; calling an ambulance, front endpapers; childbirth, 146; for children, 164; for the elderly, 227–28; for mountain climbers, 247; for travelers, 325; psychiatric, 247. See also Regional resources; Cardiopulmonary resuscitation

Employees' health insurance. See Insurance

ENT 20. See also Hearing

Epidemic kerato-conjunctivitis (EKC) 202–203

Epilepsy 185; in children, 163; treatment centers, 185

Erythema infectiosum 204–205

Exanthem subitum 204–205

Excimer laser surgery 197

Exercise 315–18; and culture shock, 235; fitness clubs, 317–19; hiking, 316; maternity, 137–38; radio, 316. See also Mountain climbing; Qigong; Sports; Tai chi; Yoga

Eye bank 209

Eyeglasses 95–96, 315; optical stores, 96. See also Vision

Eyes: See Cataracts; Conjunctivitis; Donation; Eye bank; Squint eye; Vision

F

Family planning 101–102

Fertility: balneotherapy and, 289; Japanese tips for, 107. See also Infertility

Fetal congenital disorders: testing for, 135–36

Jiairyo 144
Judo 318

K

Kalabaw no Kai 60
Kanpō. See Oriental medicine; Alternative healing practitioners
Kansai Childbirth Education Organization 120
Karōshi 192
Katakōri (stiff shoulders) 198
Kawasaki syndrome 204–205
Kendō 318
Kikō. See Qigong
King Clinic, The 33
Kobayashi International Clinic 33
Kokusai Kekkon o Kangaeru Kai 238
Kurhaus 289–90
Kyoto Birth Network 120

L

La Leche League 119, 143
Labor: calling for an ambulance, 146 ; care during, 122–24, 139; induction of, 124; pain medication for, 123–24
Laboratory tests 30; 38; included in the *ningen dokku* exam, list of, 90–91
Learning disabilities 174–75
Leptospirosis 200–201
Lice: medication, 260; pubic, 112
Licensing 25
Liver disease 196. *See also* Hepatitis
Living will 331
Lyme disease 198

M

MAC and DARC Alcoholism and Drug Rehabilitation Centers 244
Macrobiotic diet 310; health risks of, 310; mail-order foods, 309
Make-A-Wish (Japan) 331
Malpractice 22
Mammograms 93
Marriage and self encounter programs 238
Martial arts 318. *See also* Qigong; Tai chi
Massage 282–83; *shiatsu* clinics, 283
Maternal and Child Health Services Center 58
Maternity. *See* Pregnancy
Meal delivery services 307
Measles 155; vaccinations, 159–62

Medical care certificate: for infant/children 62; for the elderly 77
Medical expenses reimbursement 71–72, 76; AIDS, 60; high-cost medical fees, 71, 76; sick children, 62; tax deductions, 79
Medical specialties 20–21
Medications. *See* Drugs
Meditation 245–46
Menopause 109; clinics, 110. *See also* Osteoporosis
Menstruation: adolescent clinics for, 172–73; drugstore products, 262
Mental health 231–48
Mental health care providers: clinical psychologists, 19; psychiatrists, 25. *See also* Counseling; Psychiatric care; Psychotherapy
Mental retardation. *See* Disability
Midwives: at birth, 122–23, 139–40; clinics, 121, 128–29; home birth, 127–29; licensing of, 18, 117; traditional practices, 115–17
Milk: types in Japan, 300; calcium absorption and, 302–303. *See also* Formulas
Minatomachi Foreign Migrant Workers' Mutual Aid 83
Ministry of Health and Welfare 58–59
Miscarriage 138
Mishuk no Kai 238
Mites. *See* Allergies
Mizura 237
Mold. *See* Allergies, House cleaning
Mononucleosis (infectious) 199
Morita therapy 244–45
Morning sickness 136
Mother and Child Health Handbook (*boshi techō*) 118, 139, 145, 159
Mountain climbing 316; insurance for, 317
Moxibustion 281–82

N

Nagoya Foreign Mother's Group 120
Naikan psychotherapy 244–45
National Health Information Center 197
National health insurance. *See* Insurance
National Institute of Neurological Disorders and Strokes 136, 192
National Medical Clinic 33
Nearsightedness: excimer laser surgery for, 197. *See also* Vision
Neurology 20

改訂版・日本の医療健康ハンドブック
JAPAN HEALTH HANDBOOK Revised Edition

1998年 9 月10日　第 1 刷発行

著　者　メレデス・丸山／ルイーズ・清水／ナンシー・鶴巻
発行者　野間佐和子
発行所　講談社インターナショナル株式会社
　　　　〒112-8652 東京都文京区音羽 1-17-14
　　　　電話：03-3944-6493

印刷所　株式会社　平河工業社
製本所　株式会社　堅省堂

■ Tokyo English Life Line (TELL)

03-3968-4099; daily 9:00 A.M.–4:00 P.M. and 7:00–11:00 P.M.

03-3968-4193, fax 03-3968-4196 (office)

03-3986-7071 (in Tagalog); Tues. 6:30–10:00 P.M.

http://www.weekender.co.jp/TELL

Nonprofit affiliate of Life Line International, established in 1973 by an ecumenical group of churches to serve the foreign community's need for English-language information and crisis phone counseling. Staffed by volunteers who undergo an intensive 60 hours of training and 24 hours of practical work, it offers support, problem-solving assistance, counseling, referral, and information about resources on, for instance, organizations, doctors, therapists, support groups, crisis centers, churches, special interest groups, HIV/AIDS and resources. TELL also has links with the nationwide Japanese helpline "Inochi no Denwa" so it can answer questions on all Japan. TELL also publishes an annual information calendar listing essential services for the foreign community in the Tokyo area. For TELL community counseling services, see page 239.

■ Jhelp.com (Japan Helpline)

833, Tokyo, Japan 100-8692

0120-46-1997

http://jhelp.com

Attempts to help caller find practical information or assistance on wide range of subjects. This is also Japan's only multilingual, 24-hour, nationwide emergency service. Tries to assist caller by phone or over the Internet. If necessary, can send someone to assist on-site. Completely reliant on community support for its services. Always gratefully accepts donations as well as volunteer help with assisting callers.

■ AMDA International Medical Information Centers

Tokyo: 03-5285-8088

Mon.–Fri. 9:00 A.M.–5:00 P.M.

(in English, Chinese, Thai, Korean, Spanish, Portuguese, Farsi, and Tagalog)

Kansai: 06-636-2333

(in English, Chinese, Spanish, Portuguese)

Information on health insurance, payment of medical bills, and other aspects of the medical system. Trained interpreters and center staff work together to find specific answers to health-related questions or to provide information on doctors who speak your language. A project of the Association of Medical Doctors for Asia which cooperates internationally to improve health care throughout the world.

■ Tokyo Metropolitan Health and Medical Information Center (Himawari) Multilingual Service

03-5285-8181 Mon.–Fri. 9:00 A.M.–8:00 P.M. (In English, Chinese, Thai, Korean, and Spanish)

Information on the Japanese medical system and introduction of medical facilities with foreign-language–speaking health care practitioners. Database with 19,000 facilities, about 2,000 of which offer care in foreign languages.

■ Tokyo Metropolitan Health and Medical Information Center (Himawari) Japanese Service

03-5272-0303

Daily 9:00 A.M.–9:00 P.M.: Information on the Japanese medical system.

Daily 24-hour service: Introduction of medical facilities.

■ Foreign Nurses Association in Japan

P.O. Box 54, Ueno Yubinkyoku

1-5-12 Shitaya, Taito-ku. Tokyo 110-91

http://www.webspawner.com/users/FNAJ/

Offers classes in CPR and first aid, and the English brochure, "How to Call an Ambulance," etc. Its members have a variety of nursing and health specialties, and may be able to give information and suggestions